Console-ing Passions *Television and Cultural Power*
A series edited by Lynn Spigel and Marsha Kinder

AIDS TV

Identity, Community, and Alternative Video

Alexandra Juhasz

Videography by Catherine Saalfield

DUKE UNIVERSITY PRESS   *Durham and London 1995*

© 1995 Duke University Press
All rights reserved
Printed in the United States of America on acid-free paper ∞
Typeset in Melior by Tseng Information Systems, Inc.
Library of Congress Cataloging-in-Publication Data appear
on the last printed page of this book.

For Jim

CONTENTS

ACKNOWLEDGMENTS

I am indebted to the work, energy, commitment, and care of the group of women who are at once the focus and the creative force behind this project. I thank the women of the WAVE project—Aida Matta, Carmen Perez, Glenda Smith-Hasty, Juanita Mohammed, Marcia Edwards, and Sharon Penceal—for their insights and vision into AIDS, video, and the nature of community. I respect their courage. I value their friendship. Their work made my work possible.

I have also made AIDS video with many others whom I thank for their dedication and creativity: the HIV-Video Support Group at Woodhull Hospital, the Lay-Techs Entertainment Group at Swarthmore College, and the Audio-Video Department at The Gay Men's Health Crisis.

Of course, to write this book I have watched countless AIDS videos by friends and respected colleagues. I know that making activist video is time-consuming, undervalued, and also massively important. To all you videomakers: keep up this vital work which has soothed, enraged, and unified so many of us!

Sections of *AIDS TV* were published in earlier drafts in several journals and books under the following titles: "Camcorder Politics," *Cinematograph* 4 (1990–91): 79–86; "The Contained Threat," *The Journal of Sex Research* 27, no. 1 (February 1990): 25–46, a publication of the Society for the Scientific Study of Sexuality (P.O. Box 208, Mount Vernon, Iowa 52314-0208); "WAVE in the Media Environment," *camera obscura* 28 (January 1992): 135–52 (Indiana University Press); "So Many Alternatives," *Cineaste* 20, no. 4 (1994): 32–41, and 21, no. 1 (1995); "From Within," *Praxis* 3 (1992): 23–46; and "Knowing AIDS Through the Televised Science Documentary," *Women and AIDS: Psychological Perspectives,* ed. Corinne Squire (London: Sage Publications, 1994), 150–64. Some of this writing was generously funded by Amherst College's Copeland Fellowship and a Mellon Fellowship at Bryn Mawr College.

My gratitude to the many funders and sponsors who allowed the Women's AIDS Video Enterprise to come into existence: the New York Council for the Humanities, the New York State Council on the Arts, the Astraea Fund for Women, ArtMatters, Women Make Movies, Media Network, the Brooklyn AIDS Task Force, and Deborah Ann Light.

Many of my friends, teachers, and family directly supported the writing and rewriting of *AIDS TV.* I first thank my mother, Dr. Suzanne Juhasz, for providing both last-minute copyediting and ongoing comments throughout this five-year process. She has read this manuscript more than anyone but me; what luck to be a second-generation feminist scholar! My friends Scott Bukatman and Alisa Lebow have also read and responded to several drafts of chapters, as well as providing intellectual, personal, and practical support as my AIDS work became a dissertation and then a book. Alisa also helped me with the "frame grabs" which illustrate the book (the fancy computer to do so was generously provided by Cynthia Madansky), only the most mechanical example of Alisa's loving support. Robert Reid-Pharr and Erin Cramer gave me room to converse about all my scholarly, writerly (and emotional) woes: I needed such friendship to keep writing. Mark Breitenberg, Betsy Bolton, and Lisa Cartwright supported this work by helping me remember its value in the real world as well as the academy. My mentors Drs. Bob Stam, Paul Arthur, and most especially Faye Ginsburg, all allowed me the space to do experimental and political scholarship. In their own ways, each embodied a model for the living of a life as a committed academic. Catherine Saalfield carefully created the book's videography and then closely read a draft of the manuscript, and Petra Janopaul helped to find many of those hard-to-locate videotapes and then years later created the index with love. Finally, at Duke University Press, my copyeditor, Bob Mirandon, deserves credit for the care and attention he devoted to my messy manuscript, and my editor, Ken Wissoker, made the intimidating process of publishing a book seem approachable. He understood what I hoped to do and who I hoped to reach with this book, and he set things in place to allow that to happen.

The support of my family has always given me strength, confidence, a home. Thanks and love to Suzanne, Antonia, and Joseph Juhasz, Jenny Juhasz Schwartz and Paul Schwartz, Christina and Linda Juhasz-Wood, Meg Caddeau, and, of course, Cheryl Dunye.

AIDS TV: A History and Theory of the Alternative AIDS Media

AIDS TV is dedicated to the recognition, definition, history, and theory of the alternative AIDS media. In this book I focus on the innumerable videos and television productions about AIDS made outside commercial broadcast television, paying particular attention to my own video project, the Women's AIDS Video Enterprise (WAVE). I consider why so much video has been made, how these many tapes function and for whom, how they challenge traditional understandings of the media, and why so much of my life, as is true of many others, has been devoted to the production, viewing, and analysis of AIDS TV. As I attempt to understand how individuals and communities work to change the lived and discursive meanings of AIDS by making video, I am also concerned with the significance of low-end video itself: what is the "alternative" media?

This question is perhaps most fruitfully answered by considering what the alternative media does. The production and reception of alternative AIDS TV are forms of direct, immediate, product-oriented activism which brings together committed individuals who insist upon being industrious. No wonder so many alternative AIDS videos have been produced. In the few years since AIDS has known a name, hundreds if not thousands of media productions about the crisis have appeared, created by videomakers who work outside commercial (broadcast) television. Since the mid-1980s these projects have challenged and politicized the meanings of both AIDS and video. It is the fact of alternative AIDS video which is initially so compelling. Try as I may, I can think of no other social issue which, in such a brief time, has received this magnitude of attention using the form of video production.

Thus, my first task in this study must be to attempt to understand why. Why have thousands of AIDS videos produced by artists, community centers, public access stations, ACT UP affinity groups, and high school students come into being?[1] These videos document AIDS demonstrations, illustrate how to clean intravenous drugworks, interview longtime survivors, depict cunnilingus through a dental dam. Why this form of response instead of or in addition to marching, lobbying, or leafleting? What does the fact of the vast alternative AIDS media tell us about AIDS, video, and politics? And, for those of us who are part of the large and diverse community of makers and viewers, why do we make them? Why do we watch them? Is there a value to all of this video?

Since the invention of the motion picture camera, artists, activists, and intellectuals with ideological goals have embraced the technologies which mimetically and aesthetically record movement. From film movements of the 1920s and 1930s in the newly communist USSR, to similar movements some forty years later in the decolonizing Third World, to the movements today of rapidly organizing communities of indigenous peoples around the globe—significant production of political mediamaking occurs when fluctuations in the terrain of ideology meet with change in the realm of technology. Film or video movements (like the outpouring of tapes about AIDS) which change the face of film and political history (and, in the process, the lives of the many people who make and view them) occur when rapid changes in politics, theory, and technology align.

The coincidental and not so coincidental lining up of the new video technologies (the camcorder, satellite, VCR, and relatively low-cost computer editing) with the AIDS crisis and with theories of postmodern identity politics and multiculturalism is the founding condition upon which the alternative AIDS media is built. The overwhelming needs to counter the (mis)information about AIDS represented on broadcast television, to represent the underrepresented experiences of the crisis, to communicate with others who feel equally unheard, all coincide with the formation of a new condition of media practice, the low-end, low-tech video production made possible by new technologies. The potential of media production for those individuals and communities who never before could afford it or master it occurred just as a social crisis of massive proportions and multiple dimensions begged to be represented in a manner available to the most and the least economically and culturally privileged. The politics of AIDS—the demands for a better quality of life for the people affected by this epidemic—are well matched by the potentials and politics of video.

This said, I must continue to answer the question—"Why the alternative AIDS media?"—by building upon my framework of coinciding conditions, several more conditions specific to the history of AIDS. Because in its earliest and still most well-known manifestation this retro-virus infected the bodies of white gay men in the United States, this community's material, educational, and creative resources serve as a partial inspiration for the astonishing response to AIDS found in video and television. The artists, critics, and "cultural elite"—whose deaths were met with either cultural indifference or blame in a world which had once seemed to be based upon the security of their dominant race, class, and gender—responded in forms with which they were already familiar.[2] Then, too, a body of AIDS theory suggests that this invisible contagion is the logical culmination of the postmodern condition, *only* manageable in representation, and best managed in postmodernism's definitive discourse—television.[3] AIDS TV abounds because AIDS and television are so similar—discursive, fleeting, all-powerful. Another motivation for this massive media blitz is the lack of a cure for AIDS, making necessary a focus upon preventive education. Since no medium reaches more Americans (literate or not, English-speaking or not) than television, television is the most pervasive and persuasive form for this much-needed AIDS education.

This is what alternative AIDS TV is about: the use of video production to form a local response to AIDS, to articulate a rebuttal to or a revision of the mainstream media's definitions and representations of AIDS, and to form community around a new identity forced into existence by the fact of AIDS. Producing alternative AIDS media is a political act that allows people who need to scream with pain or anger, who want to say, "I'm here, I count," who have internalized sorrow and despair, who have vital information to share about drug protocols, coping strategies, or government inaction, to make their opinions public and to join with others in this act of resistance. Viewing alternative AIDS television—lying on a couch at home watching a VCR, sitting in church, or among friends and neighbors at a local screening— is always an invitation to join a politicized community of diverse people who are unified, temporarily and for strategic purposes, to speak back to AIDS, to speak back to a government and society that has mishandled this crisis, and to speak out to each other.

It's (Not) As Easy As It First Seems: Defining the Alternative AIDS Media

If the fundamental questions organizing this book seem simple and sometimes self-serving—What is the alternative AIDS media? What does it do? Where did it come from? What does my work within it mean?—I believe the answers are harder to come by. First is the issue of terminology. Just what do I mean by a phrase as broad and indecisive as "the alternative AIDS media"? The tapes which come under this moniker are conceived, funded, produced, and distributed in an infinite variety of ways and with diverse formal strategies, from big-budget educational documentaries that mimic the forms of commercial television and are funded by pharmaceutical companies and broadcast to millions of viewers on cable television, to camcorder recordings of AIDS demonstrations that include a critique (in form and content) of broadcast AIDS representation and are shown to small, committed audiences in art galleries, activist meetings, and AIDS conferences. In his article "Strategic Compromises: AIDS and Alternative Video Practices," John Greyson explains that alternative AIDS tapes are made for a range of reasons, by a range of producers, for a range of receptions. They are funded in many ways and are formally diverse. He lists at least nine "types" of alternative AIDS practice:

1. Cable access talk shows
2. Documents of performances and plays addressing AIDS
3. Documentary (memorial) portraits of PLWAs (People Living With AIDS)
4. Experimental works by artists deconstructing mass media hysteria
5. Educational tapes on transmission of and protection against HIV
6. Documentaries portraying the vast range of AIDS service organizations
7. Safer-sex tapes
8. Activist tapes
9. A growing handful of tapes for PLWAs[4]

These nine distinctions acknowledged, I will continue, like Greyson, to use the one word "alternative" to distinguish independently produced video from the television about AIDS produced and broadcast by the three major networks (and the national cable networks, i.e., HBO, Fox, CNN, or others). This network production I call the "mainstream media," the "broadcast media," or "commercial television." These binary terms attempt to mark a delineation between a system of media production which is standardized, profit-oriented, seemingly authorless and unbiased, and directed toward mass consumption and the many other possible systems of media production and distribution which are organized through much less regulated and standardized conjunctions of finance, ideology, artisanship, profit, and style.

I am well aware that these binary terms also serve to obscure a great deal of the cross-fertilization, mimicry, and hybridization which defines much current video production, especially because of the rise of cable broadcasting and the explosion of the home video market. Experimental form is used by *both* media, as is conventional form; conservative ideology can be espoused in either formats; "alternative" videos can have budgets larger than those of the "mainstream," and they can even make their producers a lot more money. When using this rigid binary, there is no way to differentiate between a *NOVA* program on AIDS, produced and repeatedly aired by PBS, and the one-time, at-first-censored PBS airing of Marlon Riggs's *Tongues Untied* (1989). There is no distinction between a state-funded, big-budget, moralistic educational video for teenagers preaching at them to abstain from sex and the collectively produced Second Look Community Arts' *What's Wrong with This Picture* (1991), in which diverse teenagers promote sexual experimentation, liberation, and safety. These binary terms erase the differences between television and video: one made for the purpose of broadcast and the selling of commercials and usually produced with the medium of video, the other also made in video, with the *potential* of broadcast but the primary intention of a grassroots distribution with minimal financial yield, more like art or educational film.

Yet, it does not take a Ph.D. in cinema studies to locate and articulately differentiate the two systems of representation. *A WAVE Taster* (WAVE, 1990) is a video which documents the WAVE project's production process. In a scene from April 14, 1990, the group discusses the differences between two videos about AIDS—the 1986 NBC News Special, *Life, Death and AIDS,* narrated by Tom Brokaw, and my tape, *Women and AIDS* (with Jean Carlomusto, 1988), which features a number of female AIDS professionals. In the process, the significant distinctions between the mainstream and alternative media are articulated. Our discussion proceeded as follows:

> *Glenda:* The first one was more realistic. The people were real, what they were saying is real.
> *Alex:* How do you transmit that? What about them seems real to you?
> *Glenda:* Because they experienced this. I don't know what Tom's experiences are. He was just doing his job. He got a couple of people together from Atlanta. They seemed so unattached to what was happening. The people in the first video were attached.

Alex: What kind of experts does TV choose? All these white, male scientists. But a lot of people know about AIDS from firsthand experience. TV rarely calls those people experts.

Aida: That's because we don't have a bachelor's degree, or we didn't go to ten years of college. They feel that one isn't educated enough to speak in front of people and tell them, "listen this is what I know about it." The scientists went through college, they have all these big professional degrees. That's why they're put up in front of the media as far as being able to speak, and thinking people will listen to them.

Alex: But what do they know?

Sharon: They know nothing. A piece of paper. A bunch of statistics.

Aida: They haven't really come to an experience. The way they speak is just out of knowledge.

In our conversation, we focused upon the different kinds of authority which define mainstream and alternative video: the authority of distance, education, knowledge versus experience, understanding, and attachment (figure 1). Despite the blurring of boundaries in the age of cable, camcorders, and CNN, some differences remain consistent between alternative and mainstream production. Greyson comes to the determination that despite the diversity within the alternative AIDS media, these productions function differently from the mainstream media, although they do inform and sometimes change the commercial media's representation of AIDS, because of two amorphous but critical qualities: a "confident insider's vernacular" and "effectiveness."[5] His terms, like WAVE's discussion, serve to articulate what the alternative AIDS media *is*—a use of the media to speak from within and to a politicized community—and what the alternative AIDS media *does*—to effectively construct and communicate that politicized community first to itself and then perhaps to a broader audience. Jean Carlomusto explains how the Gay Men's Health Crisis' (GMHC) "Living with AIDS" weekly cable show differs from broadcast TV:

> In contrast to network television, AIDS activist television explores the possibility of production within the context of an activist movement. Grass root media production is part of the process of constantly defining and presenting our movement. . . . We have people speaking for themselves about their experiences. They are addressing others like themselves who could benefit from a sharing of

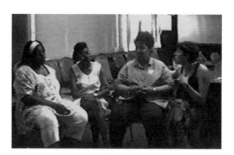

Figure 1   Marcia,
Glenda, Juanita, and
Alex, *A WAVE Taster*
(WAVE, 1990).

knowledge and survival strategies. The program's central philosophy is that we are all living with AIDS.[6]

Carlomusto describes what is a significant defining feature of the
alternative AIDS media, the positioning of producer, subject, and audience
of a video in a similar place—self-proclaimed difference, marginality, activism, oppression, distinctiveness, and, sometimes, infection. Videomaker
Catherine Saalfield calls this "'amongness' between the producers and the
audience."[7] The production and viewing of alternative media involve a willing and often sought-out dialogue among producer and audience because
the people involved *need* the dialogue; they need lifesaving information,
need to see their lives and problems represented with dignity, need to hear
politically inflected interpretations of the issues which affect them, and need
to speak to each other about what they know. People with highly specific
demands and opinions use alternative media because it can "narrowcast"
crucial information among a limited audience of like-minded people, this in
an accessible form which is quick and inexpensive to make. To do all this
work, normally with little or no money involved, the producer working from
a self-proclaimed position of marginality must necessarily be passionate—
another defining feature of alternative AIDS media. Experience, understanding, attachment, and passion define the form and content of alternative AIDS
video because its primary purpose and effect are self- and community expression and communication. This depiction does not mean that the work
is touchy-feely, but in fact the exact opposite. Alternative AIDS media is explicitly political, necessarily critical. By claiming a self-identified position
of anger or love in opposition to the "objective" norm, community identification and building begin.

Faye Ginsburg has labeled the distinction between the two media
the profit/prophet motive.[8] The prophet motive of alternative media inspires

producers to challenge the normative mode of broadcast television production and distribution. The urgency of getting out a certain message overrides the financial motivations of mainstream production (although certainly the mainstream media has a range of motivations which fall second to its profit motive, and alternative mediamakers are always pleased to make money). The creation of media work that comes from within a movement or experience and which has an urgent, explicit, and committed purpose (what Greyson calls effectiveness) is different from work that is produced because a time slot must be filled, a commercial sold, and an audience placated. The viewing inspired by these diverse systems can be understood in similar terms: watching a video because you struggle, desire, or need to see it is different from watching a television show because it happens to be on when you happen to be in front of the tube. This difference between alternative and mainstream AIDS media comes from an explicit (or sometimes newly developing) political, educational, or personal commitment to prophesizing about the AIDS crisis.

A most consistent feature of alternative video production about AIDS is not just the relationship between, but the *position of,* the mediamaker and the viewer—a position of self-identified difference created in direct opposition to a mainstream practice which insistently and consistently constructs images by and for protected outsiders, who are immune from HIV and who are distanced from the people infected with it. Timothy Landers, in one of the earliest studies of AIDS media, suggestively labels this structure as one of "Bodies/Anti-Bodies." "The Body—white, middle-class, and heterosexual—is constructed in opposition to the Other, the Anti-Body—blacks, gay men, lesbians, workers, foreigners, in short, the whole range of groups that threaten straight, white, middle-class values."[9] Alternative AIDS media could therefore be considered the video work of individuals who proudly take on the negative mantle assigned to them—"anti-body." The voice and body of an "anti-body" organize and assume responsibility for a tape's production. And as importantly, the work assumes that an "anti-body" will also be watching. Carlomusto has said in a group interview with the AIDS activist video collective Testing the Limits that "everything I don't consider video AIDS activism addresses a 'general public,' as if there is one homogeneous general public that doesn't allow for diversity."[10] The particular power of alternative media production is its unique capacity to allow individuals from the "minority," "disenfranchised," and "marginal" communities of our culture to extract and distinguish themselves from the "general public" by making and seeing diversified, individualized media images. The camcorder has equipped people to make politics in a way rarely, if ever, available to them before: in a "dominant" cultural form, yet in a personal voice; by, for, and about themselves, but easily available to outsiders.

For reasons economic and political, the possibility of low-budget alternative AIDS media alters the function of the media—producing differentiated selves with politics, histories, opinions. Because alternative media is so inexpensive, it need not be watched by millions of people to pay for its own production. Because alternative media is often funded as "art," or "education," it often need not pay itself back at all. Because alternative media targets its voice to speak to particular bodies, the processes of distribution and exhibition, not simply the nature of the text itself, play an integral role in defining it. Alternative media is made to be watched, stopped, discussed. Meanwhile, the mainstream media can never serve this function. By economic imperative, a vast audience of "middle-of-the-road spectators"[11]— usually imagined to be the straight, white, middle-class members of intact families who so few Americans actually are—is constructed as the ideal consumer for broadcast programming and the products that programs sell. People rarely turn to TV for validation of lived experience on the local or personal level because, for better or worse, mainstream media has to make a profit, which means speaking and selling to the many, not the few.

While the effects of watching TV about and for middle-of-the-road imaginary people are themselves interesting, my concern is specifically with what occurs when the mainstream media attempts to communicate precise AIDS information through these generalizing structures, and then, how the alternative AIDS media responds to the problems that this clash inevitably creates. One of the most dangerous generalized positions which was claimed for this "general public" in 1980s' mainstream AIDS media was that this public was outside AIDS: the uninfected, unimplicated, safe bodies constructed in opposition to Landers's "anti-bodies." For this reason, James Kinsella concludes in his book-length study of the broadcast media's coverage of AIDS: "at least some of the blame for the ravages of AIDS in America must lie with members of the media who refused to believe that the deaths of gay men and drug addicts were worth reporting."[12] Although 1990s' mainstream AIDS media has brought "new" ideas about AIDS to the "general public"—most importantly, some attempt is being made to challenge the inside/outside structure of the AIDS crisis, and even "normal" Americans are now perceived to be at (some) risk—the construction of an apolitical, amorphous, but very moral "general public" still organizes the voice and intended reception of mainstream AIDS reportage. The mainstream AIDS media of the

1990s continues to use an us/them, bodies/anti-bodies structure (good and bad modes of transmission, good and bad PWAs), even as it attempts to include us all (we are all at risk).

Garnering AIDS education through structures which package Americans into a sanitized general public is particularly dangerous because "knowing" AIDS involves access (or lack of access) to lifesaving information. In his book on the politics of the news media, Michael Parenti writes: "The press can effectively direct our perceptions when we have little information to the contrary and when messages seem congruent with earlier notions about events—notions that themselves may be partly media created."[13] If you know better through direct experience or education, chances are you will see through much of the misinformation, or lack of information, in mainstream AIDS coverage. If you are a woman with AIDS (or her family member, or friend, or doctor), you damn well know that the mainstream media has misrepresented this aspect of the AIDS crisis. But without personal knowledge, it is hard to see through mainstream misinformation because it is reported through structures which themselves appear authoritative and objective. (In chapters 3–5 I examine how the authoritative structures of science, documentary, and sexism have framed and authorized a good deal of reportage about AIDS.) Kinsella writes of the profound effects of presenting AIDS information to generalized, middle-of-the-road spectators:

> Does it matter that most Americans get their news exclusively from the television? Coverage of the AIDS epidemic shows just how much. TV news will continue to discount minority communities, even as crises like AIDS affect blacks and Hispanics more. . . . This disease that journalists have once again become convinced won't be affecting them or their readers, is making its way into the ranks of the nation's teens. Americans aged thirteen to twenty-one are spreading the AIDS virus through heterosexual contact at twice the rate of adults. That's another story the media are missing. . . .[14]

The need to report upon the missing stories of the mainstream media becomes another defining feature of the alternative media. What commercial TV will not or cannot say is expressed through alternative video. Most of the stories central to the AIDS crisis—about poverty, drug use, sexuality, homosexuality, women, people of color, prostitutes, the Third World, the inadequate health-care system, the inadequate response to AIDS from the national government, the connections between hard science and big business—occur outside the domain of broadcast television. In their study of broadcast news AIDS coverage, Timothy Cook and David Colby find that the mainstream media has been reluctant to deal with AIDS because this story is about homosexuals and homosexual life-styles, not to mention "blood, semen, sexuality, and death."[15] Similarly, in his detailed study of the first years of the AIDS crisis, Randy Shilts emphasizes the culpability of the mainstream media:

> People died and nobody paid attention because the mass media did not like covering stories about homosexuals and was especially skittish about stories that involved gay sexuality. Newspapers and television largely avoided discussion of the disease until the death toll was too high to ignore and the casualties were no longer just the outcasts. Without the media to fulfill its role as public guardian, everyone else was left to deal—and not deal—with AIDS as they saw fit.[16]

The work of the alternative media is to represent the "outcast's" stories of AIDS—to deal with AIDS as they see fit. Sandra Elgear and Robyn Hutt, also founding members with Carlomusto of the AIDS video activist collective Testing the Limits, comment upon the power of taking the media into one's own hands: "Challenging the notion that the center offers the official explanation, members within communities affected by AIDS become their own voices of authority. We are no longer content to sit back and comment on failure of the press to understand the impact of AIDS in our communities."[17] By becoming "their own voices of authority," AIDS activist videomakers document and distribute images of the events, people, and opinions of the AIDS community and enter these images into public history. The point is not that what is represented in commercial television is necessarily *wrong* (although it sometimes is), but that it is *incomplete*. Alternative AIDS video make the range of representations of AIDS more complex, expanding the incomplete picture created by the mainstream media and, sometimes, the alternative media as well. The work of the alternative media is based upon an understanding of multiple, sometimes competing, histories, interpretations, and politics of AIDS.

Therefore, by definition, the work of the alternative media can never be standardized, as has been true for the mainstream media, because the specific needs of unique communities and producers serve to define the conditions of production: that is, what format to use, how quickly to produce, whether or not to work collaboratively, how to fund, how to distribute. For these reasons, specific extratextual information about a video is integral for "reading" its text. Thus, in the analyses that follow, my concerns circulate both around videotapes about AIDS as discrete objects ready for close analysis and with the political and theoretical importance of the processes of video production and reception. Gregg Bordowitz, affiliated at different times with both Testing the Limits and GMHC, explains about "activist video": "It is recognized that video 'is not an object, but an event,' because its production is part of a larger effort to organize increasing numbers of people to take action. . . . The production of activist video is primarily concerned with audience and distribution."[18]

Bordowitz suggests that alternative AIDS video is "radically different from network" TV, not only because of its radical form, but because it is a much-needed *event*. To better understand both the object and the event of video, analysis of activist cultural production must unify two usually isolated interpretive strategies: (1) the "sociological" consideration of the conditions which surround the production and reception of a work of art; (2) the "critical" attention to the meanings of representation. As well as focusing upon a video text such as *We Care* (WAVE, 1990) as a container which allows access to useful countersignification, artistic expression, or innovative form, I am interested in considering what the seven participants in WAVE achieved from taking action through video production—working together as a group against a cause and making our ideas and demands public. Further, I am fascinated with considering the impact, however small, upon the thousands of diverse spectators who watch *We Care*. What do they get from viewing for half an hour the expression of individuals rarely afforded the opportunity of self-representation in our culture?

In *AIDS TV* I consider the *work* of making and viewing activist video, as much as the "artwork" itself. I attempt to detail the great significance of the material conditions which surround the making and viewing of alternative AIDS media—the hard work of funding and production, the even harder work of getting tapes *used*—which will lead to a detailed description of my own video project, WAVE, in chapter 7. In the remaining pages of this introduction, I discuss how the making and viewing of four distinct videos demonstrate the defining features of the alternative AIDS media.

Alternative AIDS media distinguishes itself from mainstream representations about the crisis by using video to constitute and then communicate to a highly specific and opinionated community of viewers who need and so seek out these images. The theoretical tools currently applied to analyze the media are not well suited to understand texts produced when activists use film or video technology. In the following pages I will suggest how activist AIDS video poses challenges to three key concepts in contemporary film and media theory, specifically, ongoing debates about the potential power (or lack thereof) of spectatorship, the psychosocial effects of identification, and the viability of realism as a formal strategy to contribute to social change. These more theoretical discussions about the nature and functions of alternative video will be introduced in the following analyses and continued in greater depth throughout the book.

Make a Video for Me! Four Alternative Videos by Women

My analysis is based on four tapes made in 1990 by women and for women: *Current Flow,* by Jean Carlomusto for GMHC; *Like a Prayer,* by DIVA TV; *Women and Children Last,* the trailer for the video *Heart of the Matter,* by Amber Hollibaugh and Gini Retticker; and *The Embrace/El Abrazo,* by Diana Coryat. Although their makers are all feminists who are active in the AIDS and media communities in New York City, each of these projects targets a more select community within this larger community (i.e., lesbians, activists, HIV-positive women, Latinas). This very process—winnowing smaller and smaller communities from the larger community—raises many of the questions most central to my understanding of alternative media. How do tapes, specifically by New Yorkers, about New Yorkers, speak to an audience of New Yorkers? How do these tapes work for other Americans (in urban environments, in rural environments), or non-Americans? Does video by Brooklynites speak to people from the Bronx?

The AIDS community as we know it today is speckled with hundreds of smaller communities and is bordered by its own margins. Women in the AIDS community form a subset, or margin, with different (and similar) needs to the community as a whole. As with artists, gay white men, AIDS activists, and countless other smaller communities whose needs and issues are targeted in the video projects of the alternative AIDS media, women have learned that the specific issues relevant to women faced with HIV infection may differ from those most relevant to other communities. For instance, to teach a woman to practice safe sex has little—other than the mechanics of condom or dental dam use—to do with teaching a gay man to do so. Thus, women videomakers have produced educational work that is explicitly for and about particular communities of women. A wide range of smaller communities are focused upon within the AIDS community of women: activists, lesbians, lesbian activists, Asian-Americans, blacks, black lesbians, black lesbian activists, and others. Clearly, such a process of infinite regression could ultimately reduce every community to the individual: make a video for me! Sounds absurd, but in fact it is the point.

As I have already suggested, a most significant way in which camcorder practice counters and alters mainstream media is that it localizes the production and reception of this usually universalizing mode of discourse. This localizing does not suggest that a black lesbian activist cannot watch or learn from a video intended primarily for an Asian-American straight social worker, but that she *can* do so. The political impact of alternative media comes as much from oppositional distribution and exhibition strategies (organizing screenings *outside* the community), as it does from oppositional production (making images from *within* a community). As video production becomes more and more accessible and less and less expensive, there is no reason not to use this medium to educate our own particular and private communities *while also* inviting other communities to see the ways in which we talk about and to ourselves. Of course, film or video can be made by cultural outsiders about people or communities other than themselves, but this is a different manner of production—one of the defining features of mainstream media.

Current Flow: Learning from the Experts

Current Flow, a safer-sex porn short for lesbians, is one in a series of such shorts produced by GMHC's media department. Because most funding for this project is dependable and constant, coming internally from relatively well-off GMHC, this work's production standards are high. Directed by Carlomusto in conjunction with an advisory panel of lesbians, *Current Flow* opens by showing a white woman masturbating with a vibrator to the sounds of a televised interview with Madonna and Sandra Bernhard. As the woman moves toward climax, a black hand stops the electricity flowing to the vibrator. Although initially angered by this interruption, another flow, equally exciting, begins as the mysterious intruder joins her upon the couch, and Sinead O'Connor's "Just Like You Said It Would Be" enters the soundtrack. Long, close, and barely edited shots of safe oral sex with a dental dam and penetration with a well-washed sex toy and then a latex-gloved hand are the tape's highlights. The porn short ends with the two women kissing, the glow of the television lighting their faces. The implications of such unapologetic, unabashed images are enormous. Carlomusto explains: "Lesbian identified sex positive imagery is scarce. . . . Although many videotapes depicting lesbian sex created for straight men are available on the shelves of even the most mundane video rental stores, only a few tapes trickle in from the West Coast made for, by, and about women. And even fewer of these deal with safer sex for lesbians. This is both oppressive and dangerous because in order to educate lesbians about safer sex we have to establish what it is."[19] No one is better qualified to say what is sexy (and safe) for lesbians than lesbian producers. And what better way for the larger community to gain insight into a desire and discourse different from their own than by watching the images created by lesbians for and of themselves?

Certainly, questions of exhibition and audience are critical for understanding such work. GMHC has a specific distribution strategy to target the audiences addressed by the tape. The safer-sex shorts are to be played in bars, projected before porn features, or used during safer-sex workshops. Small chance that *Current Flow* will flow onto the TV screens of people uninterested in lesbian sex. Although making resistant straight people see lifestyles different from their own is a political tactic (Queer Nation, initially a spin-off of New York's ACT UP, stages queer kiss-ins at straight singles' bars, for instance), it is not the politics of most alternative AIDS media. Many disenfranchised producers need the certainty of an accepting audience to feel comfortable expressing the things which often in "mainstream" culture bring antagonistic responses, discrimination, and sometimes violence.

Furthermore, alternative production is about communication: a willing dialogue. In contrast to the aim of mainstream media, a tape like *Current Flow* is not made to reach a mass audience, is not made to make money, but rather it has a limited audience and agenda. When and if such a tape gets to an audience outside its targeted community, this almost always happens because someone *brought it there.* Works with a specific agenda need specific distribution: screenings at conferences, workshops, meetings of community organizations, in classrooms; and these screenings should be accompanied by literature, speakers, or other forms of contextualization. Straight people can and should see *Current Flow,* but they should see it in a context where they can discuss lesbian sexuality in a productive, not punitive, fashion.

Like a Prayer: Opening Up to Activist Video

Like a Prayer (1990) is DIVA's third tape. The tape documents ACT UP and WHAM!'s (Women's Health Action Mobilization) well-publicized "Stop the Church" demonstration against the policies of New York diocese's Cardinal John O'Connor. The tape is broken into six sections dealing with the history of the Catholic church's position on condom use and safer-sex

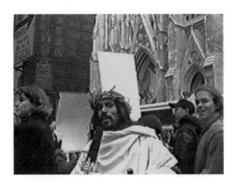

Figure 2   Ray Navarro,
Like a Prayer (DIVA
TV, 1990).

education, a deconstruction of mainstream press coverage of the demonstration, and the activities of Operation Ridiculous, an organization of clowns joined "to go where clowns have never been"—namely, to demonstrations of the militant pro-life organization, Operation Rescue. Each section of the tape was produced separately by individual members of the collective. The varied sections are held together by Madonna's song "Like a Prayer," interviews with Catholic members of ACT UP who were denied a voice in mainstream coverage of the incident, and hilarious advertisements performed by the late DIVA member Ray Navarro. Dressed as Jesus, Navarro advertises a pro-sex Catholicism: "Make sure your second coming is a safe one. Use condoms" (figure 2).

Clearly, such humor at the expense of the Catholic church does not make this a tape for everyone, and it is not intended for everyone. Similarly, not all viewers are convinced that direct action—something the tape unapologetically takes as a given—is the best response to the AIDS crisis. For instance, the women involved in the WAVE project, certainly committed to AIDS "activism," discuss feeling distanced from many ACT UP tapes, either because the demonstrators reflect the largely young, white, gay, and male constituency of ACT UP, or because the privilege implicit in the time commitment of direct action is unimaginable for workingwomen with children, or because civil disobedience is not a form of activism with which everyone feels entirely comfortable. Two important points are evident. One, anyone who does not feel invited to watch this tape, explicitly by and for AIDS activists, probably never will be a viewer of *Like a Prayer*. Two, those who *do* feel it is for them ("I'm an AIDS activist"), and then disagree with the politics or opinions found in the tape's conception of AIDS action, use this as a greatly useful learning process ("I'm an AIDS activist, but my AIDS activism does not include direct action").

This productive moment of individual and community definition can occur while people are watching *Like a Prayer* because, unlike typical mainstream media celebrating its presumed objectivity, DIVA is committed to identifying its messages as the *opinions* of individual people, just as the group is committed to showing the process of how these opinions were formed. "Alternative media are not neutral. They are, instead, highly partisan media enterprises that make no attempt to disguise their partisanship," writes David Armstrong in his history of radical media in the United States.[20] And Sean Cubitt writes of activist video: "these are voices raised in anger, seeking not to describe reality but to change it. They do not pretend to objectivity."[21]

Outside of studies like those of Armstrong and Cubitt, the effect of watching political, opinionated documentary is rarely theorized. The two most central theories of mass media spectatorship leave the viewer of alternative media out of the picture. Frankfurt School-inflected theories of broadcast television spectatorship are based upon an understanding of lemming-like viewers who, because of inability or indifference, cannot tell the difference between opinion and objectivity.[22] Although important in explaining the force of ideology in the maintenance of cultural hegemony, these ideas become less useful in a discussion of oppositional cultural production that claims its biases because it is made and received by people already motivated by a politicized critique. On the other hand, theories of the Birmingham School[23] that inflect descriptions of broadcast television with the understanding of an alienated, negotiating, or resisting viewer are inadequate for analyzing the activity of viewing a video that people *need* to see. Whereas resistance and negotiation are the key strategies of the broadcast television viewer who tries to make useful for herself TV that may be bigoted or overly general, the alternative AIDS video viewer largely can accept, support, and *identify* with the work she sees. Of course, the AIDS video viewer probably also rejects or questions material. But her criticism does not preclude her identification. Nor does it function as what Jacqueline Bobo calls "counter-reception," the critical viewing of mainstream culture by "minority" viewers who are well aware that only a slight connection exists between their lived experiences and the world envisioned on the tube.[24] bell hooks describes this strategy of reception as "critical resistance, one that enabled black folks to cultivate in everyday life a practice of critique and analysis that would disrupt and even deconstruct those cultural productions that were designed to promote and reinforce domination."[25] Counterreception, or critical resistance, is a tough pose taken up for protection against the cultural production of an oppressive society. However, TV work produced outside dominant systems and designed to challenge domination can allow for—in the right context, of course—a loosening of that protective stance, an opening up and an acceptance (which does not mean the loss of criticality). Conscious processes of identification are politically progressive strategies in response to activist television. While the viewer accepts information imparted in activist AIDS video, this does not occur because she is indifferent, uncritical, or numb but because the opinionated position claimed by a particular video rouses her into a politicized stance of her own.

Identification and Identity Politics in Alternative Media

Tapes like *Current Flow* and *Like a Prayer* exemplify how alternative AIDS media moves toward a production and audience of the specific, just as the mainstream media continues to fabricate work for a general, disease-free public to which none of us really belong. A lesbian or activist viewer of *Current Flow* or *Like a Prayer* finally sees an explicit and proud version of herself in a public forum. In *Current Flow* she sees cunnilingus performed by a woman; in *Like a Prayer* she hears a new list of the Seven Deadly Sins: "Assault of Lesbians and Gays, Bias, Ignorant Denial, Endangering Women's Lives, No Safe Sex Education, No Condoms, No Clean Needles." Unlike how she may have recognized herself previously, by having "aberrant readings" in which she "reads against the grain" of the homophobic or apolitical work usually presented to her, she may instead recognize part of herself as "lesbian" or "activist" in her similarities to, her identification with, the images constructed before her—images which insist that they come from communities with these explicit names. She can say: I've seen that before in my own bed; those sins I agree with.

Yet no identity, not even an "identity politics," is that simple, so she will also always see, in an image that is not of herself, how she *differs* from others who call themselves lesbians or activists. Maybe she is an Asian-American lesbian, or a southern AIDS activist. Such identities are complex, mobile, strategic at times, and only partially conscious. Viewing activist video provides a site where the interrogation and even potential change of one's "identity" can occur on both conscious and unconscious levels. Whether one's "identity" is as an insider or as an outsider to the position claimed by a tape, viewing alternative media that willingly identifies its construction from a position of difference, opinion, and politics can aid the spectator to challenge the stability of these positions. It is precisely in moments of *identification,* when a nonlesbian or nonactivist viewer of *Current Flow* or *Like a Prayer* sees herself and her needs in another's, the "other's," that communication—and politics—begin. "I'm a heterosexual, but that looks pleasurable to me," "I'm straight, but that's what oral sex feels like for me," "I'm Catholic, but I do not believe that the oppression of gays is condoned by God." In such moments of identification, a more complicated notion of identity is supported: as I see my own lesbianness or activistness (or blackness or whiteness or maleness), even as I am not a "lesbian," "activist," "black," "white," or "male."

Feminist film theorists have argued that the psychoanalytic mechanisms of identification inspired by viewing realist representation are one of the cinema's greatest powers and dangers. " 'Identification' itself has been seen as a cultural process complicit with the reproduction of dominant culture by reinforcing patriarchal forms of identity," writes Jackie Stacey.[26] Stacey quotes Anne Friedberg, who exphasizes that "identification enforces a collapse of the subject onto the normative demand for sameness, which, under patriarchy, is always male."[27] If the confirmation of a unified, gendered subjectivity is one most commonly theorized effect of identification within the cinema, there are many others. Paula Treichler notes many of these forms of unconscious *and* conscious identification in her reflections upon the abilities of mainstream media viewers to "identify" with PWAs:

> Questions of identification appear to involve memory, the nervous system, present goals and activities, life experience, familiarity with and pleasure in the conventions of a given narrative genre, demographic and circumstantial characteristics of the human figure (including their physical appearance, political perspective, values, real-life similarities and differences—class, gender, etc.), emotional and political connections to the text, and psychic commitments.[28]

As Treichler details, the point is not to abandon a psychoanalytic conception of identification but to supplement it with consideration of the more conscious levels of interaction which occur when film and video texts, especially politically motivated texts, are viewed by spectators who are seeking engagement with such texts as well as with the real world they represent. When a viewer identifies with activist AIDS video, while a patriarchal form of gendered identity may be reinforced, she is also being invited to imagine herself with the anything-but-normative identity of a member of an oppositional community. When engaging with activist realist video, processes of self-recognition—the naming and claiming of complex identities and identifications found outside of dominant culture—are important in constituting politicized (if still also, perhaps, patriarchal) identity.

Women and Children Last: New Centers from Old Margins

In her writing on indigenous media—video made by the "first nation" peoples around the world—Faye Ginsburg describes a postcolonial situation where ethnic or indigenous identity is affected and inflected by knowledge of, and participation in, the culture of the colonizer: "reflections of 'us' and 'them' to each other are increasingly juxtaposed." [29] The recent accessibility of video production and viewing allows a place in culture where this more fluid construction of images and identities can occur. Alternative media production allows the complicated work of identification to occur both within oppressed communities and between different communities. The possibility of self-definition occurs as that which was once the "center" is allowed to identify with the "margin:" to see itself there. In fact, alternative video allows people at the center and at the margin to see their reflection in the lives and experiences of the other.

This phenomenon is exemplified in *Women and Children Last* (1990), directed by Amber Hollibaugh and Gini Retticker. The ten-minute tape served as a trailer to raise funds for their final project, *The Heart of the Matter* (1993), a sixty-minute broadcast documentary. In their project, Hollibaugh and Retticker have redefined the "general public" for whom their work is made to look more like the public they know: working-class and middle-class black Americans. The film takes for granted that viewers from the center can identify with a marginal voice.

The tape focuses upon Janice Jirau, an HIV-positive black woman. Filmed in the close and intimate detail that only friendly relations between filmmakers and subject can produce, we hear Janice speak about the impact that AIDS has had on her life. She discusses her husband's death from AIDS and her own infection with HIV. He did not want to use a condom, and she participated in unsafe sex because she wanted to "prove she loved him . . . reassure him . . . because he was hurting." We are also privy to a moving gathering of her family. They eat, sing, and speak together about Janice's illness and their love and support for her. In conventional and beautifully shot documentary footage, we see what television rarely shows us: a strong black woman and a strong black family—not the homogenized Huxtables of *The Bill Cosby Show,* but a black family with class, ethnic, and political identity. A black woman and her family become the recognizable "center" of the tape.

But this center, Janice's interview, is framed with information which helps the viewer make sense of black, female experience, at least in a political sense. This frame is "white" representation.

The film opens with the title "1940s," which is followed by the title card from what appears to be a 1940s' film *Easy to Get*. In the appropriated images from this film, we see a white military officer talking to a black man, also in military attire, although clearly with lower rank. The white officer quizzes the black man about where and how he met his girlfriend: "Was she a pickup?" No, he met her on the street. "And you had her that night?" No, after a few dates. "And you didn't use a rubber?" "She looked clean." "Where you touched her she was filthy and diseased." Then another title appears— "1990s"—followed by a cut to Janice who explains: "I don't like the good girl/bad girl syndrome. I'm not good or bad, I'm just Janice."

This framing asks all viewers, white or black, male or female, to understand the subject of the film—the contemporary phenomenon of a black woman's experience with AIDS—in relationship to a long history of racial and sexual oppression, in and out of representation. To understand how critical it is for Janice to *not* understand herself as either a good girl or a bad girl, the viewer must try to understand a complicated history of racial and gender oppression as well as a complex black identity created from that history. The viewer must understand a long legacy of feelings of guilt and responsibility, especially among black women, for the spread of disease. The viewer must consider how white people have constructed blacks and how black people construct themselves in light of the legacy of such images.

Most activist AIDS TV, like *Heart of the Matter,* takes the form of documentary and the conventions of realism to transfer their respected subjects from marginal to central status. This new position is necessary for performing the tasks of education and self-identification central to the politics of AIDS video. Yet because activist producers rely on conventions that mimetically record reality does not require a lack of sophistication, as so much feminist film theory has suggested, about the fact that this representation of reality is *constructed* for clear and conscious ends. Feminist film theory has conceptualized how patriarchy replicates and perpetuates itself through the formal mechanisms of the cinema as much, if not more so, than through the overtly sexist stories, roles, or stereotypes found in Hollywood films. In the seventies, using critical theory as their guide, influential theorists created a decidedly feminist set of interpretations which began to explain the structural basis of the maintenance of patriarchy through dominant systems of representation. Realist style was understood to be one of these devices:

"Realism as a style is unable to change consciousness because it does not depart from the forms that embody the old consciousness. Thus, prevailing realist codes . . . must be abandoned and the cinematic apparatus used in a new way so as to challenge audiences' expectations and assumptions about life." [30]

As was true for my brief discussions about prevailing theories about both media reception and the effects of identification, the majority of feminist discussion about realist form has been developed through analyses of dominant culture. What has continually lacked theoretical attention are the effects of using conventional structures like realist style to represent oppositional content, which may be nothing more or less radical than using the camera to testify to the reality of an individual's underrepresented existence. As I have explained, activist film- and videomakers—people who are drawn to media production because they have something urgent and opinionated to say—often use the camera as a tool for defining for themselves their identities as individuals or members of minority or political communities. People hitherto represented only in the punitive or oppressive manner engendered by mainstream media can begin to confront how they want to see themselves and their concerns. Amy Taubin insists that an important lesson of the realist documentaries of the women's movement in the early 1970s is that "the way to insure marginalized people a place in history is to record their stories on film." [31] Realist codes and talking-head conventions are most typically used to do the political work of entering new opinions, new selves, or newly understood selves into public discourse. A political act founded in an awareness of what hegemonic representations typically include and censor, the realistic representation of new centers of expertise is necessarily a self-conscious process.

The Embrace: Distribution and Reception Organize Alternative Production

Mainstream media flows quickly through our lives, is broadcast, and then is gone. Because alternative media is not necessarily made to be broadcast, each project can develop its own plan for distribution and reception, which often organizes the project's mode of production and formal strategies. Take *The Embrace/El Abrazo: A Video Performance* (1990), the documentation of a theater piece. The tape was produced by the Pregones Touring Puerto Rican Theatre Collection, a group which uses an interactive theater technique known as "Forum Theater." Directed by Diana Coryat, the video version fulfills the same innovative educational function as the live performance.

Pregones produces bilingual Spanish/English theater to educate people of Latino communities about AIDS. The actors perform a scenario raising issues about AIDS which are common to the East Harlem communities for whom they perform. In the performance documented in the tape, an apartment-dwelling married couple with a child decide to kick out the wife's brother who they believe is using drugs and who, therefore, they believe must be infected with HIV. At a critical juncture, a character dressed like and identified as a joker stops the action and asks the audience to decide who is the most oppressed character in the scenario. The audience is then instructed to consider how they would behave differently to resolve the confrontation. The scene is enacted again on the tape, with an audience volunteer playing the part of the oppressed character. The new performance can be interrupted at any time by other audience members at the performance if it is decided that the situation could be handled still differently.

The video sticks to this interactive format, "encouraging critical thinking and audience participation," by using the joker character as a narrator who instructs the video spectators to turn it off and, whenever he gives the word, to discuss or even enact their solutions. When the video spectator turns the video back on, documentary footage of the solutions of two actual audiences are presented. Question-and-answer sessions from live performances, interviews with participants, and sections which provide accurate safer-sex information are also included in the tape.

Clearly, this tape, which is funded as AIDS education and not through media or arts organizations, challenges many expectations about the purposes and possibilities of media. Unlike broadcast television, which asks for the limited interaction of a maximum and universalized viewership, *The Embrace* is made to be used in small groups from specific communities and to incite audience action, education, and participation. Imagine a network-televised educational program that asks the viewers to turn off their sets! How would the home viewer catch the commercials? Unencumbered by TV's mode of financing, *The Embrace* entirely refashions the uses of the television screen for local, specific, interactive education.

We have found over the course of the AIDS crisis that education is most effective when it comes from, and is made specifically for, the diverse communities who most need to be addressed. An entire chapter of the Panos Institute's analysis of the effects of AIDS on international ethnic minorities, *Blaming Others: Prejudice, Race and Worldwide AIDS,* is devoted to the necessity of minority communities educating themselves: "AIDS prevention can only be effective if it changes people's sexual behavior. In the Third World, and among ethnic minorities in the North, this is unlikely to happen if AIDS education is perceived to emanate from the predominantly white, relatively privileged, outside establishment." [32] The chapter then documents innovative global programs where Zambians are educating Zambians, where prostitutes lead safer sex workshops for other prostitutes, where churches educate their parishioners, where Latin Americans produce AIDS educational materials in Spanish. "We don't believe in translations," says Dr. Jane Delgado, president of the National Coalition of Hispanic Health and Human Service Organizations. [33]

In the production of educational AIDS video, a similar trend has taken place. Jose Guiterrez-Gomez and Jose Vergelin, producers of the telanovela educational AIDS video *Ojos Que No Ven* (1987), also criticize translation: "Effective AIDS education directed at minorities requires a show and tell medium that can also role model positive behavior change while reflecting the language, culture, values, and lifestyles of the target audience. . . . Government agencies will often translate materials in order to save money and the result is, almost inevitably, a useless one. People simply cannot relate what they are being taught (to their lives), and the educational message falls on deaf ears." [34] Guiterrez-Gomez and Vergelin call for a move toward producer/audience identification in the production of educational AIDS media. Appropriate and useful education demands a specific voice and form of address—an explicit acknowledgment of what unifies, and identifies, maker and audience. This connection between audience and producer occurs in the "artist's response" to AIDS as well, according to Jan Zita Grover:

> An accurate reading of audience became particularly important here; AIDS activist groups and service organizations now spend as much time defining and addressing questions about audience—i.e., appropriate language, idiom, graphic style, literacy level and circulation for different "markets" of AIDS information—as any art director or account rep at DD or Chiat-Day. Many young artists have had their first introduction to their own marginality as speakers and audiences (e.g., as gay men, as lesbians, as sex workers, as artists) while working on these projects. They have also learned the salutary lesson that it is difficult to speak effectively for or to people unlike themselves. [35]

The educational work of the alternative AIDS media in this way is forced to contradict the legacy of ethnographic film, where the "other" is represented by an outsider. With the democraticization of camcorder technology, the culturally disenfranchised who are most typically the victims of the curious gaze and cameras of outsiders can for the first time afford to represent themselves using video. The camcorder offers a practical response to the theoretical dead ends of ethnography and multiculturalism. Ethnography is most typically an unreciprocated will to know some disempowered "other," while multiculturalism, according to independent media producer Ada Gay Griffin, often belies "the diversity of the self-determined points of view of the disempowered."[36] With a camcorder, a marginal community is able to represent itself cheaply and easily. The representation of the most pressing issues of our time by people from within affected communities emphasize the "self-determination of the disempowered," documenting the experiences and needs of the disenfranchised because *they* want them to be imaged.

This lesson about a different relation to subject, maker, and audience has been learned before. In the 1970s, feminists were making committed media: "the relationship of commitment between filmmaker and subject, and between these two and the audience, provides a little-discussed dimension to the issues of how women are 'represented' in (feminist) documentaries."[37] It does not surprise me that the comfortable and explicit relationship among filmmaker, subject, and audience is also invoked by Bordowitz as he tries to give words to the new cultural production by gays and lesbians, especially AIDS activist video: "A queer structure of feeling can be described as an articulation of presence forged through resistance to heterosexist society. Cultural work can be considered within a queer structure of feeling if self-identified queers produce the work, if these producers identify the work as queer, if queers claim the work has significance to queers, if the work is censored or criticized for being queer. A particular work is queer if it is viewed as queer, either by queers or bigots."[38]

Something akin to "a queer structure of feeling" is there to be seen in AIDS activist video, by, for, and about women. As a woman who has been moved to act because of the tragedy of AIDS, what I see when I view women in these videos are communities, both similar and different from myself, who also have been moved to act. I see lesbians making love in *Current Flow,* women protesting in the street in *Like a Prayer,* Janice and her family in *Women and Children Last,* the women in the audience participating in the theater workshop in *The Embrace.* I see myself in them: in their strength, and purpose, and politics—in the common struggles we have shared as women. I do not see myself in them in our differences of language, needs, ethnicity. Yet I see that I have a community around me, even if these women will never know me, nor I them. Through these video representations and video communities, I find power to go on as I learn what has been done, what still needs to be done, and that I am not alone.

The Politics of AIDS Work

As has probably become clear over the course of this introduction, I occupy several positions and traditions at once as I attempt to document the importance of alternative AIDS TV. I am an academic, artist, activist. My writing traverses these positions, sometimes commenting upon the theoretical importance of an event, the political potential of an image, the aesthetics of an interaction. The unification in this book and in other forms of "AIDS work" of these typically disparate fields of cultural action is not uncommon. In fact, the tangling of approaches and positions which defines this book also defines a good deal of activist AIDS TV, as well as AIDS poetry and theater, the analysis of AIDS literature, and AIDS demonstrations.

This straddling of art, academics, and activism has been much celebrated and debated in the writing about AIDS of the early 1990s. A large body of writing now attempts to validate or disqualify why and where the authors and others do their "AIDS work." In his introduction to a collection of essays on AIDS "art and activism," James Miller goes to great lengths to explain this odd coupling.[39] Meanwhile, Lee Edelman bemoans an increasing dogmatism coming from activist quarters, supporting only "an *AIDS activist* cultural practice"[40] (emphasis mine). Grover insists that cultural analysis bears no effect on the lived experience of AIDS. "But I can honestly say," she writes, "that sophistication around critical discourse, theories of representation, power and knowledge, appear to have played *no* role in the ways people know or have arrived at personal treatment decisions."[41] And then, in direct opposition, Stuart Hall reflects upon what he sees as the contribution of cultural studies to AIDS. "In addition to the people we know who are dying, or have died, or will, there are many people who are never spoken of. How could we say that the question of AIDS is not also a question of who gets represented and who does not?"[42] Only marching in the street counts. Teaching is best. Volunteer before you read. Write, write, write. "It is certainly true that writing about AIDS for pleasure would be ghoulish, yet it would be worse, by several degrees of magnitude, if there were no writing at all about the epidemic or the dead."[43]

I focus upon others' preoccupation with the legitimizing of their own AIDS work because it is my preoccupation as well. We all worry about what is the *right* work because although our lives and careers continue, so does AIDS. Can we do AIDS work where we do our other work as well? If we are academics in our "real" lives, can we do our AIDS work in the academy? Should we? Would our time be better spent as buddies of PWAs (People With AIDS)? Should we give it all up and go to medical school? And why would any individual devote her life working to alter the course of a global catastrophe? Why wouldn't she? We worry about the *right* AIDS work because AIDS is so big, it makes all work seem wrong, small, weak. What is a video, an article, a book in the face of millions infected and hundreds of thousands dead?

So I conclude by sharing my worries about the right work. How do I validate the work I have done in this book and elsewhere? Like so many, I have been involved with AIDS for a long time—what seems my lifetime—and in a range of capacities. Perhaps I was lucky in 1987, fresh out of college, living in New York City, in that I came to AIDS as a *political* cause. I understood that around AIDS most of the issues vital to me (sexism, racism, homophobia, inadequate access to health care, legislation concerning the body and sexuality) were becoming heightened and exaggerated in our culture and world. So I volunteered at GMHC and then joined ACT UP a few months after it formed. It was later, in part because of my work within the AIDS community, and in part because of the unceasing expansion of HIV infection, that I was also forced to take on a more personal commitment to the crisis. Watching friends deal with their HIV infection, watching friends deal with illness and death, caring for a best friend with AIDS, worrying about my own potential infection.

Needless to say, I have been doing AIDS "work" for personal and political reasons for a long time. This work has largely defined my life-style, my friends, my beliefs, interests, sexuality, and politics, my reading, writing, and viewing choices—my world. I have made AIDS videos, written the vast majority of my scholarly publications on the subject, attended demonstrations, plays, movies, video festivals, and memorial services, volunteered at community service organizations, walked in walkathons, taught courses. As for so many others (the people of the AIDS community with whom I spend a large portion of my life), AIDS has defined the shape and work of my adult life, and it will continue to define my future.

For want of a better system, I have come to understand the manifestations of my AIDS work as structured within the triangle outlined above—art, activism, academics—this then inscribed within a circle created by the movement from despair to hope and back again. Imagine a Silence=Death button without the lettering; the pink triangle pictured on the button is constructed around the three positions and approaches I take, often concurrently, toward AIDS: as an activist doing work in the "real" world, whether this be participating in ACT UP meetings or demonstrations, or volunteering at BATF in Brooklyn; as a videomaker fighting in the world of representation, making new images, and communicating with people I will never meet across TV sets; or as an academic, teaching courses about AIDS, writing my dissertation about the representation of AIDS, now publishing this book.

I move across and through this triangle, linking its end points (i.e., organizing an AIDS support group at the college where I teach, is this "academics" or "activism"?) because of the black circle which surrounds me. This circle marks the endless and unresolvable transitions and tensions between hope and despair, from saying "I hate this virus. It is unfair that it is in my world, in my friends, during my lifetime. I can't stand it that I can't have unsafe sex. I can't make sense of the suffering. There's nothing I can do. It's too big. It's too muddled with other forms of social power. I'm not a scientist, or a psychoanalyst, or a priest, I can't make him *feel better*," to "I have to do anything I can. I'll volunteer. I'll apply my intellectual energy and skills to describing what and how AIDS means. I'll make an educational video. I'll do *anything*." Then again back to "NO! Who am I kidding, I'm just making one more contribution to academic AIDS culture, one more video to add to a list of thousands. That doesn't make anyone feel better. That doesn't bring back my friend Jim."

My movement around the triangle, from activism to academics to art production, marks a constant circling from a resolve to work for change in any and all the ways I know how, to a dread and despair that I can't do a goddamn thing. My work, my life, my pain do not matter in the face of AIDS. My best friend suffered and died, and I continually sit at a computer writing, or stand at a lectern teaching, or edit a video in a studio, or distribute pamphlets at a high school, or put another condom on another penis or vagina.

But what else is there to do? AIDS has brutally affected the lives of the individuals who have suffered from its pain and who have died from it. It leaves a wake of sorrow, confusion, dread, and anger. It profoundly affects the lives of those who continue to live, from our understandings of our sexuality, bodies, and rights, to our government's proscriptions about them. It has made the criminally poor conditions under which many people lead their lives more severe and it has reinforced systems of bias which affect us all. Thus, *AIDS TV* is theory and practice, art and academics, activism and analysis, because I mobilize as many ways of knowing and acting as I can in the face of horror.

   AIDS TV is not a history of alternative AIDS media, although *chapter 2* includes a truncated history, and I have provided an annotated videography (see Videography by Catherine Saalfield). Rather, this book is a study of video texts—most usually those by female producers—and their extratextual circumstances, so as to mark, celebrate, and examine camcorder AIDS activism to help us better understand AIDS, the media, politics, identity, and community in the face of AIDS. This book attempts to think critically about the political, cultural, and theoretical implications of the many ways in which AIDS is produced and reproduced by the alternative media. It is a handbook for organizing an AIDS video support group, or for thinking critically about the representation of AIDS in television, both alternative and mainstream. *AIDS TV* is for the AIDS community: activists, artists, academics, PWAs, care providers, doctors, nurses, researchers, mothers, lovers, and all the many other individuals who continue to challenge, and remember, and struggle, and unify. *AIDS TV* is a book for people who need to better understand AIDS so that they can continue to do whatever AIDS work they can to contribute toward changing the course of this crisis both in the "real world" and in the real world of representation.

The Alternative AIDS Media: What It Is

No mainstream effort is ever going to acknowledge that AIDS is a social crisis that has come about because of the other underlying social problems that affect women, gay men, IV drug users, people of color, prostitutes and prisoners. They are not going to take the time to explain what people are protesting and why they are willing to get arrested. — Testing the Limits Collective[1]

Many producers of alternative AIDS media, such as Testing the Limits, have decided that their mission has been to correct, augment, or politicize the paltry, timid, and incorrect representations found on broadcast television. Their goal has been to give the representation of AIDS a politics, a history, and an analysis. These mediamakers have insisted upon representing the stories, faces, experiences, and opinions that have been left out of mainstream coverage. They have insisted upon radical modes of representation, shying from the distance and judgment, the lack of connection and identification, of mainstream media. Largely, their mission has been addressed by insisting that the people who are affected by AIDS are the best, most qualified, and yet least represented spokespeople about the crisis.

People affected by AIDS have not been the first to find that their concerns are not represented to their liking by the mainstream media. In fact, a lengthy and important history exists of political people challenging dominant discourse through the production of activist film and video. Thus, to better understand the alternative AIDS media today, this chapter will first look at a small sampling of political and intellectual movements which were also highly dependent upon activism within the field of film and video. In each case, demands similar to those raised by Testing the Limits were voiced: the demand to "explain what people are protesting," coupled with the demand to explain this with a critical, political, or aesthetic vocabulary that is also absent in dominant culture.

This chapter introduces the alternative AIDS media by attempting to describe its predecessors and its short history; it then offers eight detailed descriptions of diverse alternative videomakers and their projects. What I hope to produce is a body of information that will frame the more analytical chapters by detailing several basic concepts about what the alternative AIDS media is. First, it is one in a history of committed film and video movements that have come about because of rapid changes occurring simultaneously within technology and ideology. Second, like these earlier movements, the alternative AIDS media positions itself in a dialogical relationship with what it perceives to be dominant culture and the dominant media. Third, the movement itself is as complex as the dominant culture to which it responds, and so the most useful way to understand the diversity of the alternative AIDS media is to look closely at its unique projects.

In Our Own Voices: A Short History of Politically Motivated Media

The Third World has attempted to write its own history, take control of its own cinematic image, speak in its own voice. The colonialist wrote the colonized *out* of history, teaching Vietnamese and Senegalse children, for example, that the "ancestors" were the Gauls.—Robert Stam and Louise Spence[2]

In the flowering of participatory social life we call "The Sixties" a number of previously unaccommodated and disenfranchised groups began aggressively to engage history for themselves, to make it their history.—David James[3]

Aboriginal communities are ensuring the continuity of their languages and cultures and representation of their views. By making their own films and videos, they speak for themselves, no longer aliens in an industry which for a century has used them for its own ends.—Michael Leigh[4]

Early women's liberation cinema used images of women talking in close-up to validate the concept of self-expression, a crucial concept for women used to being objectified, interpreted, eroticized and generally discounted in the mass media.—Barbara Halpern Martineau[5]

As a black woman filmmaker, my objective is to contribute to the development of our own definitions.—Alile Sharon Larkin[6]

In the face of a seemingly monolithic power structure of cops, laws, corporate media and societal standards of conformity, a little machine like
the Video 8 camcorder is capable of subverting their oppressive voice of
authority by amplifying the image and voices of those people and ideas
generally deemed unimportant.—Ellen Spiro[7]

Alternative AIDS video is indebted to a long tradition of cultural
theory and production which has insisted upon the vital significance of self-
expression, the politics of self-definition, the power of speaking "in our own
voice." The colonized people of the Third World, the minority and disenfranchised communities of the First World, and the indigenous peoples of the
"Fourth World" have shared and made this demand for decades. Although
the selves, the identities, the politics that can be defined with these newly
acquired voices are as different as only community, ethnicity, gender, and
nationality can be, the call for self-determination, specifically with the camera, is held in common by them all. The demand to "speak in our own voice"
and "produce our own images" with a film or video camera is based upon
the presupposition that "we" have been represented by someone else—colonial France or England, anthropologists, NBC Nightly News, whites, men—
in a manner that is both false and oppressive, and therefore gaining control
over representation is significant in itself.

The history of the alternative AIDS media can be traced through the
formation of a number of film and video movements rooted in a struggle for
representation: from the Third Cinema and the New American Cinema in the
fifties and sixties, to the large shifts in documentary and ethnographic film
production and the development of minority cinemas (like the feminist and
black film movements) in the seventies, into the production of indigenous
media and camcorder activism of the eighties and nineties. Each of these
film movements, rooted in real political struggle, occurred when cultural,
theoretical, and historical factors converged to give new force to the politics
of self-representation and self-determination: that is, the decolonization of
the Third World, the end of modernism, the civil rights movements of the
sixties and seventies, reinterpretations of Marxist ideology, poststructuralist
and postmodern theory.

These shifts in culture occurred concurrently with technological
developments which at once made the production of film, and later video,

available to those who earlier had had little access to these expensive and complicated formats and which also made production itself simpler. David James writes that the model of the industrial cinema was founded primarily upon its "containment" within capitalist industry: "The enabling condition of the entire system is the social division that restricts access to the means of film production to the owners of film studios, concomitantly excluding the masses from production and instating them as consumers."[8] The advent of lightweight 16mm and consumer-model 8mm cameras, high-speed film, and synchronous sound in the fifties and sixties suddenly altered these founding conditions, making the film medium a viable, if not crucial, tool for the self-construction of political culture. Julianna Burton explains about the "New Latin American Cinema movement" of the 1960s: "Film was the most indus-trialized sector of the 'culture industry,' the most massive of the mass media in its accessibility to all social strata. It was clearly 'the most important art,' the most appropriate cultural means of social transformation."[9] Later, the portapack, and then the camcorder, opened up the possibilities of media production to even more communities—making video arguably the "most important art" of the seventies, eighties, and nineties.

The Third Cinema: Decolonizing Culture

The lessons of Third Cinema are instructive. Alternative represen-tation emerges out of moments of political engagement and consciousness. The politicization and decolonization of the longtime colonial subject pro-vide a first instance in my truncated history of movements dedicated to producing film and video in "our own voice." In the fifties and sixties the colonized people of the Third World were organizing the political struggles that would eventually end (at least by law) their domination by colonizing powers. At the same time, Burton emphasizes, another, related struggle was taking place, the use of film to forge "a sense of national identity and cultural autonomy."[10]

The worldwide movements for decolonization understood cultural production as both a powerful site of oppression and a necessary position for resistance.[11] Great theoretical attention at this time was being paid to the study of "ideology." Marxist reinterpretations of the relation between the "base" (economic modes of production—the infrastructure) and "super-structure" (institutions of social ideas such as culture, the judicial process, the arts, philosophy, religion) focused new attention upon the function of the superstructure, or ideology, in social formations. Classic interpretations of Marx had stressed that the superstructure merely echoed the material and social relations of the base, a dependent sphere, which simply reflects "in ideas" what is happening elsewhere. New interpretations emphasized the interdependence and reciprocity of base and superstructure. Ideology was now understood to have a "specificity" and relative "autonomy" and, therefore, an "influence" upon "historical struggles."[12]

Founded upon this notion of ideology, the Third Cinema could propose to change the oppressive dominant culture of colonialism by altering systems of representation. Thus, the "real" revolutions occurring in Africa, Latin America, and Asia were accompanied by revolutions in cultural (and often specifically film) production. In their seminal article, "Toward a Third Cinema," Fernando Solanas and Octavio Getino use the rhetoric of revolution to define the Third Cinema: "The anti-imperialism struggle of the peoples of the Third World and their equivalents inside the imperialist countries constitutes today the axis of world revolution. *Third Cinema* is, in our opinion, the cinema that *recognizes in that struggle the most gigantic cultural, scientific, and artistic manifestations of our time,* the great possibility of constructing a liberated personality with each people as the starting point—in a word, the *decolonization of culture.*"[13] This struggle to decolonize culture was enacted in film production and theory, inspiring large bodies of work on an international level. Filmmakers and theorists described the making and viewing of the Third Cinema in terms similar to those I have used for the alternative AIDS media: making and viewing politically motivated film is a revolutionary act which can help to construct "liberated personalities."

The New American and Underground Cinemas: The Politics of Aesthetics

The Beat Generation of the 1950s and 1960s, like the community of scholars, activists, and producers who developed the Third Cinema, found that its writers' and artists' radical challenges to the dominant culture (in life-style, sexuality, politics, and aesthetics) could be expressed with the newly economically feasible medium of film (the 16mm camera as well as the 8mm home movie camera became widely available in the fifties). More an aesthetic than a materialist critique of society,[14] the challenges that came from the Beats were as much to the dominant cinema as they were to dominant American culture. A "New American Cinema" was invented that challenged the Hollywood system in its conditions of production, distribution, and consumption, in economics, and in form. This cinema is the model with which much alternative American production continues today: low-budget work that celebrates and constructs the minority culture which produces it, receives it, and which it records. This work is made by people already invested in the "community" they document; it is work financed independently (often as art, sometimes as scholarship); work distributed outside the channels of the dominant cinema to a small community of people who are similar to the filmmakers.

American film production of the late fifties began to use film for the new (and radical) end of personal expression. Films like *Pull My Daisy* (Robert Frank and Alfred Leslie, 1959) were made for little money, received honors as artistic productions, and used the personal lives of the filmmakers as their subject. These films set the groundwork for the "underground film" of the sixties, which was a cinema made for almost no money with small-format equipment, usually documenting the unscripted and unrehearsed interaction of people "performing" people like themselves, and exhibited in alternative spaces. Such films were produced outside the commercial cinema's modes of production and distribution. The Beats' politics of aesthetics, their belief that the "aesthetic could provide the basis for a minority culture of general social potential," was actualized in a new mode of filmmaking that transformed all facets of production into a "countercultural activity."[15] Many of the films of this period, like the work of Jack Smith, Ron Rice, Ken Jacobs, and Kenneth Anger, incorporated transvestitism, homosexuality, and other nonconformist sexual activities, as well as drug use, as the subjects of their films and as a means toward the creativity which powered them.

James argues that the American underground film movement of the fifties and sixties is a direct precursor to the radical protest cinema of the sixties, which documented the political activism of the civil rights, antiwar, women's, and gay liberation movements.[16] The demand for personal expressiveness and self-definition voiced in the New American Cinema became the more socially engaged, and often more militant, activism and cultural production found in the video movement and the minority cinemas of the late sixties and seventies.

Reflexivity and Participation in the Ethnographic Film

Whereas sixties' documentarists discoursed confidently about the "other"— worker, Indian, black—from a presumed superior position, seventies' docu-

mentarists began to doubt their right and capacity to speak "for" the other. —
Robert Stam and Ismail Xavier[17]

Stam and Ismail Xavier, here describing Brazilian film, lay out the
terms of the historical and theoretical trajectory which occurred in ethnographic and documentary film during the 1970s. Emilie de Brigard claims
in her essay, "The History of Ethnographic Film," that "ethnographic film
began as a phenomenon of colonialism."[18] This "colonial" film practice typically used the technical apparatus of film to record with the unquestioned
objectivity of a machine the colonized people of the Third World. Clearly,
some redefinition of ethnographic film practice was needed to respond to
the struggles and liberation of its subjects "in the field." In 1975 Margaret
Mead suggested one crucial safeguard necessary to protect the newly liberated subjects of the ethnographic camera: "the articulate, imaginative inclusion in the whole process of the people who are being filmed—inclusion in
the planning and programming, in the filming itself, and in the editing of
the film."[19] What had happened in the twenty-five years since the filming of
Karba's First Years—in which Mead's unrelenting voice-over explained "the
significance" of the gestures and habits of baby Karba and his New Guinea
family—that now allowed Mead to insist upon a radical redefinition of the
ethnographic film from a device for scientific recording and interpretation
to a device for cross-cultural interaction?
    As the longtime colonial subject of the ethnographic film became
the decolonized subject of postcolonial society, the field of anthropology
was responding to changes in academic thought incurred by poststructural-
ism and other critiques of supposed objectivity. Ginsburg enumerates these
"historical, intellectual, and political developments":

> the end of the colonial era with the assertion of self-determination
> by native peoples;
> the radicalization of young scholars in the 1960s and the replac-
> ing of positivist models of knowledge with more interpretive and
> politically self-conscious approaches;
> and a reconceptualization of "the native voice" as one that should
> be in more direct dialogue with anthropological interpretation.[20]

Claudia Springer in "A Short History of Ethnographic Film" calls the new
approach to ethnographic film and anthropology "committed anthropology,"
an approach that is newly aware of the political, economic, and cultural
ramifications of the anthropologist's presence in the field.[21] Committed an-

thropology meant, at the least, a reflexive stance (the anthropologist "speaking in his or her own voice"), as well as the possibility of the anthropologist allowing the ethnographic film's subjects to contribute their own voices to the project. In his 1977 article, "The Image Mirrored: Reflexivity and the Documentary Film," Jay Ruby begins by asserting, "I am convinced that filmmakers along with anthropologists have the ethical, political, aesthetic, and scientific obligations to be reflexive and self-critical about their work." [22] His solution is an ethnographic film or anthropological study where "producer, process, and product" are evident.

David MacDougall emphasizes the importance of the interaction of anthropologist and subject, but he goes one step further by calling for the subject's *participation* in the production of the film. Arguing that the segregating of observer and observed into "separate worlds" is "distinctly Western parochialism," MacDougall suggests instead that in "participatory cinema" the "filmmaker acknowledges his entry upon the world of his subjects and yet asks them to imprint directly upon the film of their own culture." [23] MacDougall further suggests an ethnographic film practice in which the trained anthropologist and ethnographic filmmaker make their skills available to indigenous peoples so that their subjects can bring forth what *they* think is most important about themselves: "A further step will be films in which participation occurs in the very conception and recognizes common goals. That possibility remains unexplored—a filmmaker putting himself at the disposal of his subjects and, with them, inventing the film." [24] In their later work in Australia, David and Judith MacDougall explore such a practice. *Takeover, Familiar Places,* and *The House-Opening* (all 1980), were made at the invitation of an Aboriginal community at Aurukun, Queensland. The films focus on the community's ongoing struggle to retain their culture and regain their lands. Thus, in a relatively short time, anthropologists theorized an ethnographic film practice which acknowledged their own voices as subjective, and which then called for the incorporation of the subjective voices of the "subjects."

The Portapack Lets Everyone Make TV!

In the late 1960s and early 1970s the development of the portapack empowered a range of mediamakers in the First World to make their own video. The relatively low costs of the format, coupled with the features of instant playback and easy operation, made video ideal for MacDougall's call for participatory cinema. In the early 1970s and into the 1980s national governments in countries as diverse as the United States, Brazil, Australia, and Canada developed media programs dedicated to fostering "indigenous self-determination," where Native peoples were instructed in media production and began to operate their own cable television stations. The Challenge for Change program launched by the National Film Board of Canada in 1967 is perhaps the earliest attempt to establish such "a public service directive" for television. Run by George Stoney, the program was mandated to "promote citizen participation in the solutions of social problems."[25] Indigenous communities were trained as film crews to document their own culture and struggles. *You Are on Indian Land* (1969) records a brutal land-rights demonstration by Mohawks near Cornwall, Ontario. Later, in more remote regions, similar programs were supposed to serve as a panacea against the overwhelming effects of satellites which project First World media to cultures that may have had little or no contact with the "outside world." Ginsburg calls this a "Faustian Contract," because on the one hand the media became a new mode of expression for colonized indigenous people, while on the other it "threatens to be a final assault on culture, language, imagery, relationships between generations, and respect for traditional knowledge."[26]

In the United States portable video was taken up with less ambivalence by the sixties' counterculture, allowing its members to speak for themselves in opposition to what they perceived to be the oppressive voice of dominant culture and, specifically, its mouthpiece, the tube. The conjoining of the development of portable video with the period's political and cultural movements inspired a celebratory fervor over video's potential. Groups like Ant Farm, TVTV (Top Value Television), Global Village, and Video Freaks "were all founded on a belief in liberation via the democratic pluralism of television, anyone could control the means of production, anyone could and should be an artist."[27] The utopian zeal which met the release of video was based upon a contemporary analysis of the media, influenced by theorists like Hans Magnus Enzensberger, who emphasized its one-way flow. Enzensberger wrote in his 1974 essay "Constituents of a Theory of the Media": "in its present form, equipment like television or film does not serve communication but prevents it. It allows no reciprocal action between transmitter and receiver; technologically speaking, it reduces feedback to the lowest point compatible with the system."[28] Now, with video, it was hoped that the home viewer—the receiver—could transmit back in his or her own voice.

Radical video groups, like filmmakers and theorists in the activist film movements which preceded them, again founded their movements upon the theoretical, historical, and political changes around them. The theories of Roland Barthes and Michel Foucault, newly translated into English, especially inspired the makers of "guerrilla TV." Themselves responding to (and inspiring) the radical political events in France of May 1968, these writers theorized the destabilization of political power through the operations of language and textuality. Theories which interrelated systems of discourse and politics served as a battle cry for young American video producers: if meaning, knowledge, and power were constructed, then anyone could construct them; if all that people needed was an outlet for their voices, then video would allow everyone to speak.

Like the theorists and practitioners of the Third Cinema (and often relying upon them), American video users in the late sixties and early seventies also took up the revolutionary discourse of decolonization to explain their commitment to countercultural production. Cultural production was affirmed through a language of technomilitancy, as in this selection from the portapack movement's journal *Radical Software:* "Traditional guerrilla activity such as bombings, snipings and kidnapping complete with printed manifestos seems like so many risky shortchange feedback devices compared with the real possibilities of portable video, maverick data banks, acid metaprogramming, cable TV, satellites, cybernetic craft industries and alternate life-styles."[29] Although such utopian and revolutionary ideals of the early video movement were not fully realized, Patricia Mellencamp attempts to validate the changes they did inspire: "Although a middle-class, white (although intersecting with the Civil Rights Movement), educated, affluent, youth movement in the US can hardly be labeled revolutionary, the counterculture did at least signal a generational crisis in the smooth transmission of culture through institutions, including the academy, the media, and the family. It did present alternatives, among them video."[30]

The Identity Film Movements

The promise of personal and political liberation suggested by both the video movement and the underground cinema were taken up by minority producers in the 1970s who began to challenge these earlier movements on the silences that persisted for some potential film and videomakers. For instance, debates within Newsreel—which were led largely by females and people of color within the cooperative who felt that the critique of society expressed by the collective was not holding true *within* the collective—led to the 1971 production of one of the first feminist documentaries, *The Woman's Film* (San Francisco Newsreel, 1971).[31]

At this time, as in previous film movements, the political struggles of minority communities (people of color, women, gays) went hand in hand with contemporaneous theoretical critiques of culture, representation, and politics. Alile Sharon Larkin writes: "From the moment that Africans were brought to the Americas and made slaves we lost much more than our freedom. We lost control of our images. Film and TV have been crucial in the legacy and loss, our loss of name and culture, for Hollywood has the power to re-write, redefine and recreate history, culture, religion and politics." [32]

The Ford Foundation in 1991 awarded a grant to restore a 1968 community access series called *Inside Bedford-Stuyvesant*. In an article about the restored shows, Roger House describes the integral features of this program, concentrating upon the processes of community definition and political struggle inherent in the work. He notes several unique features of the program: "a belief in local control and a conviction that the community could use the medium to help define itself and explore issues of concern in its own words," a concerted promotion plan that brought news of the show to "churches, schools and the like," an explicitly political content in the programming which reflected this "unique time in black political, economic, and psychological development," and a raw and rudimentary style. [33] The ability for blacks to shoot (and see) their own neighborhood, their own political candidates, their own artists and neighbors and anger, was integrally related to the politics of black power.

The women's movement of the late 1960s also had focused on how patriarchy was served by women's lack of control over their own images. For this reason, many of these women's works sought to take control over the representation of women's bodies. Julia Lesage wrote in 1978 that in feminist films "women look at and touch each other; they all see their own sexual organs and those of the others, probably for the first time." [34] More significantly, feminist films of the early 1970s responded to the little-tapped power of women's voices. Feminist filmmakers and theorists understood filmmaking as an extension of the "activism and consciousness-raising of the women's movement," which were based upon ending the societal prohibitions of speech by and between women. [35] The camera recorded women's newly liberated voices, and film or video were ideal to get these voices out for other women to hear. "There was an entirely new sense of identification—with other women—and a corresponding commitment to communicate with this now-identifiable audience," explains B. Ruby Rich in her history of the feminist film movement. [36]

Feminist films of the period were founded on the belief that men had controlled the construction of knowledge and history. The films women made therefore allowed new—female—voices into the field of dominant discourse. Voicing their knowledge of struggle, women provided new interpretations of events, politics, history, and daily experience. Feminist filmmakers trained their cameras on "ordinary" women, allowing them to speak publicly for the first time. For example, *Janie's Janie* (Geri Aschur, 1970–71), through a lengthy interview, documented one woman's move to collective political action. *It Happens to Us* (Amalie Rothschild, 1972), one of a number of similar films, compiled women's testimony about the phenomena which shape their lives—in this case, illegal abortion. Later, a number of talking-head women's histories, like *Union Maids* (Julia Reichert, James Klein, and Miles Mogulescu, 1975) and *With Babies and Banners* (Lorraine Gray, 1977), were produced. In these documentaries, women were allowed to collectively talk their way into history.

The vocabulary of the civil rights, gay rights, and women's rights movements, matched with advancements in 16mm and video technology, initiated the recording and distribution of images of Americans who had never been so represented in forms of dominant cultural production: angry and proud women, intelligent and industrious people of color, creative and compassionate homosexuals.

The Camcorder Revolution

The 1980s and 1990s have seen an explosion in the realm of video technology: camcorders, cable and satellite TV reception, low-cost consumer editing, an interest in the nonprofessional documents of real people. The new video technologies which burst upon the scene in the mid-1980s have radically altered the media landscape, including the face of commercial television. Consumer video takes up a significant portion of broadcast airtime in a variety of programs which celebrate home video bloopers or the camcorder documentation by eyewitnesses of tragedies, violence, slapstick, or national disasters. The video recording of the Rodney King beatings is now only one well-known example of the new mass-cultural significance of "amateur" video images: broadcast again and again, slowed down, analyzed, then finally purchased and projected by Spike Lee for the opening credit sequence of his epic *Malcolm X* (1992). In 1995 one out of eight U.S. households has a camcorder, many have home editing equipment, and at least 80 percent of U.S. homes have cable or VCRs.[37] For the most part, people use these new technologies for what they were sold to do: to make home videos of weddings, vacations, and babies, to view Hollywood movies, or to consume tens of channels of programming selling hundreds of hours of superfluous products.

Yet some consumers have understood a more radical potential for these now readily available media technologies. In her "A Camcorderist's Manifesto," Ellen Spiro insists that "camcorder footage contributes to a broader analysis of an event by offering an alternative to broadcast media's centrist view. It has the power to add a dimension to the chorus of voices heard, providing a platform for seasoned activists and concerned community members, rather than the same old authoritative experts giving their same old scripted raps." [38] The use of this technology for camcorder activism makes the most of video's unique strengths: the possibility for the inexpensive production of video art, documentaries, and education, and the use of satellites and cable to broadcast this work to thirsty and underserved audiences.

Many videomakers believe in the potential powers of low-end video production as a contemporary forum for the political activism of the marginal and disenfranchised in our society, regardless of the issue around which they communicate. Karen Hirsch, the director of the Greenpeace video department, discusses the possibilities with words as idealistic as Spiro's: "There may be no environmental network on U.S. television, but there is a network of environmentalists making extraordinary television, video and film. This kind of media isn't trying to sell you anything other than a voice in the debate about the future of the planet. It is produced for the express purpose of getting you off the sofa and into the political process by clamoring for a cleaner planet. And it is working." [39]

Through the community-access movement, programs in media literacy and efforts like Deep Dish Television, which transmits alternative video across the country by satellite, a small number of highly committed Americans are using the camcorder for its most radical purpose, the one suggested in all of the movements documented in this history, to make the media an interactive rather than one-way flow, media which expresses the distinct needs of individuals or communities. Meanwhile, if the activist AIDS movement was the first contemporary movement to utilize the camcorder, it is hardly the last. Political movements from those endorsing abortion rights to labor unions and environmentalists have embraced the camcorder as the communication mode best-suited for the media-saturated, postindustrial age. For example, the Video Witnesses Festival of New Journalism, a 1991 program which included hundreds of alternative videos, screened diverse works that included, among many, a tape made by a group of female citizens of Israel, "The Women in Black," which documents the protests they stage in support of the Intifada each week (*Women in Black*, Marie-Hélène Cousineau and Chez les Vivants, 1990); a cable access show which documents the demonstration "HEXXON EXXON: An Action for Change" (*Hexxon Exxon*, Jenny Clark in cooperation with the Center for Environmental Responsibility, 1989); a video made by two artists in conjunction with local activists which deconstructs the use of the word "terrorism" in political struggles (*Counterterror: North of Ireland*, Annie Goldson and Chris Bratton with Anne Crilly and Brendan McMenamin, 1990); and four 28-minute programs sponsored by Paper Tiger Television and Deep Dish TV, which organized video responses to the Gulf War so that they could be broadcast nationally and internationally on satellite (*The Gulf Crisis TV Project*, 1991).

In review essays about the Video Witnesses Festival several elements were identified which differentiated these committed and low-end video projects from typical broadcast journalism. Among the characteristics of these projects were their explicit point of view, their passion, their intention to create an interactive dialogue with the viewer, the commitment of their makers to distribution, their explicit function as community-building tools, their capability of providing alternative information, and their focus upon self-representation.[40] Each of the political movements represented by these videotapes have their own histories of media representation. Yet because in each case the urge to create witness with video was most likely motivated by underrepresentation and misrepresentation in the mainstream media, the history of AIDS media that follows can exemplify all political movements which have embraced the camcorder. The desire to use the media to speak in your own voice is initiated by the knowledge that if you do not do so, it will never happen to your liking.

A Short History of AIDS Video: 1981–88

The following history[41] of the representation of AIDS in the media is selective rather than comprehensive. Although I make no attempt to ferret out every broadcast or alternative media representation from this period, I do seek to give representative examples of how the media covered the first years of the crisis. In these early years the role of the alternative media was largely corrective. Thus, my brief history will alternate between the work of the mainstream and alternative media, setting the stage for detailed accounts of the eight alternative video projects which themselves will serve to nuance the binary I use here as much for reasons of expediency as for accurate description. For the most part, a binary understanding of the media serves its purpose, describing a relatively straightforward history of AIDS media. The AIDS activist movement has been built upon just this perception of the binary nature of the power of representation—both the negative consequences of misrepresentation and underrepresentation by dominant institutions and the positive significance of resistant, critical, or alternative representations.

Medical journals in 1981 began reporting on an unknown disease affecting sexually active gay men, although many of the "symptoms" (generalized lymphadenopathy and rare cases of Pneumocystis Carinii Pneumonia and Kaposi's Sarcoma) had been noted in gay patients as early as 1979. At this early date, in response to a December 10, 1981, article in the prestigious *New England Journal of Medicine,* the first "expert" appeared for forty-five seconds on mainstream television, talking about the epidemic on *Good Morning America.* Yet after the first six months in the public eye, James Kinsella reports that only five stories about this new epidemic had appeared in the national press.[42] He compares this coverage to that of Legionnaires' Disease, for which the first week of the epidemic brought seventy-three reports.[43]

In 1982 the disease was given the name AIDS. Yet since the "home viewer" of broadcast television was not thought to be at risk, almost no mainstream press coverage dealt with the crisis. "Some reporters have claimed," Kinsella notes, "that until the epidemic began moving beyond gays, drug abusers, hemophiliacs and Haitians—that is, into the larger population— it wasn't a story that interested the average viewer. . . . The networks did not want to see stories about junkies or homosexuals."[44] In the minimal broadcast coverage at this time, AIDS was depicted as a "mysterious disease" affecting gay men. "Implicitly, these reports characterized gay men— because of their 'habits' or their 'sexual intimacy'—as responsible for their illness," explain Cook and Colby.[45] In response to this biased and dangerous misrepresentation, the gay press picked up the story, largely reporting about AIDS "in medicalized terms."[46] These early articles provided critical information to an answer-starved body of readers, filling in the gaps left by the mainstream media's virtually utter disregard. Equally important, in 1982 the first two AIDS service organizations were formed: the Gay Men's Health Crisis in New York and San Francisco's Kaposi's Foundation.

The mainstream press did not "discover AIDS" until 1983. At this time, according to Kinsella, mainstream press coverage increased by 600 percent, based on the release of a report in the *Journal of the American Medical Association* that the virus could be contracted casually, as well as by reports that the virus could be contracted through blood transfusions.[47] Although the major networks reported on AIDS only a few, scattered times in 1982, a year later NBC *Nightly News* aired thirteen stories, ABC eight, and CBS six.[48] Kinsella writes that this peak, like others, occurred when the virus appeared to be "creeping toward 'average Americans.'"[49] Cook and Colby call this first rise in mainstream AIDS coverage a cluster of "epidemic of fear" reporting, which capitalized upon, without dispelling, unnecessary hysteria about casual contact.[50] Grover and Treichler both suggest that the mainstream representation of AIDS from 1983 until 1986 was marked by a sort of willful blindness about the disease's larger ramifications. According to Grover, two accounts of AIDS held sway during this period: stories which judged and blamed the mostly gay male "victims" of the disease, and reports that ferreted out "innocent victims," still few in number.

In response, Grover explains, the gay and lesbian press and AIDS service organizations were motivated to provide alternative images of AIDS and PWAs. As early as 1983, PWAs understood that they "needed to 'humanize' themselves for a public that viewed them as a threat to 'the general population.'"[51] Thus, early alternative media images depicted PWAs differently from the mainstream press, which "collapsed the PWA into his illness."[52] Instead, such alternative counterimages represented PWAs as whole people with lives outside HIV, as people who were not guilty for their own diagnosis, as people who were to be identified with, not shunned, abused, or judged, and as people living with, not dying from, AIDS.[53] These representations constructed positive images and began the necessary work of building the idea and image of an AIDS community rather than an AIDS epidemic. In 1984 the first alternative AIDS videotapes were produced, largely by AIDS service organizations, providing much-needed information about caring for PWAs (i.e., *Caring for the AIDS Patient* [Hospital Satellite Network] and *AIDS: Care Beyond the Hospital* [San Francisco AIDS Foundation]). Stuart Marshall's *Bright Eyes* for Great Britain's Channel 4 was an anomaly at this time. The show attempted to place the AIDS crisis within the history of gay oppression and an analysis of representation.

In 1985 when the movie star Rock Hudson "came out" with AIDS, and then died of it, the mainstream press became intensely involved in reporting the crisis. Again, the mainstream media dealt with the potential of "heterosexual risk"—which Hudson's infection by some sort of bizarre logic confirmed—by either subjecting him to punitive reportage or finding an acceptable PWA to be kind to. In 1985, *60 Minutes* produced a segment on Pat Burke, "a heterosexual with hemophilia who became infected through contaminated blood products,"[54] although hemophiliacs represented only a tiny percentage of the population infected. "The outpouring of official attention to the handful of heterosexual cases in early 1985 proved a crucial event in determining the direction of AIDS debate in the next two years," Randy Shilts wrote. "It instructed health officials and AIDS researchers, who had had such a difficult time seizing government and media interest in the epidemic, that nothing captured the attention of editors and news directors like the talk of widespread heterosexual transmission of AIDS. Such talk could be guaranteed air time and news space, which, in the AIDS business, quickly translated into funds and research."[55]

In 1985 the first made-for-TV movie about AIDS was also aired, NBC's *An Early Frost*. The alternative press responded with tapes like *A Plague on You* (Lesbian and Gay Media Group, UK), which attempted to provide accurate information and expose the distortions of the mainstream press; *Buddies* (Arthur Bressan), a personal story of a man dying of AIDS; and *AIDS: A Bad Way to Die* (Taconic Video Team), produced by and speaking to prison inmates.

In 1986 reports were released that stated that women could be at risk of AIDS, which meant that HIV could be transmitted heterosexually. This radically altered the representation of AIDS, even though it was not a dramatic change in knowledge about the disease. Several news specials in 1986 attempted to address the panic around heterosexual transmission. These included NBC News' *National Forum: Life, Death and AIDS* in January, and CBS's *AIDS Hits Home* in October. PBS screened a *NOVA* sequence on AIDS research, *Can AIDS Be Stopped?*, and the independently produced *AIDS: Changing the Rules*. *The Ryan White Story*, a made-for-TV movie about "an innocent counterpart," was aired.

According to Grover: "the increasing divisiveness of mainstream coverage in 1985–86 was countered in gay communities by massive campaigns to affirm the values of gay liberation: re-sexualizing gay men by redefining sexual pleasure and sexual acts."[56] For instance, GMHC released *Chance of a Lifetime*, the first safer-sex erotic videotape. Educational materials of this kind (specifically GMHC's "Safer Sex Comix") were what brought about North Carolina Senator Jesse Helms's successful amendment banning federal funding for gay-specific AIDS educational materials in 1987.[57] At this time, the first significant number of AIDS tapes made by artists and AIDS activists were produced: *The AIDS Show: Artists Involved with Death and Survival* (Peter Adair and Robert Epstein), *A Virus Knows No Morals* (Rosa Von Praunheim), *Snow Job: The Media Hysteria of AIDS* (Barbara Hammer), *An Individual Desires Solutions* (Larry Brose). Also, several tapes were produced which documented the courage and humanity of PWAs: *Living With AIDS* (Tina DiFeliciantonio), *Hero of My Own Life* (Tom Brook), *Chuck Solomon: Coming of Age* (Mark Heustis and Wendy Dallas), *The AIDS Movie* (Ginny Durrin). *If I Don't Live to Be Tomorrow* (Health and Hospitals Corporation), also produced in 1986, documents the fears and biases of health-care workers.

In 1987 ABC's Nightline did a special sequence on AIDS, *A National Town Meeting,* in which a number of AIDS "experts" discussed and debated issues concerning the epidemic. The sense of fear produced in mainstream media coverage continued to inspire punitive reporting best evidenced in a PBS Special called *AIDS: A Public Inquiry.* The program documented the producers' manhunt for Fabian Bridges, a gay HIV-positive man who continued to have sex and was "hiding out with AIDS."

This kind of oppressive relationship to AIDS and PWAs by public institutions, including the media, was a significant motivation behind the formation of ACT UP (the AIDS Coalition to Unleash Power), a collective of individuals dedicated to altering the course of the AIDS crisis through direct action. At this time, GMHC's "Living with AIDS Show" began weekly broadcasts on New York City cable television for similar reasons, and Testing the Limits, the first video collective dedicated to documenting the AIDS activist movement, was formed in response to the rapid escalation of AIDS activism. The mediamakers involved with these organizations, all early members of ACT UP, believed that the mainstream media was not reporting the crisis responsibly but rather in a homophobic, sexist, racist, manner.[58] Their response was to take matters into their own hands and represent the crisis as they saw fit.

From 1988 until the present, an entirely different picture of mainstream and alternative representations of the crisis has come to the fore. Although Kinsella shows that coverage in 1988 had gone down since the peak during the heterosexual panic of 1986 and 1987, the amount of press coverage in 1988 had steadied at a rate close to the amount at the time of Rock Hudson's death.[59] According to *The TV News Index and Abstracts,* more than a hundred stories about AIDS appeared each year on the nightly news in 1988, 1989, and 1990. These reports covered a range of issues from the appointment of the President's Commission on AIDS, to the death of Ryan White, the teenage hemophiliac who became an AIDS activist, the fate of infected Romanian babies, protests against AZT, and PWAs who claimed to have contracted HIV from dentists. In the early 1990s an expanded acceptance of AIDS information in mainstream cultural production seems to be evident, even if this acceptance often takes the form of AIDS mega-stories like those of Kimberly Bergalis, purported to have been infected with HIV by her dentist, Magic Johnson, the basketball star, or Arthur Ashe, the tennis pro. In its handling of AIDS stories the nightly news now uses more graphic language as well as often including AIDS activists as a factor in AIDS stories. Whether this change indicates that the mainstream press and their imagined home viewer are more tolerant of AIDS information is open to speculation. Nevertheless, AIDS continues to make forays into the realm of mass culture, signaling its move into the shared reality of "mainstream America." To date, three Academy Award-nominated feature films about AIDS have been released: *Stories from the Quilt* (1989), *Longtime Companion* (1990), and *Philadelphia* (1993). The play *Angels in America* by Tony Kushner was awarded a Pulitzer Prize in 1993. Television dramas now sometimes include characters and plot lines which involve PWAs and AIDS. wGBH Boston began (and ended) a quarterly news magazine on AIDS called *AIDS Quarterly*, which covered topics as varied as AIDS in Texas and Poland, the slow death of a gay man with AIDS who disavowed his gay lifestyle to please his father, and the government's experimental drug protocol system. PBS produced a segment, *Other Faces of AIDS,* in October 1989 on the impact of AIDS on minorities. And *Nightline* produces three or four segments a year on topics ranging from the Roman Catholic church's stance on AIDS education to HIV home testing.

In 1987 and 1988 the number of alternative AIDS videotapes rose into the hundreds.[60] As the face of AIDS changed and diversified, so did the work of the alternative AIDS media. Video began to be produced from the many communities profoundly affected by the virus: PWAs, people working in the field, AIDS activists, IV drug users, prostitutes, people of color, gays and lesbians, women. Such work began to take account of the range of experience encompassed by the term "AIDS crisis" as well as to reach out to the range of people affected. The task of responding to mainstream representation became a less crucial inspiration for the alternative AIDS media. Instead, the countless tapes made from this time onward took on a full range of more specific goals and audiences, themselves reflecting the diversification of the people affected by AIDS. Thus, a myriad of production strategies, formal devices, funding and distribution plans, and target audiences began to structure the distinct projects of the alternative AIDS media. From 1988 until the present, a history and description of the alternative AIDS media can best be undertaken by closely examining the history of specific alternative

AIDS video projects. In so doing, I hope to highlight the differences *within* the alternative AIDS media, itself a changing and complex movement.

This chapter, therefore, looks closely at eight alternative video projects based within the New York alternative AIDS video community. B. Ruby Rich, writing about the feminist film practice of the seventies, discusses how analysis of the conditions of production is as integral to feminist film criticism as it is to feminist film production: "Feminism has always emphasized process; now it's time that this process of production and reception be inscribed within the critical text. How was the film made? With what intention? With what kind of crew? With what relation to the subject? How was it produced? Who is distributing it? Where is it being shown? For what audience is it constructed? How is it available? How is it being received?"[61]

Rich's questions are equally significant to criticism attempting to make sense of the alternative AIDS media—what it is. To answer such questions, I will describe in detail how eight alternative video projects based within the New York AIDS video community were conceived, funded, made, distributed, and received—how these individual projects are positioned in relation to both the mainstream *and* alternative media. When I pose such questions, several important and common features become clear about this "movement," even as the great diversity of these tapes is also evident. They range in budget from $2,000 to $1.3 million; they range in form from art tape to traditional documentary; they are shot on camcorders, Betacam and 16mm, by camera people who are self-identified as amateurs and professionals; they range in distribution strategies from a smattering of screenings at high schools to airings on PBS. But their similarities are also telling. Most significantly, all eight of these projects explicitly position themselves in some relationship, however diverse, to the form, reach, or agenda of the mainstream media. The close-knit nature of New York's alternative AIDS video community is also revealed—several names appear in more than one of the detailed histories (as do the names of institutions and organizations which have consistently supported this work, i.e., Downtown Community Television [DCTV], ArtMatters, GHMC, BATF). And as an alternative AIDS mediamaker since 1987, I am connected to all of the makers interviewed; they all belong to one of the several "AIDS communities" I am a part of.

This connection itself signals two important points. The first is the high level of commitment to the *issue* demonstrated by so many alternative AIDS video producers (and the institutions which help to support their work), even as our ideas change about our video productions. None of these projects would have been completed without great passion, devotion, and tenacity by the producers or collectives who made them, all of them primarily and consistently motivated by their commitment to altering the course of the AIDS crisis. Two, as much as alternative AIDS producers respond to the largely inadequate representations of the mainstream media, we as often respond to the work of peers, friends, and colleagues who produce *within* the close-knit alternative AIDS media community. The alternative AIDS media is itself large enough—and the participation of individual makers within the movement is lengthy enough—to encourage self-critique.

One final note: as someone who uses video again and again because I want to represent my image, the images of people I respect, and the analyses of issues that are important to me, I greatly respect others who do the same. Making video may be empowering, but it is also challenging, time-consuming, intimidating, and sometimes even dangerous. I wish to acknowledge, then, that this book's greatest limitation is my difficulty in being overtly critical of the video of the alternative AIDS media community whose work I so profoundly respect, endorse, and celebrate in these pages. I hope that I have created a history and critical vocabulary from which such criticism could be based, but my identification with this cause, community, and process does not make me the right candidate for such objective, critical work.

GMHC's Audio-Visual Department: "The Living With AIDS Show"

Jean Carlomusto was hired by the Gay Men's Health Crisis (GMHC) as an audiovisual specialist in 1987. At that time, the organization had "a TV set and one VCR and a need for information to get out." Today the Audio-Visual Department is staffed by two full-time employees (Chas. Brack and Juanita Mohammed) and several part-time staff members (including Alisa Lebow, Gary Winter, Gregg Bordowitz, and Carlomusto); it has its own ¾" production studio and on-line editing equipment and is responsible for the production of more than fifty tapes, including *Women and AIDS; Doctors, Liars, and Women; Seize Control of the FDA; The Safer Sex Shorts; Thinking About Death; Work Your Body; Prostitutes, Risk, and AIDS; It Is What It Is,* all of which are widely distributed at inexpensive prices by GMHC's Publication Department and are seen in arts and educational venues; it also produces hundreds of more volatile, transitory shows—maybe "good for a month"—made for cable broadcast and never distributed, including *Medical Update; Focus on Women; Caring; Mission Nutrition;* and *HIV Portraits.*

The many tapes and shows made by GMHC are highly varied. It is impossible to generalize about a GMHC look, tone, or content because work is made by individual staff members, who themselves have different styles and interests (as well as by freelancers, like myself, who are invited to produce segments or shows on issues of importance to those individuals). GMHC's video production strategies have continued to change, as does the crisis they cover. Thus, *Women and AIDS,* a tape I produced with Carlomusto in 1987, uses a conventional documentary style to relay the then unconventional information that women suffer from HIV. The tape consists of talking-head interviews with female activists, educators, and health-care providers who articulately present the distinct issues which affect women within the AIDS crisis: the potential dangers of negotiating safer sex, safer sex as birth control, the effects of racism, poverty, sexism, and homophobia upon HIV-infected women, and the scapegoating of prostitutes as an attack upon all women. The tape also includes detailed information about safer sex and about cleaning IV drugworks. *It Is What It Is* (Bordowitz, 1993) is a scripted, stylish, educational tape made for and in association with teens— MTV, not PBS, is the style being cribbed. The hour-long tape is divided into three sections which stand on their own so as to be used in workshop settings: identity, homophobia, and safer sex. It features a multiracial group of lesbian, gay, and bisexual HIV-positive and HIV-negative teen performers. In the tape's signature direct-to-camera scripted statements (as well as in the teens' confident self-presentation) they express the importance of self-respect both to acknowledge and embrace a gay identity and as motivation for always engaging in safer sex. Meanwhile, *The Safer Sex Shorts* are pornographic trailers which coordinate explicit safer-sex images to music and are made for bars and porn theaters, while *The Caring Segments* are talking-head portraits of care providers, which feature in-depth interviews with parents, siblings, and children of HIV-positive people. One week the segment of tapes on caring will highlight a Jewish family organizing within its community, followed the next week by an interview with the friends and family of porn star Veronica Vera or a black, female pastor explaining her AIDS ministry.

The show performs a variety of functions in a variety of formats because it is made to fill the gaps in the media landscape. When Carlomusto was hired, the agency was already using cable television, paying Gay Cable News to produce and air a five-minute talk show, "Outreach," which featured whatever was new at GMHC. Yet Carlomusto knew that a great deal more needed to be done: "So much of the stuff on TV was horrible. There was a total exclusion of PLWAs in its audience. Instead, everything was reported in terms of a panicked public. I wanted to do a half-hour show devoted to people living with AIDS. And that sent me out onto the streets."

Six months later, in June 1987, largely through the support of New York City Department of Health grant (which still funds a significant portion of the cable show), Carlomusto had her weekly cable show. She did not have a staff, equipment, or editing facilities—those would come later—but she began covering the rapidly escalating AIDS activist and PWA self-empowerment movements. From "a need to fill a half-hour show" she met many of the AIDS video activists with whom she would continue to collaborate and network. For instance, shooting at ACT UP's first Wall Street demonstration, she met David Meieran and Gregg Bordowitz, who were documenting the event for Testing the Limits, the activist video collective which she would later join. The following year she became a founding member of DIVA TV, ACT UP's video affinity group. "A lot of work was made because people started networking," explains Carlomusto. "Collectives aren't perfect. They are a hard way to do work. But it's also the way to get work done fast."

Carlomusto acknowledges that a different media landscape exists today. In the "early days" of AIDS video activism there was "simply a lack of stuff out there." Activists devoted themselves to the fast-and-furious production of tapes that filled the enormous gaps of coverage, information, documentation, and self-representation. Although some voices still have not been heard (women living with AIDS, for instance), Carlomusto believes that a much broader range of media information is now available. Therefore, she plans to move the show in new directions. She is now working part-time, dedicating some of her time to her own video work. Working on a cable show is exhausting. Work constantly needs to get done, with no time to sit on things and think or to do detailed research. With an altered AIDS video landscape, Carlomusto says she would now prefer to work more slowly on well-publicized specials which reach a targeted audience, maybe one every three to four months. Yet she also acknowledges the importance of the nation's first weekly show on AIDS, since it was and continues to be true that "there is new information all the time, and a real need for that information to get out."

GMHC's extensive production history demonstrates the value of consistent institutional support to remove many of the hurdles that typically confront the production of alternative AIDS media: salaries, benefits, in-house equipment, and distribution. Yet the Audio-Visual Department's infrastructure and production style are nothing like those of the mainstream media. GMHC receives a fraction of the funding of the nightly news, and they remain connected to the issues upon, and the community to which, they report. This means burnout—Carlomusto and Bordowitz have taken leaves of absence—even as it also always means creativity, intensity, and anger.

The New York City Commission on Human Rights AIDS Discrimination Unit and *Heart of the Matter*

The AIDS Discrimination Unit of the New York City Commission on Human Rights (NYCCHR) produced two AIDS educational videotapes as part of a larger preventative campaign: *The Second Epidemic,* an hour-long, made-for-public-television documentary about AIDS discrimination (1987, Amber Hollibaugh), and *Hard to Get: AIDS Discrimination in the Workplace* (1988, Alisa Lebow), a short tape made to be screened within training workshops about AIDS discrimination in the greatest cross-section of working environments. *The Second Epidemic* movingly covers actual discrimination cases taken up by the unit (a young boy forced from school, a gay male couple who may lose their apartment), intercut with interviews with Human Rights Commission staff members. *Hard to Get* uses newsreel-style segments to suggest the hysteria of much mainstream AIDS coverage. The steady, wise, informative voice of actress Ruby Dee counters this misinformation with the many reasons (medical, legal, ethical) not to discriminate in the workplace. To reach people who were not necessarily open to AIDS education (not just people already affected by AIDS, but those who are *not* and more inclined, therefore, to discriminate), the tapes use conventional documentary style to coat their more radical messages about tolerance and justice.

Unlike most alternative AIDS media, these tapes were produced slowly, carefully, and with (relatively) large budgets and a paid staff. They look like what they are—city-sponsored health education films with a PBS flair. (*The Second Epidemic* was courted by PBS, but never aired nationally because of legal issues which arose from the real-life discrimination cases it covered. *Hard to Get* has been picked up and used by several trade unions and human rights agencies throughout the country.) However, like a good deal of the AIDS work produced outside the broadcast media, the makers of this work believe that they espouse a "sophisticated AIDS politics" founded in years of radical cultural politics.

Lesbian-rights activist and sex radical Amber Hollibaugh was hired by the unit in 1986 with the specific mandate of producing educational video. She eventually worked with two assistants, Alisa Lebow (who came on in 1987) and Chas. Brack (who was originally an investigator in the AIDS Discrimination Unit). Lebow explains that "two white lesbians and a black gay man with relatively radical politics were the force behind a video from a city agency. This was state funded propaganda by people who are marginalized by that very state. We were in a unique position and tried to be responsible." These responsibilities were contradictory—to the individuals' political and critical beliefs and to their employer—demonstrating the clash of power and powerlessness which defined much of the work of the AIDS Discrimination Unit during its short life. Lebow explains that they were "in some way a part of the system of mainstream media and in some ways subverting it. Like it and not like it at the same time."

This position inside and outside the establishment accurately describes the unit as a whole, an incredibly vital force in the New York AIDS scene during its short tenure in the late 1980s. From the AIDS Discrimination Unit's inception in 1986, video was deemed an urgent part of the work ahead. Using familiar formats, it had the potential to reach large numbers of people. In the meantime, the unit also was getting out its message in other mass forms such as poster campaigns, training sessions, brochures, and publications. Although the unit's videos comprised one of its most successful endeavors, an unwieldy and apolitical city bureaucracy and creative video producers with explicit politics proved to be strange and difficult bedfellows, largely regarding issues of timing, funding, and equipment. Despite the fact that the two videos were fully funded by the commission, the staff consistently fought with the purchasing office to pay for the unheard-of services and equipment involved with video production. Meanwhile, the commission had no production or postproduction equipment of its own, although it had an arrangement with the New York City PBS affiliate, WNYC. Almost all of *The Second Epidemic* was shot with WNYC's equipment, and a good deal of the preliminary, "off-line" edit was done there. For both videos, the majority of their budgets went to the final, "on-line" edit.

Although such a process is certainly what Lebow calls "an inefficient way to make video," this system has benefits, the most considerable being the real clout and sanction given to work produced within the structure of a New York City agency. The tape can go places, and can be considered official, where most "alternative" work can never go. Yet this connection also was the videos' greatest limitation. "We didn't have an infrastructure. Everything was what you made it," says Lebow. Thus, although the unit sponsorship allowed the tapes to be distributed for free, because they were produced by a city agency it was difficult to use already established distribution companies to do this work (they could not make a profit on the tapes). Finally, although the producers were paid for their work, their positions turned out to be only as solid as New York City politics. The unit was shut down in 1990 because "we were making too much noise, we were too effective. They couldn't control us," Lebow contends.

No longer employed by the city, all three of the AIDS Discrimination Unit's video producers continue to work in some capacity in alternative AIDS video. Lebow and Brack now work at GMHC's Audio-Visual Department. Hollibaugh also works at GMHC as the director of the Lesbian AIDS Project. She also completed *The Heart of the Matter,* intended to be the first feature-length, wide-release documentary film about women and AIDS. Funding difficulties forced the makers to take on less lofty but still wide-reaching goals. Now a sixty-minute video, *The Heart of the Matter* premiered in 1994 on PBS's esteemed *"POV"* series and won the "Freedom of Expression Award" at the Sundance Film Festival. The film focuses upon the life, family, and political transformations of Janice Jirau, an HIV-positive black AIDS activist who contracted the virus from her husband who refused to practice safer sex. Jirau acknowledges how the burdens of racism, sexism, poverty, and violence made her unsafe sexual behavior seem at first like an expression of love rather than a lack of self-respect. In both private interviews and public statements to the National Commission on AIDS and to her church and family, Jirau cautions other women to struggle with the personal and cultural barriers which keep women from taking care of themselves (figure 3).

Co-conceived, directed, and produced by Hollibaugh (along with Gini Retticker), the film project shares most of the philosophies of the documentary work of the NYCCHR. Retticker, a commercial film editor who has worked on broadcast documentaries like *Roger and Me,* approached Hollibaugh after seeing *The Second Epidemic.* The two filmmakers felt that with a feature-length documentary film they could reach the largest number of somewhat-resistant audience members with their feminist-inflected analysis of the story of women and AIDS. To reach American women who need to understand AIDS and who yet would never feel they were part of the smaller, usually already politicized communities typically addressed by alternative video, Hollibaugh and Retticker felt that they needed to produce in film and to get outside the limitations of form and distribution of alternative video. This approach meant a large budget, a large crew, and then, ultimately, a larger release than ever hoped for with an educational or documentary video. In its first period of fund-raising (1988–89) the project did exceptionally well,

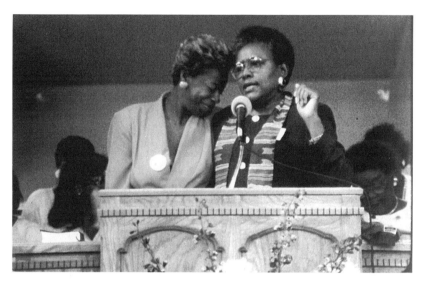

Figure 3   Janice Jirau and the Reverend Audrey Johnson, *Heart of the Matter* (Amber Hollibaugh and Gini Retticker, 1993).

getting support from various funding agencies, including the American Film Institute, the New York Council on the Humanities, the Northstar Foundation, the Paul Robeson Fund, private foundations, and private funders, for a total of approximately $150,000. A lot of money, but not the $500,000 necessary to shoot a feature film. And sad, but true, big bucks like those are not readily available for work which focuses upon women, let alone AIDS, and is based upon an explicit feminist analysis, to boot.

Precisely these difficulties served to alter the film from its intended ninety minutes and its format. The move from film production reveals the most about the production of alternative AIDS *video:* it is cheap, it can be made without the sanction of capital, it can espouse radical politics, it does not move in the realm of mass culture. The project proves one regrettable truth as well; to date, feminists are not privy to the kind of capital necessary for mainstream documentary film production about AIDS, or much else for that matter.

Tom Kalin

Tom Kalin is a film and video artist who has made at least eight videotapes and films about AIDS since 1985, although he believes that all of his work is impacted by the crisis, even if it is not explicitly about AIDS. His AIDS work has been financed, produced, and distributed in a variety of ways—from personally funded, individually produced, montage-based experimental "art tapes" to collectively produced, glossy television—yet if some kind of model is to be found to describe all of this work, it is his unique hybridization of the "heroic artist" giving form to the issues and feelings which mark his own personal/political landscape, and the "collaborative activist" who makes work which struggles to signify a collective interpretation of experience and ideology.

This tension between the intensely personal and the public and political defines Kalin's work, both in mode of production and distribution. For Kalin, the function of his work is simultaneously the articulation of his individual experience, which perhaps then speaks to, for, or about the experiences of others and his own need to search for and create community in the face of disaster. Thus, the motivations for his AIDS video range from the death of a friend, to his own anxiety about infection, to the political discourse and strategies of ACT UP.

As a gay white man coming into adulthood and artisthood in synch with the AIDS crisis, Kalin understands that there is no way his art could fail to confront the grief and pain, the difficulty of living, which has been his generation's legacy. Yet more than ten years into this nightmare, he also acknowledges that there are more "universal" themes to his AIDS work, for he now sees that humanity has always confronted and attempted to make sense of mass death, whether it be death through warfare, genocide, or disease. Furthermore, Kalin admits that even before AIDS gave his work a focus, his art was riddled with melancholy and memory. His father's death when Kalin was fourteen abruptly moved him from an idyllic childhood to an adulthood which included death, sorrow, and grief. The AIDS crisis amplified and focused this pain.

Kalin produced his first AIDS tape, *Like Little Soldiers,* in 1985–86 while getting his M.F.A. at the Art Institute of Chicago. The tape marks, for Kalin, his initial response to AIDS, a personal and profound fear with no interest in organizing or politicizing with others. He explains that the tape's abstract images are motivated by a fear of his own body: the routinized search for swollen glands in the morning, an investigation of passing, covering, othering a gay male body which can no longer hide beneath its flesh. The tape intercuts the brutal image of a pair of hands washing and picking off the white paint and then brown paint which coat them with the image of a burning shirt. In 1987 Kalin produced *News from Home* in collaboration with Stathis Lagoudikis, marking his first attempt to work through his own fears about AIDS with another. Also art school fare, the tape both implicitly and explicitly represents the anxiety of disclosure of sero-status within a relationship and within the society at large. Late 1987 also brought the death from AIDS of Kalin's first close friend. Because of this death, he fled Chicago, wanting to be in a community where the AIDS crisis was "discussed, palpable, visible."

This search for and move toward community define a second stage in Kalin's AIDS work, where even while working alone, he understood his art for the first time to be in dialogue with a community of gay men and AIDS activists. When he moved to New York in the autumn of 1987 he immediately joined the still-fledgling ACT UP. This association highly influenced his 1988 production, *they are lost to vision altogether,* which he believes is heavily inflected by an "ACT UP vocabulary" about AIDS. Kalin received his first grant for this tape, $1,000 from ArtMatters, which he used to re-edit the tape on a sophisticated, computer-controlled on-line editing system in 1989.

At this time and until 1991 he also produced work with the ACT UP artists' affinity group, GranFury. In 1990 the group produced four thirty-second public service announcements about AIDS, *Kissing Doesn't Kill.* These public service announcements, shot to parody Benetton fashion ads, are produced to promote racial and sexual diversity and tolerance in the face of AIDS; the philosophy about culture implicit in them is shared by Kalin, namely, that although culture generates from many places, the mainstream media sets the global and national agenda about AIDS. Therefore, Kalin believes, to reach people and to reach for change, you have to speak to people where they listen and in a language they understand. Thus, Kalin insists, "the ideal distribution" for even "alternative" AIDS video is television, "plop in the middle of the marketplace." Kalin explains, "you need to work to engage in the politics of Michael Jackson, Madonna, Benetton. There is no outside the marketplace in relation to art production. The best you can do is to tease the margins of the mainstream marketplace."

This Kalin attempted to do in his own short television spot, *Nation,* shot on film with a professional crew and cast and produced in 1992 with a $5,000 grant from the Whitney Museum and the American Center in Paris. Made for broadcast television, it was shown on MTV and French television. It shares the tone and rhythm of commercials and much of GranFury's style: fast-paced, sexy, didactic. The production and distribution of his first feature film, *Swoon,* took up most of Kalin's life from 1990 until 1992. Produced with approximately $100,000 of arts grant money, he freelanced to support himself throughout its production. Yet this move toward a much larger public was marked by a quick return to the private. Kalin is completing a series of "music videos," *Three Known Most.* Although they are most explictly about migration and movement, they are, according to Kalin, a diary of this one man's life in the time of AIDS.

Kalin makes tapes for ghosts: the people he has lost to AIDS, the faces he has seen on city streets or at AIDS demonstrations. He says that "they mark the terrifying feeling of being a person among many people. They are a lullaby I sing to myself to reassure myself and they are also a cry for help." Originally, Kalin distributed his tapes on his own. They are now handled by the Video Databank; V Tape; Drift; Electronic Arts Intermix; and London Video Access. Although they show primarily in an art world context, Kalin stresses that his tapes are also frequently used within AIDS activist and AIDS community settings. "I don't have anything more to say about AIDS than the proverbial Latina mother of two infected babies who is also sick herself. But I do have cultural access, entitlement, privilege." Kalin uses his privilege like an artist, like an AIDS activist. He represents what he knows, how he lives, in a mass-mediated society unaware that it is dripping with infection, unaware of Kalin's fear of death or his grief and anger unless he represents it.

Testing the Limits and DIVA TV

The Testing the Limits Collective has produced five videos since its formation in 1987: *Testing the Limits Pilot* (1987), *Testing the Limits Safer Sex Video* (1987), *Egg Lipids* (1987), *Testing the Limits: NYC* (1987), and *Voices from the Front* (1992). The shape of the collective has changed since 1987. Originally a group of six artists and AIDS activists who knew each other from the Whitney Independent Studio Program and/or ACT UP—Gregg Bordowitz, Jean Carlomusto, Sandra Elgear, Robyn Hutt, Hilary Joy Kipnis, and David Meieran—TTL is now Elgear, Hutt, and Meieran. In 1995 they completed a four-part series of hour-long documentaries about the history of the gay liberation movement, *Right and Reactions.* The collective's movement away from AIDS-specific video marks an important transition in the work of its videomakers, as does the project's $1-million-plus budget, financed by the Independent Television Service (ITVS), and slated for a PBS airing à la *Eyes on the Prize.* Although this collective always had its sights on a mass-release AIDS documentary for Middle America, not until the 1995 project did that aim become a reality. The collective has faced a constant struggle between a desire to reach a mass audience, a desire to remain true to their art school training, and a commitment to the movement which they document and participate in.

In 1986 Meieran and Bordowitz conceived of a video project to represent what they perceived as a resurgence of lesbian/gay/AIDS militancy in New York City. Bill Olander's "Homo Video" show at the New Museum served as an inspiration, bringing together for the first time what was clearly a developing movement of art and activist video centered on the politics of AIDS, homophobia, and gay identity (this show also profoundly inspired Tom Kalin). In the meantime, ACT UP was forming. It was an exuberant, dynamic time. Anything and everything were happening in the just-forming AIDS community, and it all needed to be documented.

In early 1987 Elgear, Hutt, and Kipnis joined Meieran and Bordo-witz in what was now understood to be the production of the first documentary about the newly developing AIDS activist movement. "ACT UP drove us, galvanized us, gave us a focus. There was a direct alignment between the group's history and our own. We were caught up in it—documenting daily . . . constantly." In March 1987, TTL went to shoot ACT UP's first Wall Street demonstration: "Our camera was fucked up, and there was Jean from GMHC. She shared that footage with us." At the time both TTL and GMHC were working with limited financial and technical resources and limited staff, and they were chronicling the same history; the merging of their energies seemed inevitable, and Carlomusto became the sixth member of the collective.

The organizing principle for the pilot they were producing to help raise funds for their thirty-minute PBS-style documentary was to "document everything." Without money or an office and with limited equipment, this documenting occurred however it could, which most typically meant "down and dirty footage" shot by whoever had a camera, whether they were "trained" or not. This is what Meieran calls "alternative media," that approach motivated by a commitment to a social issue, where production occurs because it has to, regardless of whether it is funded or even properly prepared for. The consequences of this manner of production are significant: "unprofessional" footage, unpaid staff members working because of dedication to a cause who are tired and stressed because they have to hold jobs to pay the bills, an insiders' viewpoint on what they are documenting. These consequences contradicted the collective's other goal: accessible, professional, conventional television that would speak to a "general public" who knew nothing about the AIDS crisis except for the bigoted, limited reportage on the broadcast networks' nightly news.

Completed in the fall of 1987 for approximately $70,000 (including a great deal of in-kind support from GMHC, from editing studios, and from others) and after six weeks of grueling collective editing, *Testing the Limits* immediately began to be distributed to AIDS service organizations as well as within the art scene. Yet the documentary never had its PBS airing; the style was too rough, the politics too explicit.

It was time to regroup. Although the videomakers continued to document madly, it was unclear to what purpose. The collective needed to reevaluate its goals and strategies. Throughout 1988 TTL took its first steps toward professionalization. The group obtained a computer, two phone lines, a bank account, and finally an office where members could handle distribution, grant-writing, and the storage of TTL's already large archive of video documentation of AIDS activism. Soon their office also housed a ¾" off-line edit system (good for rough drafts of a video, but not a broadcast quality final cut) purchased with loans and grants. The office cost money (rent, heat, phone), but it brought in more (funders trust applicants with a steady address; funding applications are more easily prepared in a well-equipped environment). Also during this period of professionalization, the collective split over a variety of personal, ideological, and practical issues, its own institutionalization being a primary one.

In the meantime, DIVA TV (Damned Interfering Video Activist Television) was formed as an affinity group of ACT UP, "organized to be there, document, provide protection and countersurveillance, and participate."[62] An article on activist video collectives by Catherine Saalfield (a founding member of DIVA TV along with Ray Navarro, Jean Carlomusto, Gregg Bordowitz, Bob Beck, Costa Papas, Ellen Spiro, George Plaggianos, and Rob Kurilla) chronicles the group's history and philosophies. She writes that DIVA "targets ACT UP members as its primary audience and makes videos by, about, and, most importantly, *for* the movement."[63] The group produced three tapes in its first life (see the following section on James Wentzy for the story of the second life of DIVA): *Target City Hall* (which chronicles ACT UP's March 28, 1989, demonstration against Mayor Ed Koch's administration), *Pride* (about the twentieth anniversary of New York's gay and lesbian pride movement) and *Like a Prayer* (five seven-minute perspectives on the ACT UP/WHAM! demonstration "Stop the Church" at St. Patrick's Cathedral on December 10, 1989).

While TTL was the inspiration for DIVA, it differed from TTL in

significant ways. As TTL was attempting to professionalize, DIVA was remaining staunchly *anti*-professional. "Watching TTL evolve into an insti-
tutionalized organization reinforced DIVA's commitment to working as a
collective. We remain fluid, make decisions with whomever comes to a meeting, and resist assigning a treasurer by dedicating any income to buying
tape stock."[64] Saalfield writes about how DIVA's commitment to "the quick
and dirty approach" of alternative production both inspired and limited the
collective's video production; its philosophy led to a "limited audience, in-
consistent participation by collective members, more process than product,"
but also "the essential goal of inclusivity, with open lines of communication
among collective members for expressing opinions and offering analyses.
Here protest is the process, communication is our form of resistance, and
everyone has a say."[65]

A loose intersection between TTL and DIVA remained; they often
shared footage, covered the same actions, and were committed to AIDS activism, as was also true of GMHC (where Bordowitz now worked with Carlomusto). But the AIDS video scene itself was diversifying and expanding to
keep pace with the AIDS crisis. Thus, by 1989 none of these groups necessarily shared ideological assumptions about AIDS video. For instance, TTL
decided to try again for a PBS documentary, this time a sixty-minute show
to be based on the PWA empowerment movement. It was an overwhelming
project with massive quantities of footage and an AIDS activist movement
that necessarily inspired the production of more.

Two-and-a-half still unpaid years later, *Voices from the Front* was
completed, now ninety-minutes in length. The group decided to transfer it
to film in hopes of getting a larger audience and more national press that
would inspire a broadcast television purchase of the tape. This proved to be
the case. Although it took seven months to get the film onto the market, its
premiere at New York's Film Forum gained it a *New York Times* review. The
film went on to play at art and independent film houses across the country, and it was even more successful on the international market. In October
1992, for a $15,000 fee, it aired on HBO.

Nevertheless, *Voices from the Front* ran up a $40,000 deficit and
never was shown on PBS. Perhaps a roadblock was the group's continued
use of "guerrilla coverage footage, reflecting the many shooting styles of the
friends and volunteers who documented demonstrations." But Hutt and Elgear suggest another reason: "We were too close to the material. Our friends,
our lives, were in that tape. If we didn't have that type of intimacy, it
wouldn't have been made. We wouldn't have gotten those interviews." Hutt

and Elgear believe that this intimacy, another feature of alternative media, allowed them to produce an inside view of AIDS activism, one that felt right to them as members of the movement they documented, but, again, this intimacy precluded a general public interest in the project. "Everything about our involvement with the material was played out in every aspect of production. Alternative AIDS media springs organically from the community affected by AIDS."

According to TTL, the year 1992 also brought about an escalation in antigay violence and in lesbian and gay militancy. TTL was documenting the birth of Queer Nation and the response of gays and lesbians to New York City's Rainbow Curriculum, and the Oregon and Colorado antigay initiatives. The group also continued to professionalize its infrastructure, ever trying to make the transition from "alternative" to "independent" media production, that is, a transition to work that waits for funding before it is produced, work that is job- rather than issue-driven, work that is organized, structured, and neat in its form and production strategies, work that answers to its producers, work that pays its creators and that is ultimately viewed by millions of Americans. In early 1993 TTL received a $1.3 million grant. The group attempted to make its pbs documentary again. But this time around they had the infrastructure, distance, process, and professionalism that only money can buy.

Juanita Mohammed

Juanita Mohammed has made several AIDS tapes, beginning in 1990 with her involvement with WAVE. Already an AIDS volunteer, she brought together through this project one of her earliest interests, media production, with one of her new passions, AIDS education and prevention. After producing We Care with WAVE, she coproduced Homosexuality: One Child's Point of View with her eleven-year-old daughter, Jahanara. Mother and daughter shot the tape on Mohammed's camcorder (she later acquired another Hi8 machine so that her production company, Mother Daughter Productions, could perform two-camera shoots), and they edited the piece while taking an editing workshop at dctv. The video was shown at several festivals in New York City, and inspired the team to begin a tape on menstruation.

In 1992 Mohammed was hired on a freelance basis by GMHC's Audio-Visual Department and became a full-time staff member. Among other responsibilities, she produces the "Caring" segment of the show—short sequences which highlight the experiences, struggles, and issues of care pro-

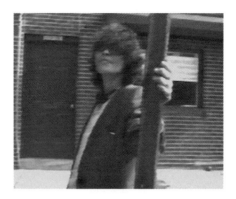

Figure 4   Alida "Lilly"
Gonzalez, *Part of Me*
(Alisa Lebow and Juanita
Mohammed, 1993).

viders of PWAs—programs about the mother and daughter of prominent
AIDS activist Iris De La Cruz, the role of religion in the health of PWAs,
and the work which occurs at Iris House, a center for homeless women
with AIDS. Mohammed's favorite "Caring" segments are *Two Men and a
Baby* (which focuses upon a black gay couple who adopted the HIV-positive
daughter of one of the men's sisters) and *Part of Me* (which tells the story
of Lilly Gonzalez, a Latina lesbian with AIDS who is a former IV drug user
turned AIDS educator; figure 4).

In the winter of 1993 Yannick Durand, director of education at
BATF, approached Carlomusto at GMHC, asking her if the Audio-Visual Department could produce an AIDS educational tape by and for teenagers. This
project had just received funding from the New York City Department of
Health. Lisa Alscott, a health educator for BATF, had worked with teenagers
at a special high school, Project Reach, teaching them to become AIDS peer
educators. Alscott had applied for an AIDS education grant from the DOH and
had received $2,500 to make a video highlighting the work of her AIDS peer
educators. Carlomusto turned the project over to Mohammed, which is how
Words to Live By (1993) was born. The tape relies mainly upon scripted and
talking-head interviews with the teen educators who worked on it and who
share their personal thoughts about HIV, safer sex, and AIDS education.
These raw statements are intercut with role plays. One role play, called
"Under Pressure," focuses upon a boy discussing with a female friend how
to say no to a pushy lover, and the other, "What If She Says No," enacts what
occurs when a girl takes on the power to resist unwanted sex.

Mohammed was brought on to handle all aspects of production,
from conceiving the project with the teens, to production and editing. She
was given $2,000, and the remaining $500 was used to pay the teenagers.

Because of bureaucratic slipups involving the grant payment, many of Mohammed's ideas about meeting with the project's students in advance had to be scrapped. In the end, much of what they used in the tape came out of their few organizational meetings. This resulted in extremely varied footage. Its quality depended upon who was there, what kind of mood they were in, how well the teens interacted with each other, and how much feedback came from Alscott, who had her own ideas about what the tape should be like. The tape ended up being shot over seven days, sometimes at school, sometimes on the weekends. It features role-plays, educational games, and talking-head interviews with the students.

These many hours of footage were transferred to ¾" and ½" video at a reduced rate at DCTV. Alscott, Mohammed, and some of the students looked at the footage and decided which scenes and interactions they liked best. Not an easy task since the kids fought among themselves, and then another difficulty arose between their needs and those of their teacher. From this footage, Mohammed created a paper edit—a written list of footage to use and how it will be edited together. She then paid Alisa Lebow, at GMHC, to do a final, broadcast-quality, on-line edit of the tape for her, which was done over the course of a crammed but productive day. The finished tape was then supposed to be screened at a premiere at Project Reach, but the event was canceled because school was out.

The tape has been screened on the "Living With AIDS" show and is used by both the DOH and BATF for teen education. Mohammed believes that the tape is effective as a means of education because it "feels like teens really made it. It's more personal than the work that comes from adults for teens. They make mistakes and correct themselves. It looks like every day, it's not lit perfectly. But kids watching it will identify. They'll know these are real kids." Mohammed thinks that the "real" feeling of this tape—signified by its *lack* of expense, professional actors, or high-end video equipment—will make it an effective educational tool.

AIDSFilms

Since its founding in 1985 AIDSFilms has produced six educational, fictionalized, "behavior-modeling" films about AIDS: *AIDS: Changing the Rules* (1987), *Seriously Fresh, Vida,* and *Are You with Me?* (1988–89), *Reunion* (1992), and *Party!* (1993). Founded by freelance film producer John Hoffman, Frank Getchell of the Children's Television Workshop, and Dr. Susan Tross from the Narcotic and Drug Research Institute, this company produces high-end, glossy, expensive, and massively distributed programs using "the vernacular of TV." All six AIDSFilms' shorts are narrative films with the look and much of the feel of mainstream TV, diverging from this model only in the communities (urban people of color) and issues (AIDS education) represented. The stories occur within a familial situation (a single black mother, her daughter and boyfriend; a single Latina grandmother, mother and daughter; three generations of a middle-class black family), which itself is embedded in a close-knit community or extended family. Focusing soap opera style upon discussions about AIDS within interpersonal relationships, the films evoke the idioms, fashions, attitudes, and environments of the communities they attempt to represent and educate to make these intense conversations believable and, therefore, effective education.

Says Hoffman: "We use the visual vocabulary that the audience is accustomed to. We believe that they trust messages that are delivered in a high-quality, professional, stylish way." Perhaps because of this high level of professionalism, in 1993 AIDSFilms was awarded a $1 million-plus competitive grant from ITVS to produce nine half-hour, magazine-format television programs, *HIV Weekly,* by and for the AIDS community. By far the most consistently and highly funded alternative AIDS media organization, AIDS-Films is also noteworthy for its concerted effort during the late eighties and early nineties to diversify its product and producers.

In 1985 Hoffman was volunteering at GMHC and thinking that he could contribute more effectively by making use of his skills as a filmmaker. Unemployed at the time, he hooked up with another filmmaker friend, Gretchell, and the two conceived of a project, *Living at Risk,* which was to document the lives of sero-negative gay men who were living and coping in the age of AIDS. Research for this project led them to Tross, who was conducting a psychiatric study of gay men in attempts to learn about effective strategies for coping with HIV. Much of the team's educational and production philosophies came from Tross's ideas of "dramatic modeling," using actors to model the behavior change that the audience is intended to affect.

From the beginning, this trio used as their model the strategies and tactics of the professional, independent television production world from which they came. They drew up a letterhead, gave themselves a name, created a board of directors, and garnered the in-kind services of a professional fund-raiser, Michael Selser. "This period was about public relations, studying how one presents oneself in the philanthropic community to gain interest and support and trust." By December 1986, AIDSFilms had gained what its founders had hoped for: the PBS affiliate in Washington, D.C., WETA, was interested in its work, and board member Aschur Edelman raised the group's first funds, $55,000, with a gala benefit built around an Alvin Ailey dance troupe performance. In the wake of this benefit, AIDSFilms received two large philanthropic grants: $30,000 from the New York Community Trust and $20,000 from the Revson Foundation. With these funds, *AIDS: Changing the Rules,* a film designed to educate sexually active straight adults about AIDS risk and prevention, went into production in January 1987.

The film aired on PBS in November 1987 to a media blitz revolving around two issues: the use of Ronald Reagan, Jr., as a host, and the use of a banana to demonstrate condom application, a banana-usage that had been sharply criticized by the banana industry. In the meantime, Schmidt Laboratories, the makers of the Ramses condoms used throughout the footage, backed the film and contributed another $100,000 for the right to distribute 20,000 copies as promotional material for its product. In the black, and with a great deal of support for its first project, the group incorporated as a nonprofit company, set up an office, and hired Tom Kalin as a full-time staff member. John Hoffman became executive director, for the first time receiving a salary.

The company continued to receive attention in the form of grants for production and distribution, raising more than a million dollars during the next two years. Much of this money was used to develop a model for distributing their tapes free to the community service organizations which most needed them. Meanwhile, over the next year, the founding members of AIDSFilms reevaluated their mission in the face of the rapidly diversifying AIDS crisis. They understood that the AIDS crisis was escalating most dramatically within black and Latino urban communities and that little media education was targeted at these groups. But how was a company made up almost entirely of upper-middle-class and wealthy white professionals to reach, educate, and represent a community that was not their own? How were they going to "quite literally, change their complexion"?

During 1988 and 1989 three new members, AIDS professionals who worked within communities of color, were recruited to join the executive committee: Ernesto de la Vega, the director of support services at BATF, Yannick Durand, director of education at BATF, and Susan Richardson, a public health educator at GMHC. This new executive board was supposed to reconceive AIDSFilms' mission, production strategies, and goals. Board members met weekly for a year, "hammering out a collective work style and filmmaking philosophy. Their task was to cut through the assumptions and presumption that color race relations, and to come up with a body of films that would address the crisis surrounding America's newest equal opportunity disease."[66]

By all accounts this was "a painful, awkward, confusing, and difficult" transition, which has been closely and carefully evaluated in a Ford Foundation-funded study, *Retooling for Diversity,* written by Renee Tajima and Ernesto de la Vega. The study details this nonprofit's attempt to complete "a critical phase in multicultural, multiracial organizational development from which other nonprofits might learn."[67] Although this process successfully engendered a new production process for the company (based on the use of advisory committees composed of people from the communities who were targeted for education, and a commitment "to a filmmaking approach where people of color are fully involved creatively and technically at every level of filmmaking from research, to scripting, production, editing and distribution"),[68] the study concludes that it is not as clear if they effectively formed "a multi-cultural organization." The report ends: "significantly, all three of the people of color on the Executive Committee have resigned from their positions, for various reasons."[69]

These important difficulties withstanding, the new executive committee did produce three very well-received films targeting specific audiences (black, urban young men in *Seriously Fresh,* black women in *Are You with Me?,* and Latinas in *Vida*); these films were written, produced, and conceived by professionals from the targeted communities of color and have been distributed, free, to AIDS service organizations across the country. Continuing the group's attempts to diversify its organizational structure, in 1990 a new executive director was appointed, Donald Woods, a gay black man formerly the director of public affairs at the Brooklyn Children's Museum. Woods immediately began work on a film targeting black men, *Reunion.* Although he was to die from AIDS before its completion, its production was completed by Laverne Berry, who went on with Charles Sessoms to make *Party!,* which targeted gay black men and was the first AIDSFilms project produced in video.

AIDSFilms is now producing *HIV Weekly.* Always committed to a high-budget, conventionally styled, and professional product, the company hopes to make quality television in its attempt to produce public programming for the HIV community. AIDSFilms also will continue to produce, using its model of a large and diverse advisory committee that shapes program content, as well as attempting to work with professionals of color on all levels of production. Explains Hoffman: "we believe and know that these films are needed at the community level. AIDSFilms identifies where there is a need, we raise money, and we fulfill that need."

James Wentzy/DIVA TV 2/AIDS Community Television

AIDS Community Television, a half-hour public access show devoted to programming "for greater advocacy, coalition building, and greater public awareness of AIDS activism," first went on the air on January 1, 1993. Twelve airing times are now scheduled monthly in all five boroughs of New York City, and many of the shows have been aired by ACT UP affiliates across the country. Since its inception, DIVA TV (or, should I say, James Wentzy) has produced over one hundred shows, including *AIDS Community Television: Introduction to AIDS Video Activism* (January 5, 1993), *Tim Bailey Political Funeral Washington* (July 6, 1993), and *Activist on Vacation* (August 30, 1994). Wentzy produces a show a week—work that is raw, angry, and thorough in its coverage of AIDS activism.

DIVA TV, the media affinity group of ACT UP, was defunct for a variety of personal, structural, and political reasons when Wentzy joined ACT UP in 1990 because he had recently learned that he was HIV-positive and wanted more information. A professional still photographer and "successfully lazy" person, who until his diagnosis had worked two to three days a week, Wentzy suddenly found "a mission in his life." He wanted to re-energize DIVA with the ultimate goal of beginning a weekly AIDS activist cable show.

In 1993 his goal was met, and he's lazy no more. Today he is either documenting ACT UP's actions (he says that he has documented 95 percent of ACT UP/NY's demonstrations since 1990), editing a new show, or dubbing old ones. "The weekly show is my life. If you want to know how I'm doing, tune into Manhattan Public Access Tuesdays at 11 P.M. or Fridays at 9 A.M." But even this is not enough. Wentzy has a new goal: a national media network devoted to reflecting the "struggles, needs, and state of mind" of people affected by AIDS.

In 1990, when Wentzy joined ACT UP, he had a Hi8 camera and no experience editing or producing video. He picked up such experience while making his first tape, *Day of Desperation* (initially telecast on June 21, 1991), which documents the first ACT UP action that he participated in and also happened to videotape. Wentzy edited this tape at DCTV for a small, reduced fee, as he did with several of his other early shows. All of them were then broadcast a few times on public access television, and they also were

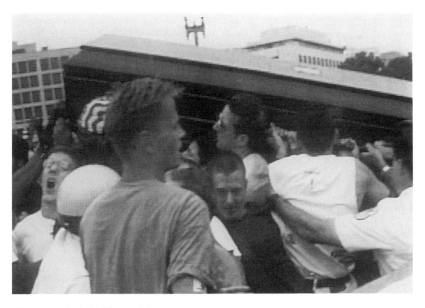

Figure 5   Political funeral for AIDS activist Tim Bailey, July 1, 1993, Washington, D.C., *AIDS Community Television* (James Wentzy, 1993).

screened for members of ACT UP across the country. Wentzy's first grant was from ACT UP for tape stock, and was approved by a vote from the ACT UP floor; for the reduced-rate editing he paid out of his own pocket. At approximately twelve hours of editing a show for his first eight tapes, these personal expenses added up. But, it is a small price in Wentzy's mind. He has gotten great personal satisfaction from this work, and he knows he is performing a vital function. Wentzy believes that he produces television which covers the AIDS crisis in the way that AIDS activists see it (figure 5). "What is unique about what I'm doing is twofold: it's the only weekly series in the world devoted to covering AIDS activism, and it's political. All activists see the crisis as a *political* problem." On the other hand, he understands that "the nature of the broadcast media is that it is fleeting, with so little chance for perspective or evaluation."

A slow accumulation of grants (approximately $17,000 since 1992 from ACT UP and funding organizations like Northstar) has allowed DIVA to purchase a ¾" off-line, cuts-only editing system, currently housed in Wentzy's living room. Here, he edits the cable show, pirates AIDS coverage from mainstream television, and makes the many dubs of his shows which are then broadcast nationally and internationally. No one who works on the show is paid, but if any of Wentzy's grant applications come through, modest salaries will be one of his primary expenditures (along with buying some vital pieces of equipment such as a computer and a sound board).

Wentzy finds it telling that the first action he documented was the *last* AIDS action covered by Testing the Limits for its second video documentary history of AIDS activism, *Voices from the Front*. I find this telling, too. Wentzy is something like a third-wave AIDS video activist in a movement that has had only the briefest of histories: re-creating a wheel with his own twist only three years after the first video collective devoted to covering AIDS activism was formed (Testing the Limits) and two years after a group was formed as a direct arm of ACT UP (the original DIVA). He seems to have come to video for the same reasons as any number of camcorder activists before him: because he had to. Whether Wentzy admits it or not, the most significant limitation of his model of AIDS video production is what makes it so compelling. It is dependent upon the strength, commitment, devotion, inspiration, and well-being of the driven but vulnerable James Wentzy. "This work is my life," he says. "I'll be perfectly satisfied when I die. Although I would like to have a few more years of programs. Since each year is fifty-two shows, that means I'll be able to do quite a bit."

Meanwhile, other individuals and organizations (from high-powered organizations like AIDSFilms and the New York Commission on Human Rights, to individual artists and activists like Tom Kalin or Juanita Mohammed) have been using both low-end and high-end video to educate diverse communities (gay teenagers, urban communities of color, artists, PWAs, care providers of PWAs, the "home viewer" of broadcast TV) about safer sex, the interpersonal, physical, and emotional consequences of HIV infection, and the politics of the representation of AIDS.

After concentrating here upon the production histories of eight diverse alternative projects, one conclusion about this work rises above the expected remarks upon the similarities of commitment, struggle, and ideology which set apart the alternative AIDS media from other media. Into the second decade of the AIDS crisis, and nearing ten years and tens of hundreds of alternative AIDS video projects, what I see is a crisis of multiple perspectives, diverse dimensions, countless communities, and limitless personalities, and a response, in video, which attempts to take this web into account. So many alternative AIDS videos have been created because a complex and mutating social crisis needs as many responses as there are forms to respond in.

As all of these projects show, mediamakers come to AIDS with camcorders and 16mm cameras, with their sights on national TV and individual video monitors, and with political inclinations which range from the left to the center to the apolitical. And it is precisely this openness of the alternative AIDS media, as opposed to the bounded and closed nature of so much mainstream television, which I celebrate and applaud: a forum as rich, open, and malleable as are the individuals and communities who have been scarred by AIDS and scared into action against it. For the AIDS community, in all its diversity, as for minority populations around the world, access to media production allows us to express our needs, define our own agenda, counter irresponsible depictions of our lives, and recognize our similarities and differences.

AIDS and Conventional Documentary Form

> During a war (which this most definitely is), should we adopt conventional
> forms (for video artists, the documentary or the music video) to reach large
> audiences who mistrust artsy experimentation, or should we develop a criti-
> cal deconstructive vocabulary that stands in sharp contrast to the smug
> distortions of the mass media? —John Greyson[1]

During the war of AIDS representations the battle plan for the vast
majority of video producers has been the adoption of conventional documentary form. Except for a surprisingly few made-for-TV narratives and the
topical inclusion of a character with AIDS on a soap opera or prime-time
drama, broadcast AIDS coverage occurs in the diverse forms of TV news: on
the nightly news, in news specials, or in news offshoots like the talk show
or news magazine. To a large extent, the alternative media has also relied
upon the conventions of realist documentary to produce issue-oriented educational tapes, archival records of civil disobedience, or portraits of people
affected by the AIDS crisis. Realist (transparent) form is particularly useful
for the range of mediamakers who capitalize upon the mimetic power of film
or video so as to testify to the *reality* of documented experiences and ideas.

During this war of meanings, conventional documentary form has
proven most useful, since what is at stake are vying interpretations of the
reality of AIDS. Alternative producers use mimetic form to give witness to
the beliefs, values, and experiences left out of or misrepresented by broadcast news programs. The ideas and existence of poor or gay people, drug
users, women of color, prostitutes, PWAs are mimetically recorded so as to
enter their images into the public record. By aping the *form* of the broadcast
documentary, even as its *content* is most likely being critiqued or altered,
the alternative media claims a level of authority that is otherwise never as-
cribed to the oppositional "realities" they choose to depict. In the process,

realist form as well as the broadcast media's vision of an acceptable reality is challenged.

In this chapter I will consider why and how the vast majority of commercial and alternative programs about AIDS rely upon reality-based footage organized in the period's prevailing realist style(s). Mimesis is so crucial to AIDS mediamakers because what is at stake is not *reality* (documentaries are representations after all), but authority over perceptions of reality. In mainstream AIDS media, hegemonic culture is authorized by its unhampered play through realist news presentation. Conventional documentary form allows for and then naturalizes distance from the recorded subject. The distance of realism—especially in the recording of the marginalized bodies of AIDS—is presented as objectivity. Meanwhile, the alternative media claims the authority of dominant culture by usurping dominant forms. In many alternative videos the distance that realism requires is used to either deconstruct the dominant representation of reality or to naturalize alternative or marginal realities. In either case, the requisite distance of realism can be self-aware. Reflexive realism makes room for a critical re-vision of what has been previously understood to be the objective truth. The mimetic representation of an alternative reality becomes a self-conscious or deconstructive act which challenges the "naturalness" of the dominant reality. However, in alternative documentaries the distance of realist style is as often self-consciously erased, just as it is in traditional documentary, so as to inspire identification with the reality being pictured. This more conventional use of the form nevertheless allows for the validation of unconventional visions.

Certainly, a range of recording and editing techniques are encompassed by the term "conventional realist form," including studio newsroom footage, the direct interview or "talking head," the cinema verité observational long take, or the montage of images narrated by a voice-over. Trinh T. Minh-ha concedes that none of these documentary styles are, in and of themselves, more or less "real": "The question is not so much one of sorting out—illusory as this may be—what is inherently factual and what is not, in a body of *preexisting* filmic techniques, as it is one of abiding by the conventions of naturalism in film. In the reality of formula-films, only validated techniques are *right,* others are *de facto* wrong. The criteria are all based on their degree of invisibility in producing meaning."[2] "Conventional" is the operative term here, as it signifies both that the clues we use to reference reality-based, or mimetic, footage *change* (what appears to be a transparent device today is the look of AT&T ads tomorrow) and that producers, both mainstream and alternative, rely upon whatever is currently the standard or customary naturalist form to gain authority. Thus, when I use the word "realist," I am actually referring to any variety of structural devices which are, at the particular moment of their use, considered by makers and viewers to allow for a relatively unencumbered passage of the real world before the camera onto the television sets which later project this world as images. Even so, this is not to imply that all, or even most, viewers and makers believe that the realist images they see are unmediated. Those who are willing to be self-aware about the constructedness—the fact that images are shot and edited by individuals making choices rather than simply appearing as if in some natural state—of realist images can be inspired by direct experience, theoretical or political knowledge, or through reflexive codes within a particular work. Still, we watch and make these images; we even need these images. How else are we to see and communicate what goes on outside our range of vision? Mainstream and alternative videomakers and viewers alike often choose to use and accept these less than entirely "real" images, even if we know better, because AIDS video is made to help us make sense of a new, real-world phenomenon involving terror, pain, horror, anger, purposefulness, and courage so magnificent as to be fictional.

The Urgency of the Said: Debates about Ideology and Documentary Form

> It is hard to be reflexive if you have something urgent to say about a pressing issue. And for most documentarists the urgency of the said takes far higher precedence than the self-consciousness of the saying. —Bill Nichols[3]

Although I agree with Bill Nichols that "the urgency of the said" of AIDS demands conventional form, I would argue that something more complex—may I suggest, even *reflexive*—occurs in the process of articulating controversial, radical, or ignored realities through a mimetic approach. Thus, this chapter's first agenda is to establish that politically motivated media which takes up conventional style does so for self-conscious ends—not because conventional style is the easiest or simplest way to get across urgent information, but because it may also be the most strategic. Although this chapter will provide a more in-depth discussion of this question, let me suggest two simple explanations for why realist style is not fully transparent in alternative AIDS documentaries. Money alone often determines that seemingly un-self-conscious works of alternative documentary demand a reflexive stance upon the "pressing issues" they represent. The alternative media's lack of capital is formally signified in their productions (in color quality, image graininess, access to special effects, performers' skill levels) and thus their distance from the forms (and industry) which they imitate is also written on their sleeve. In Trinh's words, the visibility of the lack of money (in lighting, color quality, editing technique, performance) shatters the requisite invisibility of realism, and so it is "wrong." Broadcast TV is the highest-end video; authoritative form is expensive. However, as the sophistication of low-end technology makes the distinctions between economic advantage more difficult to trace, the depiction of an alternative reality—even if un-self-consciously realist in form—itself can inspire a self-awareness about the constructedness of more customary representations of reality. Upon the viewing of usually unrepresented or unseen "truths," the mainstream media's "reality" is proven to be merely a realist representation of only *some* aspects of reality. When another world is pictured with the same formal techniques used by commercial television (lesbian mothers, capable PWAs, functional families of color) we begin to *see* all that we do not see on the nightly news. This said, it remains open for consideration whether the depiction of unpictured realities (admirable drug users, healthy PWAs, strong and intelligent women) themselves require new forms.

A great deal of film and media theory—especially that concerned with its political potentials—has been devoted to the following concerns: can radical messages be communicated through traditional forms? can the masses be reached through nontraditional forms? can sophisticated political or theoretical arguments be articulated through systems rooted in simplistic structures of knowledge, subjectivity, power, or pleasure? For the most part, these debates have been constructed on rigid dichotomies between conservative politics and realist representational forms, on the one hand, and progressive politics and reflexive, avant-garde, or deconstructive techniques, on the other. Greyson maintains this split in his remarks about the representational war—"conventional forms" versus "critical deconstructive vocabulary"—even as his words acknowledge why fighting video artists need to travel between both kinds of formal approaches. Similarly, Nichols signals an either/or choice for mediamakers: "the urgency of the said" or "the self-consciousness of the saying." Instead of considering how these approaches often become integrated (especially in political work, and more recently in mainstream media which haphazardly takes up a deconstructive *style* whenever it looks good), more rigid schema have typically organized media study. The stakes seem high, for reasons both formal and theoretical. Ongoing debates about the production of political or radical culture are raised: the relationship between form and content, the relationship between representation and personal subjectivity.

Take the discussion of realist form which inspired the formation of feminist film theory. Feminist discussions in the early 1970s associated sexist roles and stereotypes found in representation with sexism in the real world. More theoretical considerations of these issues moved these discussions toward the formal structures of the cinema itself, and it was suggested that the apparatus of film plays an operative role in the maintenance of women's oppression in patriarchy. For instance, Claire Johnston expresses a critique of the "realist codes" used in the early work of feminist film: "any revolutionary must challenge the depiction of reality; it is not enough to discuss the oppression of women within the text of the film: the language of the cinema/depiction of reality must also be interrogated, so that a break between ideology and text is effected."[4] In the seventies some British and American feminist film theorists, taking up contemporary textual theories, understood that the dominant culture naturalized the oppression of women by reproducing dominant ideology in the "real" images of cultural production. E. Ann Kaplan suggests in her influential essay on women's documentary practice that "realism as a style is unable to change consciousness because it does not depart from the forms that embody the old consciousness. Thus, prevailing realist codes—of camera, lighting, sound, editing, mise-en-scène—must be abandoned and the cinematic apparatus used in a new way so as to challenge audiences' expectations and assumptions about life."[5] Similar arguments about the dangers of a "window on the world" aesthetic were made regarding the early political work of black filmmakers as well. A theoretical certainty about the dangers of realism engendered a difficult situation where politically radical film theorists were forced to disavow or condemn most of the political documentary of the period, which was produced in the name of causes they supported, yet outside academic theory.

Yet an equally vehement response to these critiques has continued from both outside and inside the academy. For instance, Kobena Mercer, describing the "documentary realist" films of early black British producers, explains that such films "constitute the means of encoding alternative forms of knowledge to 'make sense' of processes and events from a black perspective."[6] And Barbara Halpern Martineau says in defense of the feminist films which feature talking-head interviews: "by empowering ordinary people to speak as experts, they question a basic assumption of dominant ideology, that only those already in power, those who have a stake in defending the status quo, are entitled to speak as if they know something."[7] Similarly, Marxist filmmakers in the Third World have argued that "realist" films help people see the reality that is oppressing them. Fernando Birri writes: "by testifying critically to this reality—to this sub-reality, this misery—cinema refuses it. It rejects it. It denounces, judges, criticizes and deconstructs it."[8] Although it is important to distinguish representation from reality, as most documentary theory insists, I believe that this distinction occurs self-consciously within many realist texts which use the authority of mimesis to "denounce, judge, criticize and deconstruct" reality. Further, I wish to consider the power of individual viewers to see through the pretense of transparency.

Using the term "realism," after all, is merely identifying a system of changing codes and structural devices which tells us nothing about how these codes are created, by whom, for what ends, and how they are received. Certainly, realism naturalizes the present state of affairs of the society it reflects, but this society is itself constantly changing. The prevailing meanings of AIDS, or any other cultural phenomenon, are not fixed; they transform, often in relation to challenges in the realm of cultural production. Over the course of the AIDS crisis, the alternative media has realistically attested to states underrepresented in broadcast television, later to find these phenomena brought into commercial television's image of AIDS. And, isn't that one of the purposes of alternative, realist work? If you enter images of women with AIDS again and again into a culture that tries to resist the fact of their existence, eventually the picture will change, and then political and personal realities will change accordingly. Research on women and AIDS will begin; women will be educated about HIV transmission. Alternative AIDS media production is based in both a complex cynicism and optimism about the power of the media. The mainstream will never change, so we better do it ourselves; our work will eventually contribute to real social change, that is why we do it. Activist video production must be simultaneously rooted in the belief that cultural capital is firmly entrenched and that it is infinitely dispersed.

For Every AIDS Reality a Realist Form

In this chapter I analyze two commercial AIDS documentaries from different periods in the history of AIDS—NBC's Special News Report *Life, Death and AIDS* (January 21, 1986) and *Time Out: The Truth About HIV, AIDS and You,* produced in 1992 by Arsenio Hall Productions—to demonstrate how documentary form is used to affirm and inscribe a range of AIDS realities, but also how the crisis, and thus its mimetic reportage, changes over time and across communities, to some extent *because* of changes within media representation. By countering the strategies of these commercial documentaries with the formal choices of several alternative AIDS videos, I hope to illuminate the variety of effects allowed by realist structural devices: from the perpetuation of the prevailing ideology to its contestation and re-creation. Thus, the politics mentioned in the title of this chapter are not so much those of mimesis as a formal strategy in and of itself, but rather those of the producers who use this particular form for particular ends. AIDS documentaries, both mainstream and alternative, use realist form to both create and reflect a politicized (even if often presumed neutral) vision of reality. In the process, the biases, fears, blind spots, and ideologies of the maker and the intended audience are envisioned as well. As I work to nuance what have mostly been totalizing theories of realism, I also hope to complicate clear delineations between dominant and alternative culture.

Contemporary American media is better understood by thinking about the many dominant and alternative *cultures* which are created through the marketing strategies of the mass and alternative media. For instance, if it was once true that broadcast television conceived of its audience as white, today the networks target a substantial body of programming to people of color. Thus, unlike *Life, Death and AIDS,* Arsenio Hall Productions' educational videotape *Time Out* speaks from a position of something closer to alternative dominance. The tape relies more upon the conventions of the nighttime talk show than those of the nightly news, relies upon the distribution currency of video and not broadcast (it is loaned free at video stores), and it both contests and affirms aspects of "dominant" culture; for example, it mocks the authority of the uptight white establishment even as it assumes all of the cultural and economic power of the black entertainment and sports industries. Meanwhile, alternative producers crib from the styles of dominant television, making faux-news (GMHC's *Medical Updates,* which record an anchorwoman at a desk reporting vitally necessary news, DIVA TV's Ray Navarro posing as a "news anchor"—who also happens to be Jesus Christ—to report on the demonstration "Stop the Church," in *Like a Prayer,* 1991) or music videos about condoms (*No Rewind* [Paula Mozen, 1992], *The ADS Epidemic* [John Greyson, 1989]).

Thus, throughout this chapter I will need to invoke the concept of dominant and marginal cultures that are dynamically connected to both the form and content of the mainstream *and* alternative media. *Time Out* is almost entirely different from NBC's *Life, Death and AIDS* because it mimetically records a different "dominant" reality—that of the younger, hipper,

darker, more urban MTV/BET crowd. The tape establishes its desire to privilege an alternative dominant reality by cross-cutting two discussion scenes
in its first few minutes. We are introduced to a group of eager, honest, primarily white kids from Centerville, Ohio (really), who articulate an idea
("it's like we're in a bubble here, we think we'll never get it"), only to be
immediately dissed by the ideas expressed in the group discussion of the infinitely smarter, cooler, and primarily black kids from New York City ("you
can never think you're in a plastic bubble. AIDS can get you at any time and
so you have to be prepared"). *Time Out* affirms the street smarts of black,
urban culture over the bumpkin, white suburban culture that more closely
resembles the intended audience of NBC News. Arsenio Hall Productions (a
subsidiary of Paramount) understands that there are *many* purchasing cultures, some of them eager to consume anything—including AIDS prevention
education—that is sold through the codes of hip urban hybridity.

For this reason, it should not be surprising that *Life, Death and
AIDS, Time Out,* and the host of alternative videos to be discussed here
represent almost entirely different realities with their mimetic forms. The
reality of AIDS is, in fact, a myriad of crises, each to be represented "realistically" by the variety of cameras engaged in documenting the AIDS crisis.
One example of the transformation in the politics of AIDS "realities" is the
two programs' construction of AIDS authorities. While *Life, Death and AIDS*
relies upon the expert testimony of white male doctors, scientists, and journalists, *Time Out* seeks its answers from pop stars and the teenagers who
make them rich, giving a great deal of program time to beautiful, smart,
HIV-positive young people (including Magic Johnson), whom it positions
as the real experts on AIDS—in the process taking up one of the alternative media's long-standing political goals, giving PWAs primary authority
about AIDS.

Constructing or Dismantling Control in the AIDS Documentary

This chapter aims to investigate the ways in which diverse AIDS
documentaries use transparent form to construct or dismantle control, distance, and command over their content. *Life, Death and AIDS* was only one
in a flood of broadcast media programs produced in 1986 that were concerned with alleviating (and at the same time fanning—a certain amount of
panic *sells*) the general public's escalating heterosexual panic. This program
wielded all of its authority to reflect and confirm the endangering but prevailing attitudes of the period. AIDS was a crisis affecting "others"; "normal"

Americans had no reason to panic because they were distanced from AIDS by their whiteness, by their sexual preference, by their class. It is a complicated feat that this program at once succeeded at feeding the public's fears while ultimately positioning this same general public on the peripheries of the crisis. Although a spirit of alarmism colors the program, by show's end an ambivalence between fear and distance has been straightened out, and Brokaw reminds us that: "if you're heterosexual and don't live a freewheeling lifestyle . . . your chances are 1/1,000,000." Therefore, the show ends by confirming two seemingly contradictory prevailing misconceptions about AIDS: panic is appropriate when focused upon a fear of others, and the general population need not be concerned enough about personal risk to take precautions against infection.

In the 1992 worldview of *Time Out,* the reality of AIDS has changed on both counts; neither panic nor distance are deemed appropriate responses to what has so clearly become a massive and enduring global epidemic. Historians Elizabeth Fee and Daniel Fox note that in the 1990s the social understanding of AIDS has radically shifted. "We are dealing not with a brief, time-limited epidemic but with a long, slow process more analogous to cancer than to cholera."[9] This view of AIDS necessitates long-term and universal behavioral change—safe sex and clean works for all. Since the early years of the crisis, AIDS activists, educators, and researchers have demanded that Americans see that race, sexual orientation, gender, and class do not protect people from AIDS transmission, as so much early press had maintained. *Time Out* reflects this "new" AIDS reality in its realist images. The professional basketball star Magic Johnson and many other "normal" (heterosexual, non-drug-using) Americans testify to their positive HIV antibody status, heralding themselves as the direct victims of 1986 news reportage (its whiteness, its distancing, its uptightness) because during these very years, and because of these very messages, they contracted the virus through *heterosexual* sex ("we're not gay and we don't use drugs," this new kind of HIV-positive AIDS expert insists again and again). *Time Out* wields its slightly funky but still super-hetero authority to try to reduce panic and promote acceptance over distance. If anyone, even Magic, can contract AIDS, then we must accept once and for all that normal (heterosexual, non-drug-using—the tape repeats this formula like a mantra) people can be HIV-positive—our friends, people like "us."

Although the tape clearly reflects some real shifts in attitudes about what constitutes the reality of AIDS, these shifts are underscored by a homosocial panic so intense that even with all of (straight) hip-hop culture's authority on its side, the program can't quite quell it. *Time Out* naturalizes an AIDS reality where difference and distancing are reduced with regard to who is or could be HIV-positive (rich people, straight people, white people, teenagers), while desperately trying to maintain a hold upon who is not or could not be *gay* (the show's comedian host Arsenio Hall and Magic Johnson, who carefully, but lovingly, touch each other in the image which illustrates the cover of the video's box). This video takes on the difficult task of trying to convince its intended audience that AIDS is a straight disease and that viewers must acknowledge it as part of their reality. Such an attempt brings up a great deal of male homosocial anxiety since, like paternity, heterosexual HIV transmission is only indirectly verifiable. Thus, as *Time Out* reflects the changed (representational) AIDS reality of heterosexual transmission, it also mimetically records the profound (male) homosocial panic of young, straight, hip American boys who are terrified of being labeled gay as soon as they acknowledge their proximity to HIV. Even as the tape challenges earlier misinformation about AIDS, it does so in a manner which confirms a new set of irrational fears and bigotry.

In the meantime, many alternative AIDS videomakers have been attempting to document what has consistently and increasingly been the reality of heterosexual *and* homosexual transmission of HIV *for women* (not because they are vectors to men or children, but in their own right). Many alternative tapes have been fighting the uphill battles for recognition that AIDS affects women, that it does so differently from how it affects men, and, finally, that the term "women" always includes lesbians, women of color, and female IV drug users. Many alternative feminist videomakers have consistently worked to fight not just sexism but homophobia, racism, and classism as they make educational materials that attempt to reach communities other than those of the well-to-do, gay, white men who were educated first. *He Left Me His Strength* (Sherry Busbee, 1989), a tape which documents the AIDS educational work of Mildred Pearson, a middle-aged black woman who cared for her gay son when he was dying of AIDS, is an excellent example of an alternative tape which mimetically records a reality that includes the difficult work of fighting homophobia as people in the urban working-class and poor black community begin to address AIDS. An active member of her Baptist church, Pearson understands the deeply ingrained cultural barriers that members of her community feel toward the life-styles of gay male PWAs. In talking-head interviews, Pearson, her pastor, the Reverend Walter Parrish, and a fellow AIDS educator from the Brooklyn AIDS Task Force, Ernesto de la Vega, acknowledge homophobia within the black and Latino communities. "Mildred offers a bridge between black gay men and their struggle and anger to the rest of the community which has denied their existence," explains de la Vega. Pearson argues for compassion, care, and tolerance as she speaks at churches and support groups among black Baptists in New York. "These are the same young people that loved you and cared for you; that made you happy. You can't just walk away from them," she says to her fellow parishioners after a service. Busbee's realist representation of Pearson's work does not serve to obscure and therefore authorize a community's homophobia, but rather it makes this homophobia the mimetically recorded reality which is the tape's difficult subject.

Part of Me, produced for GMHC's "Living With AIDS Show" (Alisa Lebow and Juanita Mohammed, 1993), documents the words, home, and neighborhood of Alida "Lilly" Gonzalez, an HIV-positive lesbian who is a recovering drug user. "I lived comfortably all my life with my sexual preference and I've learned to live comfortably with my disease. I have six kids; six grandkids. I'm 41, and always came out publicly with both. Take me as I am." Lilly explains how she used crack to numb herself to her fear of AIDS when she first began having symptoms. "I wanted to die and I didn't want to die. And the confusion is there. So you get high. But that's not a solution either. If AIDS doesn't kill you, the crack does. It's easier to live as a PWA than as an addict." Conventional talking-heads documentary style is used to allow Lilly the forum to describe her underrepresented experience and politicized critique. "The department of health was giving out condoms like crazy, but very rarely would they give out dental dams. The government wants safe sex but aren't willing to provide you with the necessities to do it." Lebow and Mohammed use the video camera to document a reality rarely recorded by dominant culture. In so doing, they disprove many common assumptions about AIDS, HIV transmission, and women: that lesbians do not have it, that women do not use drugs, that women who *do* use drugs are not also capable of being responsible contributors to their communities. They show an articulate Latina lesbian, who is HIV-positive and who works as an AIDS counselor and educator, explaining her story to women within her community. By taping her, they extend the reach of Gonzalez's work to teach poor urban women of color that both HIV and lesbianism are part of their community. "I don't deny it to anybody. I'm positive. It's me. It's part of who I am. I have nothing to be ashamed of."

AIDS education is difficult work, and producers of AIDS videos make complicated decisions when they choose the images which construct the realities envisioned in their tapes. These decisions are often based upon considerations about the beliefs and values of the intended audience as much, if not more so, than those of the makers. The decisions about which aspect of reality to include in a realist documentary attest to how often makers are fully conscious about the constructed nature of what is only one possible, if also true, vision of the reality of AIDS. Lebow and Mohammed discuss the difficulties they encountered making the "Lilly piece" in ways that help us better understand their work, as well as that of *Time Out* and *Life, Death and AIDS.* Since the mainstream lesbian community is in significant denial about class, and in some ways race, Lebow and Mohammed had to consider whether exposing their largely white working-class and middle-class lesbian viewing constituency to the images of a poor, sometimes drug-addicted lesbian of color would be a useful educational strategy (in that it serves to shatter a safe but untrue vision of reality and therefore enables lesbians and their allies to fight their battles against AIDS with more complex understandings of lesbians' experiences), or whether this strategy would serve to alienate or otherwise turn off the women who are the tape's intended audience (Lilly's experience is so foreign, so "other," they will not identify with the tape, and therefore not realize that it is information they need to know).

In a similar vein is *Time Out,* with an intended audience explicitly identified as young, straight, would-be urban kids, doing the *right* educational thing by implicitly confirming the homophobia which defines youth culture in order to reach these viewers in terms they understand? And similarly, if NBC perceives that the majority of their intended straight, white, would-be yuppie viewers would be alienated by discussions of homosexuality, are they doing the right thing to leave this aspect of education to the gay-identified AIDS activist video community? At this stage in the chapter, these questions will be left open to point to the complicated decisions that all of us involved in AIDS education must resolve as we continue to try to educate people about very difficult behavioral change because of a life-threatening virus that also has, by coincidence or not, attached itself to some of the most controversial subjects of our society (sex, illicit drug use, poverty, homosexuality, class, the health-care system). How do we envision reality so that we can change it?

Mimetically Recording a Wrong Does Not Make It Right

American broadcast news is a powerful form of communication that tends to present, as if they are natural rather than culturally produced, the

existing ideological structures of power, powerlessness, desire, and prejudice upon which it reports. "The news is a privileged discourse, invested
with a special relation to the Real," Margaret Morse asserts in an article
about the immense credibility granted television news.[10] She explains that
the mimetic nature of film and video is one of several forces that join to
confirm this "special relation to the Real." The news is read as an authorized reality because of shared assumptions between its makers and viewers
about broadcast TV networks' neutrality and a belief that "seeing is believing."[11] The *unnatural* authority of TV news is founded upon the pretense
of the "natural" objectivity of its recording equipment. Thus, the present
(and catastrophic) circumstances of the AIDS crisis are often presented as if
they are "natural"—that is, as they should be and always will be—through
the process of news reportage. By reporting the "reality" of AIDS with the
presumed " 'objectivity,' 'neutrality,' 'impartiality,' and 'balance' "[12] of TV
news, the political, economic, and moral history of this short-lived crisis is
disappeared.

This kind of passive reflection confirms "the taken-for-grantedness"
of how things are in our culture. Without other forms of analysis—voice-
over, editing, or political, historical, or cultural criticism—the present state
of affairs is reified. "This aesthetic rules out progress," writes Paul Willemen
about realism in the cinema. "If things are as they are, it is impossible to
even contemplate showing them as they might be."[13] Locked into a form that
is expected to report mimetically upon an admittedly horrific state of affairs,
the mainstream media is often set into a position that perpetuates, rather
than interrogates or alleviates, the most horrific aspects of the crisis. This
is exemplified when *Life, Death and AIDS* repeatedly envisions AIDS with
images which are already culturally current (i.e., gay men walking arm in
arm, a junkie shooting up, nameless Africans in nameless villages). The news
need only report "realistically" what exists in the natural world to legitimate
already current definitions of the socially "ill" and the socially "healthy."
Even before HIV, gay men, prostitutes, IV drug users, people of color, and
women were often considered impure.[14] The possibility—if invisibility—of
a "real" infection only serves to validate earlier assumptions. Thus, mainstream documentaries do not reflect the "reality" of AIDS as much as they
do our already operating discourses about marginal subcultures and their
assumed relationship to the epidemic.

Confirming the present state of affairs without correcting it seems
to be a primary tactic for *Life, Death and AIDS*. The program opens with a
tone of fear, while at the same time it sets itself up as the most likely force

against this terror. In the process, "the regime of the 'fictive We'"[15]—the generalized, purified speaker and reader of mass media news—is also set in place. Throughout the show, this "we" or "us" will include anyone, like Brokaw, who assumes distance from the crisis, distance from possible infection, distance from people who are affected. This distanced relationship to HIV structures the show's simple form and agenda: normal Americans have questions about AIDS, the show will answer them. Brokaw serves as middleman between prerecorded on-the-street interviews where Americans ask questions about AIDS and live feeds to experts around the country, who answer these questions. Interspersed through this question-and-answer format are prerecorded informational segments with a science correspondent on specific issues such as AIDS and gay men, AIDS and drug users, AIDS and children, and prescripted segues narrated by Brokaw which are illustrated by statistics and graphs.

For a good five minutes Brokaw speaks the fears and anxieties of "normal" Americans without dispelling them. "Worry about AIDS is part of being a parent now." "Police, firemen, hospital workers deal with their own fears." "Everyone agonizes over blood transfusions." "Even some of the faithful are frightened about receiving communion through a common cup." These words are accompanied by illustrative images: mothers at a PTA meeting, police learning how to give mouth-to-mouth resuscitation through a protective mask, a priest holding up the communion chalice. Brokaw expresses "our" irrational fear about AIDS; the show's images illustrate and confirm our wrongheadedness. This is a most brutal example of the way mainstream realist representation preserves the status quo, even when the present state of affairs is one of misinformation. *Life, Death and AIDS* feeds our fears and says we are right to be wrong. The show gives as much program time to its on-the-street-interviews speaking misinformation as to the deferred testimony of experts with "answers." Thus, the show focuses on reevaluating this issue as it is already evaluated—the sexist, racist, homophobic, frightened way which feels comfortable.

Interestingly enough, *Time Out* also opens with the same simplistic question/few answers structure. Yet the show's adaptation of this format, especially through its use of humor, reveals its differing assumptions about knowledge in general as well as specific changes in knowledge about AIDS. Its hybrid news form—borrowed in part from the talk show as Arsenio and Magic chat face-to-face on bleachers in a gym, and in part from the news magazine, as different minisegments hosted by celebrities are visited upon Arsenio and Magic—is not based upon the same concept of knowledge as that reflected by the nightly news. Rather, performance, humor, personal interaction, feelings, and especially *style* are given authority over abstract ideas, advanced degrees, or neat presentation. Whereas stuffy Tom Brokaw and his guests use every formal approach in the book to affirm their authority (steady shots, continuity editing, professional affiliations grafted onto speakers' chests), Arsenio and his buddies use form to pretend they have no authority whatsoever (handheld camera, pixilated video, jump cuts); they are just like the folks on MTV, who are just like the kids who watch them and then go buy the products they endorse over at the mall. If the news hides its ideology behind "neutrality," Arsenio camouflages his agenda with fun-loving entertainment mixed with the authority of heterosexuality.

The tape actually begins with Arsenio walking onto a basketball court and taking off his sweats and putting on high-tops. This occurs very quickly in fast-motion editing and concludes with the title "The Show-down." Then we see Arsenio and Magic jokingly playing one-on-one. The joke is how intimidated Arsenio is playing basketball with this superhero ("I wasn't ready. I was fixing my sock, man" [condom?]). And how he is nevertheless going to assume a cocky, macho attitude ("You can't take a man to the hole when he's bending down" [!]) as he requests "take" after "take" until he can finally score a basket against the bigger, better, realer man ("I'm a talk show host," he whines). His anxious masculinity à la the main characters in the 1992 film *White Men Can't Jump* begins the tape (he's black, but skinny), only to reach its climactic resolution at tape's end when the two men's embrace is frozen and gently fades from the screen.

After the brief showdown, Magic and Arsenio are now taking a chat break on the bleachers. First, Arsenio puts to rest any anxiety about *Magic*'s masculinity. "When the news came out that you were HIV-positive, people thought you couldn't play basketball. I'm here to say you can." Magic uses this statement articulating confusion about AIDS, masculinity, and homosexuality as a segue into discussions concerning confusion about AIDS information. "People have a lot of misconceptions about HIV and AIDS. A lot of people don't know the difference." Cut to Pauly Shore, Mr. Misconception (in this version, we are told up front that people do not know much, but then we are again forced to sit through their misconception-in-action for several minutes). Shore, wacky MTV VJ and sexually ambiguous yet aggressively straight teen idol, says (also in the signature MTV style of pixilated video and rapidly jump-cut footage which is used throughout the program), "I'm Pauly Shore, here to tell you what AIDS is. AIDS is . . . a disease. You get it through sex. Sex. Sex . . . . Sharing needles too . . . . You can't get it from a toilet seat . . . ." He is getting visibly confused, and we can tell he is running out of ideas. "Let me think. Actually, I'm really kind of clueless about what it is. Are you guys kinda clueless too? All that stuff you heard me say doesn't really make sense, so I'm going to get some help, okay?" This permits a cut to Pauly performing on-the-street interviews where other clueless young Americans in shopping malls are going to display their semi-ignorance as well. "I know that it's a virus." "Immune. Um. Deficiency. Um." "It's a disease that affects the immune system." "System, right?" "You get it from unprotected sex with someone who has AIDS." After flirting with two shy blonds who correctly answer "no" to Pauly's "do you get it from toilet seats? saliva? can I have a kiss?" he concludes his segment with the optimistic statement, "I really thought that people wouldn't know what it is. But most people are kind of on top of it. Are you guys on top of it? Do you know what it is?"

Well, perhaps these interviewees are on top of it compared to the saliva-worried, communion-cup-panicked interviewees in *Life, Death and AIDS,* but whether they know enough to protect their lives is open to debate. Whereas the 1986 documentary highlights thirty-something middle-class, Middle Americans conveying their misinformed fears, the more hip 1992 version shows that six years later teenagers have some (limited) clue about what AIDS is; at least, they are not needlessly afraid. If anything, the sequence seems to show that the teens included in the opening have accepted AIDS into their world vision and understand it in about the same way they understand the rest of their social reality (with faltering, stuttering, half-assed lack of attention). Although the rest of the tape will be populated by teenagers who are *expert* AIDS educators or PWAs themselves, the program opens with only semiaware youth affirming what it would otherwise be seeming to challenge: that it *is not* okay for teens to treat AIDS like they do the Gulf War or the budget deficit, because benign-if-cool indifference to HIV can kill you. In its opening the documentary uses its mimetic form to record what "real" kids really know: *not enough.*

Meanwhile, alternative producers need not pander so egregiously to their intended audiences because they usually screen their work to a self-identified audience which wants to be there. Documentary can also be used to help us "see" what we *really* need to know, not simply what we perceive to be true. For instance, Dziga Vertov, arguing about the possibilities of the socialist film in the 1920s, writes that "kino-pravda" (film truth) is not merely based upon a reliance on the mimetic nature of the filmic medium, but rather "kino-eye" is the documentary cinematic decoding of both the visible world and that which is invisible to the naked eye.[16] He theorizes a political documentary practice that uses pieces of mimetic documentation to construct complex and political interpretations of the reality being pictured, even if some aspects of this truth are invisible. Unlike the objective display of Americans' lack of knowledge which opens both *Life, Death and AIDS* and *Time Out,* alternative AIDS videos use documentary to see differently these truths which are usually blindly accepted. This use of mimetic form works to challenge, and potentially change, the existing state of affairs.

Many alternative AIDS videos are devoted to revealing *and then* dispelling the fears and misinformation of the "general public." Such videos crib the style of the documentaries whose information they challenge, but in so doing, the form alters accordingly. *We Care* (the Women's AIDS Video Enterprise, 1990), for example, uses a structural device throughout the program that presents pages from the book of "AIDS Myths." In on-the-street footage, people say things such as "you can tell an AIDS person from how they look. All dried up. Withered," or "People with AIDS get it from not washing properly." However, unlike the commercial programs I have discussed, these incorrect statements are *immediately* dispelled by "AIDS Facts," also articulated by people-on-the-street who are, in this case, in the know: "AIDS people don't look any different from me or you," "You get it from unprotected sex, sharing IV drug needles, and it is passed from mother to infant." And, just to make sure that mimetically recorded misinformation is never perceived as truth, the images of people voicing incorrect information are also covered by a big red "X" or the word "myth" flashing over the speaker's face.

Strategies of deconstructive montage and humor are used to mark misinformation *as it occurs* in *Hard to Get* (Alisa Lebow, 1989), *Voices from the Front* (Testing the Limits, 1992), *Like a Prayer* (DIVA TV, 1991), and *Snow Job* (Barbara Hammer, 1986). In *Hard to Get: AIDS in the Workplace,* false information is signified in the text by black-and-white archival newsreel footage, accompanied by an authoritative male narrator who conveys AIDS hysteria that is so blatant and silly that it permits the viewer to challenge all authoritative news sources. "At the Hem-ha Institute for Misinformation, experts explain to onlookers how to protect themselves from the AIDS virus. A hermetically sealed vehicle allows safety for the whole family. Now the whole family can rest easy." Such exaggerated misconceptions are immediately countered by the steady and wise voice of the tape's other narrator, the actress Ruby Dee, pictured in color over black-and-white newsreel footage.

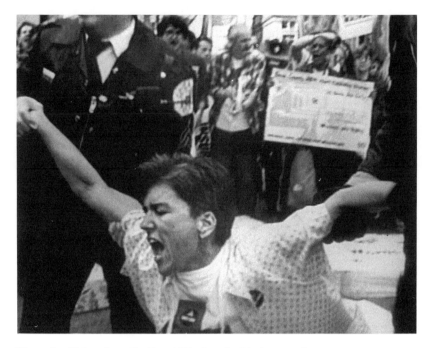

Figure 6   *Voices from the Front* (Testing the Limits, 1992).

"Before we can talk specifically about the issues that come up at work, it's important to talk about how you get the virus that leads to AIDS." The tape gives us formal clues to recognize, as we see it, "wrong" or "right" realist information. Hysterical misinformation takes the form of parodic, black-and-white retro-footage, which is immediately followed by its correction, seen in the color images of Dee.

In *Voices from the Front, Snow Job,* and *Like a Prayer* the makers use appropriated broadcast news coverage to deconstruct itself. *Voices from the Front* opens with an *analysis* of mainstream coverage articulated by AIDS activists and cultural critics who discuss how the broadcast media has misrepresented AIDS. Vito Russo, an AIDS activist and film critic, explains that "members of my family who get all their information from the mainstream media know two things about me: that I'm going to die and that the FDA and the government is doing everything in their power to save my life." This is followed by network news footage of Ronald Reagan (with Russo continuing, "I think they're lying," under the president's encouraging words about his administration's commitment to AIDS funding); then we see Reagan's press secretary and the secretary of health and human services, both claiming how much they are doing about AIDS. This is followed (implying a causal relationship through editing) by a 1985 NBC News report which claims that mainstream America "is deeply worried about AIDS" and wants people with AIDS to be tattooed, quarantined, or given special identification cards. Russo returns: "If I'm dying from anything, I'm dying from the sensationalism of the mainstream media." The reality pictured here is one made up of deceptive and lying leaders, a duped media, and observant, aware PWAs who construct alternative realities with their abilities to view critically and then act upon their analysis (figure 6).

As long as the so-called mainstream population sees, and understands themselves to be immune from (if afraid of), this infection, or the homosexual men or deviant activists who were once thought to be its sole host, then this is what the media will see every time it "mimetically" reports on the general public's knowledge about the crisis. The incorrect and dangerous present order is confirmed every time the TV camera unproblematically frames it as reality. But it is equally simple to use mimetic forms to show that prevailing knowledge is inadequate and that others know better. Documentary footage of real people saying really wrong things can be used to either reflect or counter the present state of AIDS reality.

The Distance of Documentary Form

The AIDS crisis is not merely a crisis in health, but one of authority. To claim authority over AIDS justifies distance, distance from contagion, from the "kinds of people" who are sick, and from responsibility for this crisis which may originate in biology but which is protracted socially. Documentary is also rooted in authority. The body of the narrator is one signal of how these documentaries use distance and proximity as integral features of realist style. Brokaw's staid, suit-clad, studio-situated, white, upper-middle-class male body signifies a different relation to authority than the sweaty, sporty, chatty, affectionate, homosocial bonding routine performed by Arsenio and Magic. Whereas the nightly news and its offshoots rely upon the grounding presence of an anchor who digests the opinions expressed around him and remakes them into the property of the news, Arsenio and Magic pretend to disperse authority in their tape to many and constantly shifting voices.

Interestingly enough, the absence of a narrator is almost a universal feature of alternative AIDS media. For alternative videomakers this becomes a realist convention in its own right. Thus, tapes go to great ends to structure their argument without the controlling, authoritative (but formally expeditious) presence of a narrator. Alternative tapes will use title cards to express information which is unclear from the footage alone (*We Care; Voices from the Front; Second Epidemic*), or sometimes the maker will picture herself, when necessary, to explain what the tape is about (*Prostitutes, Risk and AIDS; Free Whores; (In)Visible Women*). A most common structural stand-in for the narrator is a video organized around one well-spoken interviewee who articulates the transitions and themes of the tape through carefully and thematically edited but unscripted talking-head interviews (*Kecia; DiAna's Hair Ego; Her Giveaway*). It is only hybrid alternative tapes (high-end educational documentaries sponsored by wealthy nonprofit organizations which have a stake in traditional modes of authority) which use an authoritative and absent narrator. This conventional marker of authority functions in the work of the alternative media as it always does—to signal distance from the tape's material. It is standard in alternative AIDS media to shy away from a formal strategy which serves to signify the very thing that the content is hoping to disprove.

Other authorities appear in a program besides the narrator, and these key players typically wield the same power in the tape that they do in real life. Again, mimetic representation allows society's prevailing structures to be played out unchallenged. In *Life, Death and AIDS* authority within the program is assigned by relying upon already operating hierarchies of "health"—misinformed assumptions about who is risk-free, who is at potential risk, and who is infected. A series of iconic "healthy" Americans—cowboys, PTA moms, firefighters—ask questions in on-the-street interview footage. They are locked into a health loop legitimized by documentary form. They must be outside the possibility of infection themselves because they do not *look* like the kinds of people who have AIDS: they look healthy (they do not look gay, or black, or as if they shoot drugs). Because they look healthy, they get to ask questions. Given the slot of question askers, their good health is confirmed.

A wall of four video monitors—each displaying one head—holds the answers. But only white male experts' heads fill the monitors—men working at the Centers for Disease Control, the National Institutes of Health, and at a San Francisco hospital overburdened with AIDS cases. In the terms of documentary, that mechanical reproduction of the "real" world, this can be explained not as sexism or racism, but as the unbiased reportage of the world-out-there, a sexist, racist place where women, PWAs, and people of color are underrepresented in the ranks of experts. The biases of the medical institution (that there are too few professionals who are women or people of color) are reflected by the mainstream media which mimetically reports upon the "reality" of the professional world. But this is only one version, and vision, of reality. By organizing the show upon a taken-for-granted definition of "expertise"—one which looks for professionals only where white men work—many of the people who are working with AIDS are left out of the picture. For example, PWAs are extremely well-informed about AIDS, and they come in all races, classes, both genders, and of any age. Yet, although several gay, white male PWAs *do* get to talk during the show, these men who are themselves AIDS activists or health professionals are questioned only about their *sexual* practices and never their expert knowledge about AIDS. Gay men are not understood as experts; thus, they are not treated or *seen* as experts.

There are alternatives to this prime-time logic and its insistence on the existing, dominant structures as the only possible organizations of power and vision. In fact, another nearly definitive convention of alternative AIDS media is that expertise is transferred away from those who have wielded power so criminally for the duration of the epidemic to those who have suffered or fought against the powers-that-be. Alternative tapes give authority about AIDS to people who possess lived experience of the crisis: PWAs and people who are HIV-positive, activists, social workers, mothers of HIV-positive children. These tapes reflect the important work accomplished by individuals outside dominant systems and institutions. For example, the videotape *Women and AIDS* (1988), a show I produced for GMHC's "Living With AIDS Show" with Jean Carlomusto, locates itself within already existing, if "marginal," professional communities where women hold positions of power. Whereas *Life, Death and AIDS* perpetuates the dominant myth that women and people of color are not experts, *Women and AIDS* reflects a world where the *only* experts are women, many of them women of color. Realism is used to construct an alternative reality in which some of us often reside. Professional women easily take the seats of their white male counterparts in the tape's conventional talking-heads shots. Spectators comment upon how empowering it feels to see so many bright, articulate, intense women taking power over the crises of AIDS. Many other tapes create this all-female troupe of experts (many if not all of whom are women of color), even as they otherwise maintain traditional documentary form. Some of them are *Her Giveaway* (Mona Smith, 1990), *Women and Children Last* (Amber Hollibaugh and Gini Retticker, 1991), *I'm You, You're Me* (Catherine Saalfield and

Deborah Levine, 1993), *(In)Visible Women* (Ellen Spiro and Marina Alvarez, 1992), *Grid-Lock* (Beth Wichterich, 1993), *Doctors, Liars and Women* (Jean Carlomusto and Maria Maggenti, 1989). Imaging women discussing their work and all that they know informs viewers that these female professionals exist. Compare this reality to *Life, Death and AIDS* and similar broadcast programming, which create and quote a "real but untrue" world that appears to be one from which these women are absent.

Many people, besides female professionals and articulate PWAs, are left unaccounted for in shows like *Life, Death and AIDS,* people who are not allowed even the pretense of speech: poor people of color (especially women) who have never been granted the authority of discourse in dominant culture and who are referred to, nominally, in *Life, Death and AIDS* by blurred images of "ghetto" streets; mothers of infected children, who are infected themselves, but who are represented only vicariously by the doe-eyed images of sick babies; prostitutes and IV drug users whose status as "criminals" ensures not their invisibility, but voyeuristic, confrontational, and only sometimes "consensual" images; gay teenagers who, like all teenagers, are at real risk for infection, but who have always been silenced. The trajectory of control over AIDS is governed by access to speech and control over images: the power of defining, naming, showing, speaking.

This is a primary motivating force behind the massive production of alternative AIDS videos—define, name, show, and speak AIDS to gain some control back. It is interesting to see where control has shifted and where it remains the same in the 1992 AIDS-scene of *Time Out.* Gay teens have some voice in this program. Also, several of the female PWAs discuss their own infection and then, later, the HIV infection of their babies. This occurs *after* the audience gets to know the young women by themselves, a progressive strategy which works to alleviate the blame which is commonly felt towards HIV-positive females who also happen to be mothers. Poor people, drug users, and prostitutes are not represented in this show; they are not yet part of the hip agenda. Even in 1992 class difference is still not interesting to the young. Should it be? How *could* it be?

Although some empowered producers are brave enough to break the silence imposed on them by broadcast television, rectifying such imbalances of authority is never merely a matter of recognizing who does not speak and making it possible for them to do so. Social constraints more deeply imbedded than TV withhold the possibilities of speech from many individuals. Thus, prostitutes' rights activist Carol Leigh speaks for a large community of women who (like IV drug users) are silenced because discussing their concerns and needs regarding AIDS also identifies their illegal behavior. And most mothers are hesitant to speak publicly about AIDS because they are worried that their children will face discrimination if their mothers are recognized on television. The project of the alternative media becomes the complicated task of being at once sensitive to, while striving to alter, the power relations which limit public speech in our society.

For this reason, several alternative AIDS media projects have shied from the documentary altogether, using the more familiar format of the soap opera or *telenovela* to communicate AIDS education. Projects produced for disenfranchised communities of color, typically denied speech because of linguistic, economic, and cultural barriers, have used scripted narrative to displace the complexities of finding "real" men and women who are willing to publicly discuss their experiences with AIDS. Tapes like those produced by AIDSFilms (*Vida, Reunion, Are You With Me?*) represent how AIDS affects minority communities by dramatizing difficult encounters between family member or lovers. *Se Met Ko* (Patricia Benoit, 1989) is produced in Creole and creates through scripted narrative a safe space for dangerous conversation about how Haitians are discriminated against in the United States and how this hostile treatment is similar to the homophobia which occurs within their community; the video also discusses how to put on a condom and how to ask a male lover to use one. Similarly, Bebashi's dramatizations of scenes involving the connections between battering, drug abuse, and HIV infection in poor, urban communities of color (*Final Decision, Grandma's Legacy*) would have needlessly endangered already endangered women if "real" women were interviewed in the tapes. Instead, the producers met with affected women in focus groups and then worked with this information to develop scripts. *AIDS Is About Secrets* (AIDS Institute, 1989) dramatizes the complex issues faced by female partners of male IV drug users. And the AIDS Institute's *AIDS: Not Us* (1989) dramatizes the experiences of urban, black boys.

All of these narrative tapes create their scripts by working directly with affected communities. "Real" needs and problems are voiced safely through the words of actors. These tapes make difficult information palatable and "function concurrently as advocacy and sympathetic, seductive narratives." "They employ entertaining forms, primarily that of episodic narrative built around dramatic encounters between simple character types," according to Catherine Saalfield and Ray Navarro in a review of alternative AIDS media made by and for communities of color.[17] In these videos, alternative producers claim the authority of a different system of conventional forms—those of narrative television and Hollywood.

While it is true that it is particularly difficult for women, people of color, prostitutes, or drug users to speak in white, patriarchal culture, it is also true that under the right conditions disenfranchised people can and do speak powerfully. Alternative media can prove that the dominant reality is not the only reality by creating safe spaces from which women feel comfortable speaking. In *Women and AIDS,* for example, the voice of a woman, identified as "Anita: A Woman Who Is HIV Positive," is accompanied not by her face, but by images of women walking around city streets with children or shopping for groceries. This approach allows the hitherto invisible HIV-infected woman to be involved in the production while still respecting the predicament she faces by exposing her image. Another strategy used—for example, in *The Heart of the Matter* (Amber Hollibaugh and Gini Retticker, 1993)—is to find one powerful woman who is willing to speak in front of a camera and interview her openly about how she made the difficult transition into the world of the dominant, and possibly punitive, culture. Why was she willing to speak? In this tape, Janice Jirau, an HIV-positive black woman whose husband died of AIDS, explains the process of her own empowerment from self-recognition to social action. Suddenly "society's victim," a "sick" black woman is nothing like a victim at all, but she is instead a woman powerfully in control of her own situation through self-articulation. The tape does not empower her by pretending that the oppression of minority women does not exist. Rather, it creates a space where Jirau can comfortably confront, and by doing so challenge, these societal imbalances.

Documentaries See the Prevailing Ideology Wherever They Look

In the few cases where the mainstream media does train its cameras on the disenfranchised, it assumes that this gesture is sufficient compensation for the imbalances of public discourse. However, the "realistic" images created by TV cameras usually perpetuate, rather than contradict, the real power relations they record. This is largely because the mainstream media aligns already constructed codes—which signify authority in themselves— onto bodies which themselves signify varying degrees of authority (female bodies, black bodies, gay bodies, sick bodies). Many of the codes of documentary label, categorize, and imply understandings of authority—for example, how an interview is framed, the proximity of the camera, titles, the positioning of participants within the interview setting. Dai Vaughan offers some detailed examples. "If we switch on our sets and see a man addressing us directly, we know he is a narrator or presenter. If his gaze is directed slightly off-camera, we know he is an interviewee, a talking head. If he is turned away from us by an angle of more than about 15 degrees, he is a part of an action sequence. It is clear that there is a hierarchy of authority implicit in this code." [18] In the case of AIDS reportage in *Life, Death and AIDS,* the power of formal presentation neatly aligns with the social hierarchies already in place in the "real" world. The program assigns the representational strategies for picturing "normalcy" to Brokaw, the doctors, and the Americans on the street; they are pictured in deferential, steady medium shots and in-synch voice track. The filmic strategies for picturing those outside the mainstream—anything from ragged, handheld, crisis coverage camerawork, to the picture-blackened voice-garbled imaging of the "criminal"—are given to the PWAs (and people *assumed* to be infected) in the program. For instance, it is clear that the prostitutes (seen but not interviewed) are different from the other participants who are caught in on-the-street footage (PTA moms, etc.), because the camera keeps at a cautious distance from the sex workers. The look of the footage, as well as the words of the accompanying voice-over, imply the infection of these women and confirm misconceptions about prostitutes' risk. Meanwhile, one special lady gets to introduce herself: "Hi, I'm Amy. I have AIDS." She is also allowed a steady, tripod two-shot (a medium shot slightly distanced to include two bodies in the frame) with her husband. The IV drug users are never allowed a name. Their images are accompanied by the science correspondent's voice-overs. When they are allowed to talk, it is only in response to one of the crew members who shouts questions at them from a safe distance. In this sequence on "Drugs and AIDS," the camera is either too close, or too high, shooting these subjects as distinct body parts (arms being shot up, the backs of faceless people walking out of places where drug users gather to take drugs). The prostitutes and Africans imaged in the program are not even granted the privilege of an interview, let alone a steady shot in which they are centered in the frame. Instead, they are caught unaware by a camera positioned as far away from them as possible. The words we hear with these images are, of course, the science correspondent's controlling voice-over. Thus, prevailing assumptions about race, class, gender, and infection are confirmed by the form of the television footage alone.

The talking-head interview is another case in point. This documentary staple is never, in fact, merely the head of a person uttering words. Talking heads belong to people who have professions and ranks which are flashed over their features as titles. They are filmed in rooms, houses, and offices which reflect social standing and position. They are gendered. They have facial features which identify ethnicity. They are garbed. They have diverse relationships to spoken English—accents, lingo, vocabularies. In a society where authority is more often gauged by the trappings of class, race, and gender than by the content or quality of one's argument, authority or lack of authority can be deduced as soon as a camera records a particularized head talking within its reality. In this fashion, the nonauthority of PWAs is confirmed, even as the program grants them talking-head interviews. Over the course of the TV special, several PWAs are pictured within their "real," but coded, talking-head backdrops. Amy is the show's "innocent victim," a married suburban woman who received a contaminated blood transfusion. She is interviewed seated next to her husband by a picturesque fire in the hearth of their suburban home. Unlike this woman, the first gay male PWA presented is not depicted in his home. Rather, as he begins to speak in a live interview, seated in a hospital room, a still image of him appears, as his voice continues, and covers his real-time image. Now he is pictured in one frozen image, dressed in a hospital gown. He stands in a sterile gray room surrounded by steel medical equipment. A doctor is examining his eyes. Certainly, the image is "real," but why is this space of discomfort used as the natural space for the not-so-innocent gay man with AIDS? The IV drug users in the tape, "honestly" depicted in their world, are interviewed in an empty, burned-out city lot—their home the dirty, fenced-in desolation where they shoot drugs. The mainstream media seems to picture IV drug users, like black men, almost exclusively "on the streets."

Contrasting alternatives could have been chosen rather than the biased but "true" reflections of reality created in *Life, Death and AIDS*. For instance, the crew could have sought a different place for interviewing the gay male PWA: his suburban house, as tidy and attractive as that of any straight blood recipient. Similarly, the IV drug users could have been interviewed when they were feeling their most safe, comfortable, and in control— not when they were sick and shooting up to feel better, but when they were in their own apartments. Yet the images selected serve a higher function— "to confirm the patterns of the world we seem to know"[19]—a world where cultural outsiders (gay people, IV drug users) inhabit spaces which seem to reflect their cultural differences.

The alternative media has worked hard to picture realities that other groups who call themselves *we* "seem to know." *The Forgotten People: Latinas with AIDS* (Hector Galan, 1990) devotes its first section to Latinas who have contracted HIV through contaminated drug needles. The narrator begins the show by explaining that half of HIV-infected Latinas are infected in this manner. (This show is another hybrid, so not surprisingly we find a narrator; coproduced by Galan's company and KCET, a public broadcasting affiliate, it was funded by the Centers for Disease Control.) The video then introduces us to Paula and her two sons, who are seen entering her apartment with groceries. We are told that she has used intravenous drugs for most of her life. Through Paula, we meet her mother, Louisa, and her sisters, Marta and Brunhilda. All three sisters are HIV-infected; all three sisters were addicted to drugs from their teenage years into their thirties, often sharing needles with each other. Two of the sisters each have two sons. None of the four women lives with a husband or lover; all of them are pictured in their homes, cooking dinner, braiding each other's hair, taking care of their children. Louisa has been separated from her husband, an alcoholic, for decades and has raised her eight children alone. However, the narrator concludes the segment by explaining that the three sisters are lucky. Although they are infected with HIV, unlike the majority of poor Latinas who are using drugs, these women are recovering from a life of drug addiction through their family's support. Louisa says, "they are my children. When they are sick they need me the most. I support them, help them, encourage them, watch over them."

Tapes like *The Forgotten People* attempt to realistically portray worlds that a legitimate and underserved "we" know only too well. The tape's structure—the sympathetic oration of a narrator corroborated by talking-head interviews of affected women and their families—although somewhat condescending, still manages to allow women whose experiences have been largely invisible to explain themselves. The women who are interviewed are given respect, authority, and a home in the tape. The narrator does not judge; the information she provides gives historical, economic, and cultural background to the women's words. Women, who are ignored or mistreated in broadcast television, here are given the time and safety to explain their versions of complicated life stories which are structured by poverty and, therefore, sometimes include drug use. To educate other poor Latinas before they too become HIV-infected (through drug use, or through having sex with currently active or former drug users), the reality of their world and experience needs to be caught in educational materials directed to these communities. This world is rife with drug addiction, as well as the many other consequences of poverty, including low self-esteem, abuse, female-headed households, and poor medical care, but *also* well-cared-for apartments, supportive family networks, and people who have given up drugs.

Using realist form to reflect already operating understandings of social hierarchies is a prime example of how the distance of realism naturalizes the world it reflects. The issue of interview consent is another example of the way in which real cultural and economic power relations are reflected in the operations of documentary production. The camera and the news industry are seen as sexy, attractive, and mysterious to most Americans outside the industry. Furthermore, the big budgets of some news shows often provide monetary incentives to convince individuals to appear on camera against their better interests. In *Life, Death and AIDS* several consensual interviews are shown that do not represent the interviewee to his or her best advantage. The drug users probably signed a waiver for their images to appear, and maybe they made a few bucks. Their losses cannot be calculated in dollars, however. Such tactics occur frequently in victim-centered documentary so that the immoral tactic of the filmmakers paying the "lead" of *On the Bowery* (Lionel Rogosin, 1955) enough to keep him in liquor but not enough to allow him to get off the Bowery is repeated in *AIDS: A Public Inquiry* (WGBH-Boston, 1987), where the TV crew pays the down-and-out PWA Fabian Bridges enough for a hotel room, but never enough so that he can go home and try to get better.

Because of interactions like this one, many alternative media producers arrive in "AIDS communities" to find, too late, that the most comfortable speakers have already been interviewed by the mainstream media, feel abused or manipulated, and are unwilling to give further interviews.[20] Furthermore, although alternative makers may strive to partake in a different morality of interviews—for example, they might share opinions or a political agenda with their interviewees or guarantee the way in which footage is used so that it is acceptable to the interviewee—the apparatus itself often makes this ideal a difficult one to live up to. Whatever the intentions, after the interview is over the mediamaker "owns" the material, plays and re-plays it, edits it, and archives it, while the interviewee is left at home.

How does the alternative media respond to the ethical challenges of consent? In *Prostitutes, Risk and AIDS* (1988), a tape I produced with Carlomusto for GMHC's "Living With AIDS Show," we made countless attempts to arrange interviews with sex workers, but we failed for obvious and important reasons. Women were reluctant to have their faces shown. They were worried that children or family might see them. We could not and did not wish to force these women to be interviewed, nor did we want to take up the mainstream's strategy of quick-and-easy on-the-street interviews, the glamour of the camera convincing people to speak, even though they could be endangered. But how were we going to get their stories on to the tape? The dilemma became the organizing principle of the tape, which is largely about social control over the speech of prostitutes, about why it is so difficult to get

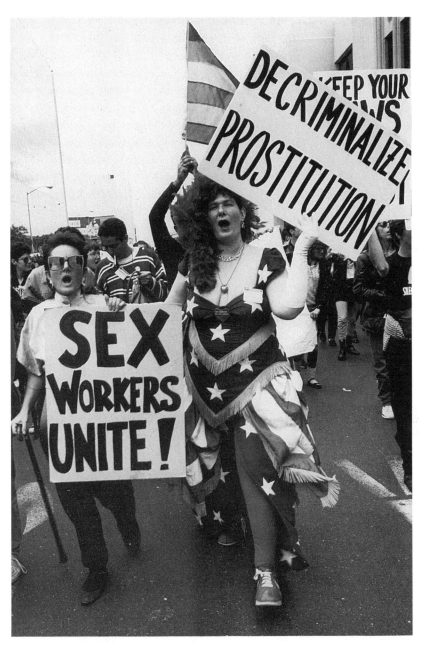

Figure 7   Carol Leigh.

this story on ¾" broadcast videotape. Instead of replicating the real problems faced by sex workers, the tape focuses on these problems.

Needless to say, the self-critical strategies that Carlomusto and I chose as outsiders to a community working to represent the issues affecting this community are not necessary when sex workers make their own tapes. The video work of Carol Leigh is important here. According to her promotional materials, Leigh since 1987 has prolifically produced videos on everything from prostitutes' issues (*Daisy Anarchy at Klub Kommotion, Just Say No to Mandatory Testing, Mandatory Testing Demonstration—Hall of Justice, Whores and Healers, Safe Sex Slut, Outlaw Poverty, Not Prostitutes*), to women's studies, gay and lesbian issues, and politics/sociology. As activist, videomaker, prostitute, poet, and media celebrity, Leigh gracefully handles the issue of consent by herself articulating the connections between money, sex, AIDS, drugs, and government inaction (figure 7).

The Prevailing Ideology Changes

But what of the talk show, what codes of authority does *Time Out* use, and to what ends? Unlike *Life, Death and AIDS,* there is an antihierarchy established in *Time Out.* All speakers, performers, and sequences are shot in the same style; everyone is given the same level of authority, from stars to PWAs. This is a world vision which pretends to picture an America with *no* hierarchies, where blacks, whites, those who are HIV-positive or HIV-negative, doctors, rap singers, straights, gays, scripted actors, and on-the-street interviewees all deserve the respectful lack of respect of the MTV camera. But even as the tape stresses this rhetoric in style and script—"It doesn't matter if you're gay, straight, bi, whatever. I'm proof it can happen to anyone," says Magic—the show constantly *slips.* Before this remark (clearly the show's intended feel-good position), Arsenio says: "Lots of people only think it affects gays and drug users." "I thought that too," responds Magic, "only gays and drug users could get it."

The repetition of the phrase "gays and drug users" within ten seconds of airtime sounds a little strange, and in fact such phrases litter the program, signifying who is acceptable and who is not in this highly constructed reality that pretends to have no hierarchies of authority. The precise statistic that heterosexual sex is responsible for 75 percent of HIV infection is repeated twice as well, first in a comedy narrative sequence, then three sequences later as Paula Abdul reinforces the danger to heterosexuals. The reinforcement by repetition of straight sex as the real site of concern protects the program from sliding into the questionable support of "gays and drug users." To insure this from being the take-home message, the tape triumphantly concludes with heterosexual romance. In a sequence titled "Boy Meets Girl," we are introduced to a clean-cut, white 22-year-old boy who is lifting weights in a gym and who we also learn is HIV-positive. We learn that Jason met a cute, equally clean-cut and white young girl at a group for teen AIDS peer educators. They fell in love. We see them walking arm in arm in a mall. She buys shoes, as he restlessly waits. Girls . . . Then we are informed, "Boy Wins Girl." He says: "I bought her a ring." The married couple kiss on a beach and ride through L.A. in a sporty convertible. They discuss their fears and the other difficulties they face in knowing the boy is HIV-positive. They have safe sex, and the girl worries about what will happen when the boy dies. A perfect heterosexual romance, with one melodramatic hitch.

I am certainly not suggesting that a problem exists with educating straights about the dangers of HIV, the reality of heterosexual transmission, or the possibilities of sex, love, and romance when a partner is HIV-positive. However, I do suggest that reemphasizing the real homosocial panic which has arisen in the face of a changing AIDS reality does not help a cause where a large percentage of affected people are gay men, lesbians, and their allies. If this tape were actually trying to break down operating hierarchies, we would see gay and lesbian couples negotiating sex and romance, and other couples dealing with issues of addiction and HIV transmission. But the only two men who are pictured together in this show (considering the possibilities of sex, love, and romance, even when HIV is a factor) are Magic and Arsenio. As their words reinforce the authority of heterosexuality by trying to distance (with a rhetoric of acceptance) homosexuality, they keep *slipping*. When Arsenio tells Magic how he lost out on a night of lovemaking when he asked a girl he had brought home to use a condom, and "she copped an attitude and left," Magic says: "poor baby . . . ." Although the surface meaning of the sequence is that talking honestly about sex is more valuable than a one-night stand, there is a mocking, loving tone that implies something more, like losing a girl is not really the loss that Arsenio is pretending. Then, when the boys are listing slang words for condoms—"jimmy-hat, raincoat, rubber, space-suit for the littlest of astronauts"—Magic turns to Arsenio and says, "You're not the littlest astronaut are you?" "Oh man, why are you dogging on me?" Arsenio pleads. Yet another example: Arsenio wonders if people treat Magic differently now that he is HIV-positive. No, he still gets "high-fives and hugs, brother." "Well, you look good." "I *know* I look good." And then the two buddies break into worried and somehow still suggestive giggles.

Their artful, fearful, and perhaps even self-conscious flirtation signals one of the greatest difficulties of current AIDS education. Is it the responsibility of Magic and Arsenio to fight homophobia while they fight the transmission of HIV? Is it the work of *Life, Death and AIDS* to acknowledge the racism, classism, sexism in the society upon which they report while they educate the racist, classist, sexist audience which they intend to reach? Although I am trying my best to acknowledge how producers of all manners of AIDS educational video are forced to make complicated decisions to best reach their intended audience, I will continue to insist that this work can be done without pandering to the lowest common bigoted denominator. Realist style can be used to perpetuate the status quo or to work toward changing it. *No Rewind: Teenagers Speak Out on HIV/AIDS Awareness* (Paula Mozen, 1992) provides a useful counterexample to the panicked world envisioned in *Time Out.* Similar in both form and content to *Time Out,* this tape attempts to speak to teens "in their own language," that of "lively and accessible" MTV footage. But, produced as a master's degree final project by an independent artist, the tape lacks the financial and cultural resources found in *Time Out.* Like *Time Out,* the tape relies upon teen AIDS educators, fast cuts, rap songs, and teen PWAs, but *No Rewind* substitutes the talking-head interviews of a gay, black, HIV-positive teenage boy and a straight, white, HIV-positive teenage girl for the narrator roles played by Arsenio and Magic. Although much of the tape attempts the difficult work of convincing its teenage audience that this is a straight disease, in *No Rewind* this agenda is not promoted through the denial or unallayed fear of gay male sexuality. When we first meet the male narrator, he says, "All the men who were getting AIDS were gay and old, I thought I was immune to this." This leads the audience to believe that the boy is straight and young. But his next comment begins, "When I first came out to being gay was in 1991." Ready to incorporate homosexuality into teenhood, the area of denial being brought to the forefront in this tape for urban teens is not male homosexuality, it is age; teens think their age protects them, but teens can be straight, gay, or bisexual. Thus, the section "Teens Educate" begins with a black female teen saying, "the first wave was homosexuals, the second was IV drug users, and the third is teenagers." No special emphasis is placed, in this chilling progression, on categories like straight, gay, or non-IV drug user; the third category is simply "teens," who are all of these things and more.

In this example, Mozen imitates the style of Arsenio Hall's television production to reach teens. She sees in fast-paced, slick, music-soaked video footage an effective strategy to reach teens of the MTV generation. However, in her piece there is no necessary connection between this style, or the intended audience of media-savvy teens, and normative attitudes about male homosexuality (however, it is critical to note that this tape makes no references to lesbian sexuality). By using conventional form, Mozen and her teen educators sneak in their less-than-conventional message. Thus, I conclude where I began. What, if anything, is the relationship between conventional form, "reality," and AIDS?

Conclusions: The Making and Viewing of *Safer and Sexier: A College Student's Guide to Safer Sex*

I taught at Swarthmore College in the early 1990s. Like college students at similar institutions, Swarthmore undergraduates are young, very smart, mostly wealthy, largely white, and extremely naive. Like most Americans, they know the so-called facts about AIDS. They know it is not easy to be infected with HIV, so they are not worried they will catch it in the dining hall. They know that they should be having safer sex, and they even have a fairly good idea about what the latest understandings of safer sex are—that you should not have anal, oral, or manual intercourse with another individual without the protection of a condom, dental dam, or latex glove. These are people who have come into their sexual identities during the AIDS crisis. They do not know sex outside the ominous and devastating parameters of STDs (sexually transmitted diseases) and AIDS. Yet, like most Americans outside the gay male community, they do not practice safer sex with any consistency. In fact, the frightening and definitive characteristic of their sexual behavior is that they *sometimes* practice safer sex, depending upon the circumstances and the partner. This half-assed incorporation of the ideas and rules of safer sex, of course, is not much safer than never practicing safer sex at all. Is there a video we could show them that would make a small contribution toward changing this situation? How do students watch sex, and does watching safer sex necessarily contribute to behavioral change?

As we try to help people begin to live their sexual lives in a manner that has never been lived before, many have hoped that video representation is a useful place to expand our imagination about sexual practices so that we can envision, and then perhaps include, the use of condoms and dental dams *every time* we have anal, oral, or vaginal intercourse. Carlomusto writes about her work on such a tape for lesbians: "saying 'use a dental dam' is not the same thing as saying 'use a condom,' since many women don't even know what a dental dam is."[21] Clearly, the production and dissemination of realist representations of people having safer sex would be an important intervention into a sexual/media landscape where safer-sex acts are rarely represented.

For the most part—in fact, somewhat systematically—college students see *only* images of heterosexual unsafe sex, and it seems they do *not* challenge what they see. According to *Women, AIDS and Activism,* published in 1991 by the Women and AIDS Book Group of ACT UP/NY, a 40 percent increase in adolescent cases of AIDS has occurred since 1990, a full 70 percent of teenagers have sex before they are eighteen, one in ten gets a sexually transmitted disease each year, and one in ten females becomes pregnant. Only one-third of high school girls use contraception regularly, and less than one-quarter use condoms. All of these statistics seem to indicate a largely uncritical audience which learns much about being sexual in the unimaginative, unprotected ways that are imaged in the mainstream media. Furthermore, the horrifying number of my female students who are anorexic, bulimic, or simply obsessed with their bodies to a point of personal harm clearly reveals a profound inability to separate the lived experiences of their bodies from the stupid, punitive, and powerful pictures of slim, taut female bodies which surround them.

Yet, unlike some feminists, I have confidence in the abilities of readers (even college students) to negotiate alternative meanings from the limited sexual representations of the dominant culture. For, although it seems clear that much of our lived sexuality is produced in reference to Hollywood's and broadcast television's images of sexuality, countless examples of resistant sexualities exist that do not conform to dominant representations. For example, lots of people are gay in a society that rarely represents homosexuality in its dominant discourses; many men are not abusive in a society that represents sexuality and violence as if they are the same thing; and some people do have safer sex, even if they never see it practiced in Hollywood films. People learn about and construct their sexuality through a range of both dominant and local forms of meaning. Safe sex is, after all, not merely a matter of sex, but according to Cindy Patton a more complicated cultural construction that joins science, fantasy, group histories and identities, and varied logics of health. She writes that we use a range of "decoding strategies" to come to personal definitions of sexual identity:

> Sexual expression is learned through communication and observa-
> tion in both public and private social venues as well as through
> mediated observation and communication, including medical texts,

the popular press, how-to-books, and pornography. . . . A range of subject-positions in a range of social fields creates for each person a set of registers, or decoding strategies, or a hermeneutic, which in turn positions him or her in a network of policing, advice, sexual possibilities, style, erotic "preferences," and closets.[22]

According to Patton, people acquire their ideas and practices about sexuality from a range of both selected and proscribed representations. Viewers of both dominant and marginal images of sexuality form a complex system of "decoding strategies" through which personal meanings and practices about sexuality are produced. The question then becomes, as it was for the producers of *Time Out, Life, Death and AIDS,* and the many other videos considered in this chapter, how to make an AIDS educational video which effectively speaks to a particular audience about sex in a way which actually serves to help them construct a new sexual reality? Can your work be familiar enough to reach people and yet new enough to promote change?

During the school year 1992–93, I worked with eight of my students in a time-consuming extracurricular project to produce an AIDS educational video for college students which would attempt to intervene in the unsafe reality which organizes most college students' sexual lives. The HIV-peer educators at Swarthmore College decided to develop a video for use during the safer-sex workshops which are given each year at all the dorms on campus; we then also worked to distribute the video to colleges and universities across the country. To date, we have distributed more than two hundred copies of the tape nationwide, and it went on to win second prize in the documentary category of the Academy of Television Arts and Sciences' College Television Awards. The peer educators feel that using video is an integral part of their work. They say that video provides both a form of authority that they cannot have as peers educating their peers, and also that it serves as a break from the heavy, interpersonal focus of their presentations. Using video, they can show things they cannot show in real life, such as how to put a condom on a real penis or how to put a dental dam on a real vagina. Finally, we organized the project after finding that none of the safer-sex educational videotapes that were available reached our particular audience, who were either shocked by or dismissive of the safer-sex videos intended for other audiences.

We learned in the process that when educators show Swarthmore College students safer-sex education tapes made for drag queens, Latinos, urban women, or lesbians (even if one or two members of the crowd are from these particular communities), the audience members say they do not "identify," which results in their simply turning off. They use a tape which demonstrates particular sexual and ethnic identities which are *not* their own as a means to clear themselves from risk. Since they do not see themselves or their peers there, they see the tape as a confirmation of the distance they already believe separates them from the crisis and from safe sex. This also holds true for the mass-release, mainstream videos and television programs that have attempted to address generic teenagers through broadcast television. The moralistic images of teenage sexuality offered up by television are laughable, imprecise, punitive, and distanced. If it is felt that images of safer sex come from the outside, people who view them feel either ridiculed, attacked, distanced, or judged.

Instead, educators and viewers agree that most students feel most comfortable seeing people like themselves talking about and performing sex. Carlomusto explains that "material has to be culturally relevant, rendered in ways meaningful to specific audiences."[23] Thus, her safer-sex porn tapes are all produced with focus groups, which are made up of people from the communities being represented and addressed, and they are seen in carefully chosen sites like gay bars, porn theaters, and community centers. College dorms are not the intended screening sites of these tapes, and college students are not the intended audience. When we do show students the explicit sexual imagery in GMHC's tapes, it does not work as AIDS education because their fears and bigotry get in the way. By accepting that showing 18–22-year-old, mostly middle-to-upper class, mostly white, mostly straight kids the sexual images from GMHC's safer-sex porn tapes does not work because their homophobia, racism, and other hostilities get in the way, are we pandering to the lowest common bigoted denominator? Shouldn't we insist that college students look at these images so they can see that white, straight, Hollywood sex is only the tip of the iceberg? Shouldn't we insist that when you talk about and show sex, you do so in the many varieties, positions, and configurations that diverse people use? Isn't this *real* safer-sex education, after all? The answer to these questions is "yes," to a large extent. Educating college students about safer sex by showing them white-bred, prudish, cute Hollywood images of "boy meets girl," gets you somewhere, but not far enough.

What *does* work are the strategies of realism and identification as formal methods which prepare people to be open to new ideas (realism can be used to confirm the status quo or to produce alternative visions of reality). Realism in this case refers to people on the screen looking and acting like

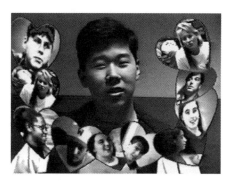

Figure 8   Ho Yang, *Safer and Sexier: A College Student's Guide to Safer Sex* (Lay-Techs Entertainment Group, 1993).

the viewers; if they wear similar clothes, use similar lingo, perform similar sexual acts, then the *resistance* of viewers from particular communities begins to come down. In fact, my students feel that realistic specificity—current fashion, popular songs, today's slang—and the localization of identity—so that class, race, sexual preference, location, and age are claimed—are the most important factors to begin helping people listen to and see safer-sex information and imagine themselves performing safer sexual acts (figure 8). They do not want one safer-sex video for Swarthmore, but ten or twenty, to play for and be made by the variety of social, ethnic, and extracurricular identities that students take up. That is, one video should be available for African American students, one for frat boys, one for women's center types. Only by seeing themselves on the screen will they begin to take the educational message seriously, and personally. Only by *identifying* will they begin to imagine that they themselves could incorporate these new messages into their lived experience.

Our video, *Safer and Sexier: A College Student's Guide to Safer Sex,* used these realist strategies. All the bodies in the tape were Swarthmore College students. They sound "right," authentic, real. They talk about sex in the way that college students did in 1993. They choose the right music and wear the right clothes. Yes, the tape is dated, but it was also cheap to produce. Another could easily be made when this one becomes obsolete. And with our concerted effort, we represent a variety of body types (fat, thin, tall, black, white, Asian, male, female) and a variety of sexual proclivities (from asexual to homosexual, from no-risk behavior to risky but protected interactions like vaginal and anal intercourse). We accepted the premise that to educate college students, we needed to speak and look like college students, and then we drew a line about how far we would go to reach this intended audience of liberal arts students. If our viewers are homophobic, we decided that they will have to deal with it, leave the room, or turn off the tape. If our viewers are afraid of explicit sexual images, our video is not for them. We created a vision of a safer-sex reality for college students that also reflects our own biases, ideologies, and beliefs. Ours is a pro-sex, multicultural, hetero-, homo-, bi-, and safer-sex reality captured on tape by our camcorders. College students who do not agree with this depiction of reality can create their own, and, because of camcorders, they probably will.

4 THE PLEASURE AND POWER
OF SEEING SCIENCE

Envisioning Pleasure and Power in
the Science Documentary

Pleasure and power do not cancel or turn back against one another. They
are linked together by complex mechanisms and devices of excitation and
incitement. —Michel Foucault[1]

A car is moving down a dark, isolated country road. It brakes at a
security booth. With bumpy and sloppy movement a cinema-verité camera
catches an officer's back as he says, "Driver's license, please." A loud "BOOM"
is heard on the soundtrack, and a cut is made to the face of the driver, gro-
tesquely lit so that his white but bearded features are barely outlined. He is
probably the *Halloween* man, escaped from a mental hospital, sneaking by
the unsuspecting officer with a stolen license so as to rape and maim the
woman at road's end.

A narrator's voice enters: "U.S. Army, Fort Dietrich, Maryland. Once
renowned for its biological warfare experiments." The car pulls forward. In
slow motion, mist wisps about mysterious storage tanks. "More AIDS virus
is produced here than anywhere else in the world." Danger! They're creating biological AIDS warfare at Fort Dietrich. This is worse than *Halloween!*
Those tanks are full of deadly AIDS virus!

But no, this is quickly revealed to be a setup. The narrator's voice
returns. He explains that at this place "an intense scientific effort to unravel
the complexities of this strange and deadly virus" is being waged. Only then
does the camera cut to a clean and well-lit scientific laboratory. But why the
mysterious car and driver? Why the buildup with its threat of apocalypse?
Why all the codes, entertainment devices, pleasures, and excitement of a
blockbuster horror film in what is—surprise!—the opening sequence of "Can
AIDS Be Stopped?," a 1986 PBS *science documentary?*

In this chapter I analyze two PBS science documentaries about AIDS
("Can AIDS Be Stopped?" and the Winter 1990 segment of WGBH's *AIDS Quar-*

terly, "The Trial of Compound Q"), along with several alternative tapes, all of which attempt to represent the science of AIDS. This analysis is done so that we can gain a better understanding of the reporting of science in documentary: how the pleasures of viewing, knowing, and controlling are all invoked by viewing AIDS science. In my analysis (and the tapes I describe), only minor distinctions are made between discussion of science as a discourse and of medicine or basic research as distinct scientific practices. This approach both reflects my debt to the feminist theoretical tradition which uses medicine as the best example of a more pervasive phenomenon of sexualized and distanced control and an elision made less critically in the programs that I analyze. Science documentaries about AIDS switch, without missing a beat, between coverage of medical treatment and basic scientific research. Thus, when I refer to "science," I do so in a manner which loosely joins any number of practices that systematically study, treat, control, and attempt to cure AIDS. This "science" is practiced in both corrupt and moral ways, by people who are well-paid and by those who are volunteers, by experts with advanced degrees and by activists who teach themselves what they need to know. And these many varieties of science are the subject of a range of evidence-seeking cameras and systematic documentary explications.

I am interested in how the authority and distance which I have already established as integral features of documentary production are also essential components of "good" science. Science, in all its forms, is at once the science documentary's subject and its method. Brian Winston in an article considering the "Documentary as Science" makes three points about the mutual dependence of the two institutions: "(1) The camera emerged from and was situated in the realm of science. (2) A dominant thrust of this science was the systematic observation of nature via many apparatuses of which the camera was just one. (3) The scientific heritage of the film apparatus is critical to the documentary."[2] The documentary, so steeped in the history and authority of science, sometimes also takes science as its subject. In science documentaries like the two PBS shows discussed in this chapter, the power and pleasure they acquire in their study of AIDS science is naturalized and sanctioned by both science and documentary. The scrutinizing gaze of science is condoned by the scrutinizing gaze of the documentary camera; the control of the televisual narrative authorizes the control of scientific inquiry; the technologically enhanced vision of the scientist is infinitely reflected in its technologically enhanced recording by the documentary camera. Both the form (documentary) and content (science) validate each other by taking for granted their similar underlying structures.

Much recent theory about science and documentary has focused upon revealing the usually transparent ways that the cultural power of these institutions has been constructed and implemented. Theorists of documentary have argued that this use of the filmic apparatus has no greater claim upon truth than does fiction film.[3] Documentary "truth" is discursively constituted and is a social relation like any other form of culture. Similarly, it is argued that science and documentary are subjective and political because scientists and filmmakers have their own opinions, because the institutions themselves embody dominant "concepts, values, and ideologies," and because these institutions are often big business motivated by economics and politics.[4] In a book on press coverage of science, Dorothy Nelkin explains: "The coverage of technology is mainly promotional; the dominant message conveyed is that the new development will give society the magic to cure economic or social ills."[5] Not surprisingly, the corporate sponsors of "Can AIDS Be Stopped?" were Allied Signal, an electronics and engineering firm, and Johnson & Johnson, a health-care products manufacturer.

Promotions from big business withstanding, the two PBS science documentaries I examine here gain great power and pleasure through knowing the subject of AIDS. They take up the same truisms that organize both the institutions of science and documentary.

> To see is to know.
> To know is to control.
> To control is a pleasure.

Science and documentary rely on visualization technologies—the microscope, the film camera, the computer—to gain access to knowledge about the invisible virus which perhaps causes AIDS. Both institutions claim the authority of rationalism and therefore are authorized to control what they see. This control brings satisfaction and mastery—it feels good. In *The History of Sexuality: Volume 1,* Michel Foucault writes of the particular kinds of pleasure which arise from visual conquest: "the power which thus took charge of sexuality set about contacting bodies, caressing them with its eyes, intensifying areas, electrifying surfaces, dramatizing troubled moments. It wrapped the sexual body in its embrace. There was undoubtedly an increase in effectiveness and an extension of the domain controlled; but also a sensualization of power and a gain of pleasure."[6] In the science documentary the path from seeing to knowledge to power and pleasure—so common as to pass unnoticed in many cultural institutions—becomes twice transparent and so, perhaps, twice as good.

What are the representational effects of this doubling of distance, this multiplication of authority? Taking up the analytic project of Foucault, feminist theorists of science think critically about the ways that the pleasure and power of looking have been used by men who have historically held the privilege of vision. Emily Martin writes: "some have singled out reliance on vision as a key culprit in the scrutiny, surveillance, domination, control, and exertion of authority over the body, particularly the bodies of women."[7] The envisioning of AIDS is used in the science documentary to wield a further "domination, control, and exertion of authority" over the body with HIV, a body like a woman's—already disenfranchised, already presumed ill, already punished. Although feminist interpretations of science often focus upon the medicalized gaze—the male doctor's privilege to look at his unclothed patients—the more fundamental question is the gendered power relations of science in general. Who looks through microscopes? What questions are asked in biology? How do the paradigms of scientific method reflect the needs of the men who invented them? The historically gendered structures used in the work and representation of science mean that AIDS is usually conceptualized within already current, oppressive, and nearly always sexualized rubrics.

When men scientifically scrutinize nature, other men, HIV, or knowledge in general, this activity is already codified by tropes of gender, sexuality, and power. "One of the most common metaphors in Western history for such (scientific) mediation has been the sexual relation," Evelyn Fox Keller maintains. "Knowledge is a form of consummation, just as sex is a form of knowledge."[8] Thus, I would suggest that perhaps the most profound consequence of the doubling of distance through the amalgamation of science and documentary is a relatively intractable gendering of the positions of production: the viewer is male (video camera, narrator, scientist, home audience), that which is seen is female (biology, microscopic retro-viruses, KS lesion, PWA). Must science and documentary look at AIDS' bodies in an already codified position of subjugation—as if they were women? What other systems of power and pleasure (outside of gender or sexuality) could structure the curious, information-hungry gaze? And, then again, what occurs when these often-dominated and controlled bodies wield visual mastery themselves? Can the object of the gaze decide to see, and if so, what does the AIDS community see when it looks at science?

Ambivalent Authority in the Alternative Science Documentary

Alternative AIDS documentaries are founded in an understandable ambivalence about science. AIDS activists distrust science, even as they must learn how to talk its talk and walk its walk. They must fight the medical and scientific establishment to insure that the needs of PWAs take precedence over the intricacies, rituals, and profiteering of science. Yet they must also befriend science so that their voices and needs are heard in the development of research, health care, drug development, and sales. Thus, as I went to great lengths in chapter 3 to discuss how the authority and distance of documentary are in fact constructed (or dismantled) for particular ends, I will do the same in this analysis of "science." The transparency of science and documentary is capitalized upon, but sometimes also challenged and revealed, in the variety of documentaries produced about AIDS science. There are any number of reasons why AIDS activists, PWAs, and AIDS researchers need to distrust, challenge, scrutinize, and then control *for themselves* the AIDS science which is at once their enemy and one of their potential saviors.

This said, the distinctions between mainstream and alternative media representations of science (and the use of documentary to do so) are not so neat. While PBS's "The Trial of Compound Q" is explicitly about the moral and factual ambiguity behind much basic AIDS treatment research, the majority of alternative tapes about AIDS science, while invested in critiquing the authority and control of establishment AIDS science, do so to stake an alternative position of expertise from which to speak. For the most part, AIDS activists who challenge authority also need it themselves. AIDS activists who challenge scientific facts—not just raw data, but objective knowledge itself—also rely upon them. Reality-based movements— especially those which depend upon scientific advances (a cure for AIDS), upon exact and authoritative information (correct doses, careful diagnoses), and upon clear and concise systems of expression (listen carefully, this information could save your life)—are not allowed the epistemological luxury of deconstructing away reality, facts, knowledge, or direct systems of communication. While arguments about the necessity versus the inaccessibility of radical form have always split political documentarians wishing to articulate critiques of hegemonic systems, AIDS science documentaries, motivated by a need to get out important information quickly, seem to enact a pragmatic ambivalence. Although it is easy enough to critique the realist style of broadcast documentary, it is rather difficult to express really important information about the world without the familiarity of realist style. How do alternative AIDS videomakers pick up and break down standard documentary style to negotiate their complex relationships to AIDS science? In their science documentaries, as they attempt to criticize the commonly accepted authority of the scientific establishment, do they make other realms of power and pleasure appear natural?

With all these hard questions to answer, it may not seem surprising that AIDS activists have made relatively few documentaries which picture AIDS science. When AIDS science is represented, it is most typically through the talking-head interview of a progressive health-care provider, scientist, or AIDS activist who explains in lay terminology the "facts" of AIDS. This interview is then intercut with the information of nonexperts who display other kinds of knowledge about AIDS. For example, in *We Care* we felt it was important to have a doctor provide "expert" testimony about what was and was not, in her scientific opinion, medically safe when caring for a PWA. For better or worse, people trust the information of a medical doctor in different ways from how they respond to the knowledge of a person actively caring for a PWA. Scientists and doctors know science. There is no way of avoiding them or the highly specialized knowledge they have, nor should there be. Yet the black female doctor we chose is afforded no more time or deference than any of our other interviewees. Her information is one voice in a series of interviews focusing upon the information of AIDS volunteers, PWAs, social workers, and family members of PWAs. While AIDS activists and videomakers must challenge forms of institutional authority like documentary form or the scientific method, they also depend upon them just as they do other forms of expertise.

The second way that AIDS science is typically represented in alternative AIDS video is in tapes produced with highly practical goals and/or extremely narrow intended audiences. Such tapes are made to perform a complicated analysis or explication of AIDS science information for viewers in need of this particularized knowledge. For example, in 1987 the Testing the Limits Collective taped Michael Callen as he pretended to be Julia Child addressing the hundreds of people who were to receive from the PWA Health Group in New York City the experimental AIDS treatment A-Lecithin, or egg lipids. This cooking lesson focused upon how to divide AL-721 into portions, freeze it, and then use it. Callen explained: "We made this tape so that you wouldn't ask us millions of questions when we deliver the A-Lecithin to you. The PWA Health Group is about self-empowerment. We take our health into our own hands and take control over our lives." The tape was played in the courtyard of Judson Memorial Church. As PWAs came to the church to pick up their portion of AL-721, they were instructed to watch the tape. Video was used to its best advantage. Callen did not have to show the same setup procedures over and over; his scripted and rehearsed humor served to relax and inform a stressed-out audience.

A final example of how AIDS science is most typically seen in alternative AIDS video is in the documentation of AIDS demonstrations which are often waged against drug companies (Burroughs Wellcome), research centers (the CDC, the FDA), or particular hospitals or medical institutions. An enormous amount of the AIDS activist agenda has been devoted to challenging the medical and scientific establishment which has operated largely without scrutiny for generations. These efforts have meant that many AIDS activists have trained themselves (formally, through advanced schooling, as well as informally by reading books, talking to people, and attending conferences) to be as knowledgeable as the researchers and doctors who control many aspects of their lives. Thus, in *Seize Control of the FDA* (Gregg Bordowitz and Jean Carlomusto, 1988) an AIDS activist who has participated in the demonstration states, "We are the experts when we go there. We can speak to them as equals."

As the line between AIDS expert and AIDS activist diminishes, do the structures which documentaries use to report AIDS science become blurry as well? I would suggest yes and no. The ambivalence about science felt by PWAs and their supporters seeps into their videos in slightly schizophrenic documentaries which both contest and create authority, which mock experts as they model new forms of expertise. In the science documentaries analyzed in the following pages, different strategies are chosen for different kinds of information and different ends. There are alternative science tapes which entirely refuse authority through humor or dispersion; there are tapes which take some authority to then give some away through performing a self-critique; there are tapes which claim authority by equalizing power distinctions between the subject and object of knowledge. Regardless of the choices made by individual producers, what becomes clear in all of these tapes is the dilemma faced by most mediamakers attempting to articulate a radical critique of structures of power using a form that is itself dependent upon these same structures. While a great deal of feminist film theory decides that women cannot represent themselves, their desires, or their difference through film, most alternative AIDS mediamakers simply go for it. Maybe this is because life-or-death information is at stake and someone needs to refute the misinformation flowing from the mainstream media as quickly as possible. Most broadcast AIDS science documentaries are produced as entertainment, not direct-action, are produced with the distance of "good" journalism, not the proximity of day-to-day needs, and can enjoy a relatively straightforward trust in, and pleasure and power from, the seeing of AIDS science. Therefore, the alternative AIDS media intervenes with images created from a different position: using cheaply, quickly, and matter-of-factly whatever available forms are the most viable for their educational agenda.

The Three Routes to Pleasure and Power

Scientific truth, like other versions of reality, is socially constructed; the maintenance of our belief in its truthfulness is socially accomplished.— Susanna Hornig[9]

In "Can AIDS Be Stopped?" the spectator is offered three related routes to the pleasures of knowledge and power, all constructed through the privileged relationship to sight which defines science and documentary: (1) the powers and pleasures which are associated with control over the subject of study, (2) with participation in a narrative which follows a vanquishing superhero, and (3) with taking up a permitted gaze over the "other." All three of the structures set in place in *NOVA* rely upon gender: the metaphor of sexuality organizes scientific study and its authority; gender roles underlie narratives of power and control; and women's bodies are continually allowed to be looked at in compromising ways in our society.

The three routes to power and pleasure are set into place in the science documentary with little self-consciousness and a great deal of cultural conditioning paving the way. First, *NOVA*, like most documentaries, invites the viewer to identify with its own controlling vision over its weekly program's content. The viewer can take on the role of the omnipotent and omnipresent, unnameable and unseeable force—what Bill Nichols calls the "voice of documentary"—which constructs, organizes, interviews, makes music and images, and tells it like it is. Second, the structure of the horror film is appropriated to order the program into a narrative about scrutiny, knowledge, and conquest. *NOVA* allows the spectator a second site for power-and-pleasure-through-vision: the adventures of the superhero/scientist out to conquer the monster AIDS. Finally, a third system of delight is produced by taking on the gaze of the narrative's protagonist, the conquering scientist, in the permitted and uninterrupted study of others. In "Can AIDS Be Stopped?" and to a lesser degree in "The Trial of Compound Q," the spectator can assume the scientist's gaze as he stares, probes, examines, and ultimately knows the monster AIDS in all of its cultural manifestations: sexually exotic Africans, prostitutes, homosexual men. Unlike Christian Metz's discussion of voyeurism at the cinema, however, the science documentary *informs* its pro-filmic subject that he or she is being watched, studied, and scrutinized.[10] With this in mind, the printed scroll read by the narrator at the *NOVA* program's beginning can be seen less as a warning than as a tease of the good stuff to come: "The following film contains graphic illustrations of human anatomy and sexual behavior. Viewer discretion advised."

At the head of "Can AIDS Be Stopped?" before an image appears, there is a deep, clear voice which booms, "Tonight, on *NOVA*." Speaking out of the blue with no name, no face, and no identity, the voice embodies a verbal register for the returned presence and ongoing authority of *NOVA*, of television, of documentary and science. *NOVA*—the voice, the program— will introduce, organize, explain, and confirm the content it so judiciously chooses and then presents. Stuart Hall describes the organizational function of the media as a necessary making-sense of the jumbled modern world it presents. "What has been made visible and classified begins to shake into an *acknowledged order:* a complex order to be sure. . . ."[11] AIDS, in particular, demands the ordering hand of documentary because it is one of modern culture's most frightening sites of purposelessness. "Nothing could be more meaningless than a virus," suggests Judith Williamson, explaining the tremendous energy expended trying to define AIDS. "It has no point, no purpose, no plan; it is part of no scheme, carries no inherent signification."[12] AIDS is a scientific puzzle unsolved, a frightening example where nature has yet to be contained by science. Yet in this episode *NOVA* makes a coherent flow out of its collection of AIDS footage: interviews with scientists, trips to labs, images of beakers and test tubes, national statistics about infection, and scientific explanations of AIDS. Thus, the show's basic documentary structure—its certainty in itself as a coherent and authoritative source of knowledge—becomes a first example of the trajectory from visualization to pleasure and power. The authority and success with which the program organizes its own sound and image bites somehow stand in as compensatory coherence for the real incoherence of the phenomenon upon which the program reports.

An alternative to this incontestable and tautological force can be seen in *The AIDS Quarterly.* This science documentary takes a different approach to the construction of authorial control. Rather than relying on an unidentified and omniscient narrator, the program is written and narrated by a well-known TV personality, Peter Jennings. Before each episode of the magazine format show, Jennings walks into a darkened room, and the lights rise with his introduction, "Good evening. I'm Peter Jennings." Compare this to *NOVA*'s faceless, nameless host. Jennings stands in a carpeted studio and chats with the home audience. He embodies—anthropormorphizes—the show's authority, its voice. The feeling is familiar, friendly, informal, human—manly. He explains that tonight's show will include three segments on topics related to AIDS.

As Jennings introduces the first segment—"this is the story of desperate and defiant people"—the frozen image of a young man appears in a screen suspended behind him. Jennings turns toward the picture and labels both the segment and the face, "The Trial of Compound Q." The words appear written on the face behind him at his call. The camera then enters the space of this second screen, as if at his bidding, as if in relation to Jennings's movement, as if he is seeing it. Jennings's voice carries over into the sequence, anchoring the program to himself: a real and nice guy standing in a real room. Unlike *NOVA,* which constitutes through its invisible narrator a single, logical narrative for the disparate events in its hour, *The AIDS Quarterly* suggests that the issues raised by AIDS are complex and interrelated but not subsumable under one overarching and oversimplifying plot. Like the nightly news, the magazine format mixes diverse forms of discourse into one cohesive program. Narrative coherence resides in Jennings's position as anchor. The program returns to him after each segment, and his presence is the necessary segue into the next AIDS story. The authority and logic of the program resides in Jennings; if one disagrees with the show, one disagrees with this man.

Although this method of documentary narration seems more ideologically "honest" than that of *NOVA* because it locates and identifies the source of its opinions, it is not outside the powers and pleasures of authority. Of course, these are not really Jennings's ideas alone, but those of a news team itself embroiled in issues of corporate and political sponsorship. And Jennings is no simple man. Rather, he commands the tremendous respect that nightly news anchors are afforded in our society, and more. For he is not working for ABC News here; he is *volunteering*—one of President Bush's "thousand points of light." On his day off, he does not answer telethon calls or walk in a walkathon, he works on this show. Thus, we like him (and rightly so) for what he appears to be doing. We like ourselves for participating in this benevolent act, yet another manifestation of what structures PBS— highbrow, back-patting funding drives. We trust him because his heart is in the right place *and* because we already trust the news. This system of seeing, emanating from Jennings, although different from *NOVA*'s impersonal stare, is in this case difficult to contest because of the emotional and moral pulls of loyalty and philanthropy.

Whereas the two PBS science documentaries I study depend upon a male voice or body to provide coherence to their content, the alternative AIDS documentaries which cover science use other structures to impart their scientific knowledge. Their choices are often made in direct opposition to these forms of male authority. As I explained in *chapter 3,* alternative AIDS documentaries rarely use narrators to structure their content. This formal device reeks of a kind of authority and control that such programs are inevitably attempting to contradict. For this kind of control is most frequently used to silence and delegitimize the words and knowledge of most PWAs and AIDS activists. But imagine trying to make a coherent show without a narrator! It is necessary to edit together into a consistent and directed flow a train of unrelated thoughts spoken extemporaneously by a host of interviewees. Then there is still the question of how to impart precise information quickly and efficiently through the testimony of unscripted speakers. Inevitably, such tapes must rely on the talking-head interview with a doctor, researcher, nurse, or AIDS activist to explain technical knowledge. This information is then contextualized within a series of interviews which place their scientific detail into a broader discussion of its history and politics and its relation to the lived experience of PWAs.

A segment of GMHC's program *Living With AIDS* called "Medical Update" provides an interesting exception to this rule. As the segment begins, we see a young woman seated like a news anchor at a desk. She reads from notes on the desktop, "Good evening, my name is Mary Beth Caschetta. I'm the editor of '*Treatment Issues,*' GMHC's newsletter for experimental AIDS therapies. This is what's new in medical information in AIDS." For the next five minutes she (somewhat falteringly, thus signifying that she is no news anchor) reads highly technical information about new drug research and trials. She imparts much-needed information with authority. Yet the dissimilarities to the network news far outweigh the similarities. Most notably, the segment provides no visual or other relief from her dense and complicated narration. No cuts to graphics, illustrative images, corroborating interviews, or words of a friendly coanchor. The image is stark: a blue cloth is the backdrop to her virtually immobile face. This form allows for the quick, immediate, no-nonsense imparting of information—less like television and more like a textbook on tape. GMHC uses this segment of their cable show to get highly specific information to a targeted audience that needs it enough not to want fluff and already educated enough not to need basic background. However, it is no coincidence that a nightly news show format (however distilled) is taken up to impart complex information. When Caschetta explains, "A new drug called DaunoXome manufactured by Vestar, Inc., was reported to show a clinical benefit in 95 percent of a small cohort of men with Kaposi's Sarcoma. The drug is a lyposomal version of a classic chemotherapeutic agent. Lyposome is a fatty substance that the drug is encapsulated into allowing the agent to be more specifically targeted to cancer cells," we need to believe that Caschetta knows what she is talking about. We need to believe in her control over this technical knowledge. We need to trust—not challenge—her expertise. Borrowing the form of a news show gives her this necessary authority, just as it proves a most effective style to quickly express dense scientific information. Yet this style also gives authority to her *critique* of the scientific establishment's authority. "On a related note, AIDS activists were successful in pressuring Daichi Pharmaceuticals to move forward on a drug that has potential in treating KS and breast cancer." *Medical Update* uses standard documentary narration to authorize GMHC's simultaneous embrace and challenge of the scientific control over the lives of PWAs.

Seeing It Makes It So; or "The Map Precedes the Territory"

A second example of *NOVA*'s adept construction of its own authority through mastery of vision is its creation and presentation of random but fancy computer-generated images of science. At the show's beginning the narrator describes a "strange and deadly virus." The image which accompanies his lecture is a fuzzy sphere, a bit like a tennis ball. For no reason other than for its scientificity, a thin horizontal line descends on the field of the image, making a beep, beep sound like an electrocardiograph monitoring the heart of a patient in intensive care. The image moves closer and closer, the lines move faster and faster, and the beeps get louder and quicker. Then, there is a cut in image as the voice says, "Littering its surface, hundreds of virus particles are budding forth ready to spread disease. This is how AIDS begins." With "magnification," we see "how AIDS begins": the tennis ball is covered with countless, symmetrically placed pimples. This is only the first example of a series of four such computer generated science illustrations which play again and again during the show. Simply by repeating these random and imaginary computer constructions of invisible and hypothetical events, their status and authority as "real" depictions and "real" explanations of "real" events is constructed. Through their constant repetition, the viewer becomes familiar with these meaningless graphics and grants them a credibility by virtue of recognition: ah, yes, the T-4 cell's outer membrane. . . .

NOVA establishes a privileged relationship between itself and the world it reports upon through its technological mastery over vision. For the lay audience, tuning into NOVA with the explicit agenda of learning about a topic with which they are unfamiliar, with little reason not to trust NOVA, and probably possessing neither the skills nor the information with which to contest it, this tautological system of science presentation is somewhat bullying: image confirms voice, and voice confirms image. This is also Jean Baudrillard's vision of the postmodern world: "The real is produced from miniaturized units, from matrices, memory banks, and command models— and with these it can be reproduced an infinite number of times. It no longer has to be rational, since it is no longer measured against some ideal or negative instance. It is nothing more than operational. In fact, since it is no longer enveloped by an imaginary, it is no longer real at all."[13]

These less-than-real images are authorized by an obligatory statement which follows from a doctor or scientist who, in turn, confirms the information and image produced by NOVA. Knowledge is confirmed by vision; vision is empowered by knowledge. For instance, Dr. William Haseltine says, "What we're finding is truly astounding. It's as if this virus comes from the depths of the seas encrusted with new biological organisms that we've never seen before in all of biology." Midway through his interview appears the previously seen rotating image of the blue orb, symmetrically dotted with pulsing white pimples. NOVA lets the home viewer see what "we've never seen before," what even Dr. Haseltine cannot—the new, encrusted, biological organisms of AIDS. The first truism of science and documentary—to see is to know—is thus artificially, but forcefully, assured in NOVA by computer-imaging technology that simply manufactures "images" of the things that NOVA says it knows. "The territory no longer precedes the map, nor survives it. Henceforth, it is the map which precedes the territory."[14]

What would an image of the territory preceding the map look like? In DHPG Mon Amour (Carl George, 1989) and Silverlake Life (Peter Friedman, Tom Joslin, Jane Weiner, Doug Block, 1993), the diary-like representation of a PWA's daily life requires the inclusion of images and information about medicine, treatment, sickness, and science because the real bodies of AIDS require it. These documentaries, attempting to chronicle the mundane

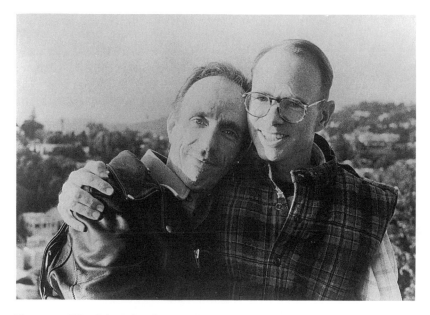

Figure 9   *Silverlake Life: The View from Here* (Peter Friedman, Tom Joslin, Jane Weiner, and Doug Block; Zeitgeist Films, 1993).

details of life with AIDS, must in the process focus closely upon AIDS science. Pills, visits to doctors, acupuncture, holistic teas, hospitals, difficulty sleeping are some of the many scientific details which play an immense role in the life of the PWAs chronicled in *Silverlake Life.* Purportedly made for a mainstream audience, the video evidences the tedious, maddening, and overwhelming control of AIDS science in the life of one PWA. The "mainstream" viewer—presumably the viewer who has no first-hand knowledge of AIDS—learns that the lived experience of AIDS is dependent, to a large part, upon science: how adeptly the PWA can control it, and how strongly science controls the PWA. Real pain requires real medicine. Real medicine is not always so easy to acquire and then, healing does not always come from pills, anyway (figure 9).

In a real world of health care dependent upon politics, economics, and bureaucratic confusion, *DHPG Mon Amour* lovingly and clinically demonstrates the infusion of the experimental drug DHPG Gansiclovir into the body of the filmmaker's lover, David, to combat his infection with CMV retinitus. The film is produced to make public what the science of AIDS entails in the lives of PWAs. "Hi, my name is Joe Walsh. We made this film to tell you about DHPG and its side effects." It is art and activism for PWAs to let others know about the drugs that control them, about the drugs which they control themselves. We watch David carefully mix vials of DHPG with water and other solutions. We see him sterilize the medi-port catheter under his chest before he pierces his skin so that he can inject himself with the drug. (The filmmakers inform us that they fought the doctors to get this slightly submerged, and therefore hardly visible catheter, as opposed to the Hickman catheter the doctors were prescribing without consideration to how wearing a visible catheter would make David feel about his body.) Over the images of this slow, grueling procedure, the two men narrate information about the drug, their lives, and their political opinions of AIDS science. "I want the world to wake up to the fact that AZT is not the only fucking drug. Be aware. Fight everyone. This drug wasn't even approved when we went into it." They explain how little doctors told them about the drug, and the many "lies" which doctors did impart. Yet they also want to make sure that the audience understands that although the painstaking course of DHPG looks as if it is a hassle and appears painful, and the insistent fighting with doctors that is necessary to get to use experimental drugs looks taxing and frustrating, the film also celebrates the drug and science because "it's keeping David alive." A complicated vision of AIDS science is constructed through documentaries which image the bodies of people who are living with AIDS day-to-day. This is a vision of dependence upon science to make the pain go away, to cure the opportunistic infections, as it also is a vision of resistance—distrust, the need to push doctors to explain honestly and clearly what they are doing, the activist agenda of fighting for and then using alternative and/or still-unapproved treatments.

The Pleasures and Powers of Narrative

Dr. Haseltine's "depths-of-the-sea" rhetoric serves another function besides its descriptive detailing of the visage and personality of HIV. It is part of the second system of pleasure through vision and knowledge which is put into place by *NOVA:* the AIDS-as-monster-that-ate-Manhattan narrative structure of the program. This second strategy makes sense of the incoherent or unknowable (unseeable) phenomenon of AIDS by fabricating, and in the case of documentary by making visible, a story. Narrative gives coherence, structure, and pleasure to the random and frightening phenomenon of AIDS because it permits closure and it allows conquest. According to Nelkin, this coupling of closure and conquest is often the form that the media takes up in its coverage of science. "The message is our ability to win over the forces that besiege us. Order is restored."[15]

It is specifically, and importantly, the narrative of the horror movie (although science fiction, romance, and the detective thriller are also invoked) which organizes, visualizes, and makes pleasurable the acquisition of knowledge about AIDS in "Can AIDS Be Stopped?" For the horror film is not only a structure where good ultimately triumphs over evil, but one in which the distinction between good and evil, scientist and monster, self and other, is clearly and carefully delineated. In fact, the function of the horror text is to construct a body, an other, a MONSTER, that embodies what is not wanted in the self. "The monstrous which narrative splits off from the self is a projection of unacceptable parts of the self—and indeed, of society."[16] Then, the horror narrative allows the scientist, or any other good guy, to kill the monster and thus purge the potentially polluting projection.

Early AIDS media performed a similar function. Reports were quick to isolate risk for HIV infection into communities—"risk groups"—of others. It seemed clear who was safe and who was sick, who was to purge, who was to be purged. Yet by the 1986 production of "Can AIDS Be Stopped?" it was evident that *all* people, depending upon their behavior, were at risk. Boundaries were dissolving, and, according to Williamson, this made people anxious. "The virus threatens to cross over that border of Other and Self; the threat it poses is not only one of disease but one of dissolution, the contamination of categories."[17] Gay men have been considered "border cases"[18] as well, threatening otherwise "stable" boundaries of gender and sexuality.[19] Narratives like "Can AIDS Be Stopped?" reclarify boundaries in a confused and illogical real world where borders are not nearly so simple. With perhaps too much simplicity, too much finality, *NOVA* identifies the good guys and the monster.

At the opening of the show all of the dramatis personae are introduced in preparation for the drama about to unfold. The first image introduces the innocent victims—a young man and woman, ice skating hand in gloved hand at Rockefeller Center. Maybe this is a musical comedy. But the narrator shoots this hope down when he says, as we watch them spin, "Bruce and Bobbie—a young married couple at the beginning of their life together. There's only one problem. Bobbie has AIDS." The voice continues as the image cuts to a graveyard. "She is only one of over 11,000 Americans with the disease. Another 15,000 have already died." We are told in so many words (images) that Bobbie will die. Can't anything be done to save Bobbie? Who will come to the rescue?

"In the face of this new and deadly epidemic," answers our narrator, "science is engaged in a desperate fight to understand and overcome the AIDS virus." The comic book language is accompanied by the metonymic images of science that will be used throughout the show—test tubes, white-coated backs leaning over microscopes. There is a cut to Dr. Haseltine, who makes his sea-monster comparison. "What we're finding is truly astounding. It's as if this virus comes from the depths of the seas. . . ."

NOVA has set its narrative strategies into motion. Here is a horror film, complete with the innocent, threatened heroine Bobbie, superhero Science, and AIDS, the creature from the Black Lagoon. The narrator wraps up the introduction. "The scientists, society, and the victims, are drawn together by a single haunting question"—innocent Bobbie stands in her kitchen, pouring and drinking a glass of orange juice—"Can AIDS be stopped?" Music swells, as Bobbie and her clean kitchen fade. Will the hero save Bobbie from the AIDS monster before the lights of her kitchen and life fade to black?

I admit that my language is melodramatically charged here, but this is much less for ironic effect than to get across the ludicrous sensationalism and surreal silliness which define the structure of this otherwise "serious" program. I cannot emphasize enough how bizarre it is to watch this highbrow "educational" program, in which important and complicated information is presented, using the formal strategies of a "B" horror movie. An effective critique of the silly sensationalism used in much reportage of AIDS science is put forward in John Greyson's Zero Patience (1993), the first feature-length musical about AIDS. Greyson specifically attacks the mainstream media's illogical, hysterical focus on "Patient Zero" (the Canadian airline steward who was purported to be the first "carrier" of HIV, infecting gay men across the globe in his hedonistic travels) in the same tabloid form in which the original horror stories were told. Greyson rebuts a number of examples of bad AIDS science—in particular, the kind of paper-selling but knowledge-numbing searches for the "cause" of AIDS, i.e., Patient Zero and African green monkeys. This hilarious, intelligent, campy farce tells how Patient Zero comes back to life to block the opening of "The Hall of Contagion," which is to be mounted in Toronto's Natural History Museum, and which is to be funded by a pharmaceutical company under current attack by a local ACT UP chapter for its scandalous monopoly on a drug for CMV. Greyson's use of melodramatic and musical conventions to tell his tragic and political tale serves as both pointed critique of the style of mainstream coverage as well as a much-appreciated antidote to the understandably self-serious media work by most alternative producers. Because AIDS science is so cor-

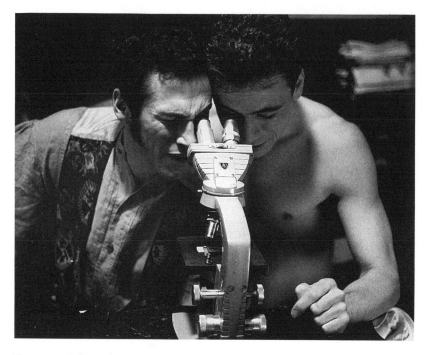

Figure 10   John Robinson as Sir Richard Francis Burton and Normand Fauteux as Zero, *Zero Patience* (John Greyson; Cineplex Odeon, 1993). Photo by Rafy.

rupt, because AIDS pain is so severe, because it is ten years and more later and little has changed, most alternative AIDS media is sad, angry, dire, aggressive, bitter, critical. And *Zero Patience* contains all of these emotions, but it also is funny, charming, loving, sexy, and witty. Greyson fights melodrama and tabloid journalism—with melodrama and tabloid journalism. However, not only are his scientist-heros smart, they are sexy and (homo)sexual, too (figure 10).

The Magic Cure

The eerie mood of sea monsters rising to snatch young skaters away from Rockefeller Center is continually constructed by means of music, lighting, and sensationalist language throughout the show. A sense of threat, fear, and mystery is manufactured to build anticipation regarding the conquest of the monster by science. But this mood is also constructed so that the resolution of the narrative (and the AIDS crisis, the show suggests) can be articulated within the discourse of horror. The show manufactures a visual image, an actual site to behold, where "answers" are stored. To see is to know. But in this mythic narrative, things can be *seen*—like answers—which are not so visible in the "real world." Answers are said to be in a "magic" place, what the narrator calls the "magic box" of possible cures. Unlike *Life, Death and AIDS*, which argues that answers do not exist, *NOVA* constructs, visualizes, and falsifies its own vision of the answers which will end the crisis.

The show is split into halves, the laying out of the problem (Can AIDS Be Stopped?), and solutions to this problem. (Yes, it can be stopped, with magic, i.e., big science.) The sequence which introduces the "answers to AIDS" opens on black. A light enters the screen when a door opens; the camera is inside a refrigerator. Unidentified hands enter the space and grab something that has been resting inside. It is a box. An Asian scientist picks it up and carries it to a table. The narrator says, "They've tested hundreds of substances and narrowed the search to the contents of what is known as the 'magic box.'" Of course, hidden behind the box's spell-encrusted top are not only the magic serums that will cure Bobbie, but the program's more economic and political agenda, which is to present pharmaceutical cures and medical research as the magic resolutions that will solve the very crisis that *NOVA* has constituted.

Not surprisingly, the following scene depicts Bobbie's experimental treatment with AZT. After having been on AZT for several months and seeing a weight gain and stabilization of her fevers, Bobbie says to her doctor, "You don't know how pleased we are. I mean we are so happy right now." Dr. Samuel Broder responds, "But you have to understand that although I'm extremely gratified about your response, I can't be sure that it's the drug that we gave you that did this." Bobbie concludes the scene with "I attribute it to the drug, though. I do. I don't care what anybody else says, it's the drug."

The scene ends with Bobbie's unfounded faith in the drug, not her doctor's more cautious advice. But this is necessary in the terms of a mythical narrative that presents easy (magical) answers to difficult problems. "The press coverage of new technological developments plays upon and probably encourages the public's desires for easy solutions to economic, social, and medical problems," writes Anne Karpf.[20] Unlike horror films, where the monster can be vanquished in two hours, the crisis of AIDS cannot be reduced to the search for a cure, nor will the problem be solved when and if a cure is found. The ills of AIDS are not just physical, but economic, social, cultural, political.

Although medical research and medicine are important for people with AIDS, the oversimplification of the search for and acquisition of medical cures forecloses accurate reportage on the complexities of medical research, the politics and economics of the pharmaceutical industry, and the negative (as well as positive) effects of particular medications. Furthermore, a focus on magical medical cures means that little attention is given to the politics of *who* is predominantly affected by AIDS and why, means that little attention is paid to holistic and other non-Western responses to illness, and means that little attention focuses upon who *does not* have access to experimental studies or expensive medication.

This is what is under scrutiny in "The Trial of Compound Q," which is specifically about the scientific, economic, political, and moral complexity of medical and pharmaceutical research. The sequence monitors two drug protocols—one legal, the other illegal—for a Chinese "abortion and cancer drug," Tricasanthin, known as Compound Q. At the segment's beginning, Martin Delaney, "one of the most important AIDS activists," approaches Dr. Alan Levin to see if he will run an illegal, speeded-up drug trial to analyze the effects of Compound Q since PWAs are taking the drug anyway without supervision and with little knowledge about it. Dr. Levin agrees to run an accelerated trial. Like a "trial," the show weighs the verbal testimony of people on both sides of this "case." Dr. Volberding at San Francisco General Hospital, who is conducting the eighteen-month official study of Compound Q, explains why in his opinion things need to progress slowly. FDA officials are also given room to discuss the history of present-day experimental drug trial regulations: why things are so lugubrious. Then we get Dr. Levin's "testimony," much less euphoric than the words about AZT articulated in *NOVA*. "The odds are good that someone is going to die. This is not a magical panacea."

The segment follows three gay men (unlike *NOVA,* here the gay subjects are named and interviewed about their feelings and motivations) through the study, interviews them throughout, chronicles the death of two of them (perhaps, the show suggests, as a result of the study), and shows Dr. Levin and Delaney making the difficult moral and medical decisions about whether they should continue the study, and at what dose level. The conclusions of the segment are presented with ambivalence. Tandy Belloo, the only survivor of the original study, is much improved (after a bout of AIDS dementia, caused most probably by the Compound Q) and is taking Compound Q for a second time. He says, "I was disappointed when it wasn't a miracle cure. . . . But I think it's working." Delaney is now leading an official protocol with the FDA. Dr. Levin says that he continues to believe that he has a moral obligation, "above the laws of the land," to save lives however he can. Dr. Volberding says that it is not a good idea to do studies in nonacademic environments, but he now understands that the motivations behind unofficial studies are similar to his own.

The speakers in the program, and the program itself, conclude that no easy answers are out there. It is unclear who was right and who was wrong, and whether the two studies got anyone anywhere. Yet if anything is celebrated here, it is the search for knowledge itself, both by the scientists, and as championed and demonstrated by *The AIDS Quarterly*. A narrative structures this program, but it is not the simple resolution of horror. Rather, the structure of the trial system of liberal democracy is engaged. Two sides are to be heard; listen to them, weigh them, draw your own conclusion, vote Levin or Volberding. This structure is also the system which most typically organizes the news: show the *two* (not the many, complex, interrelated) sides of a debate and let the viewer decide. Hall writes: "In this way television does not favor one point of view, but it does favor—and reproduce—one definition of politics and excludes, represses, or neutralizes other definitions. . . . It also, incidentally, offers a favorable image of the system as a system, as open to conflict and to alternative points of view.[21]

Unlike "The Trial of Compound Q," *Grid-Lock: Women and the Politics of AIDS* (Beth Wichtenich, 1992) presents only one agenda in its reportage on a current conflict about AIDS science. The tape focuses upon women's long fight to alter the CDC's list of opportunistic infections which define AIDS so as to include the gynecological disorders which plague women with HIV. The tape features a number of articulate female AIDS activists, health-care workers, and community organizers who carefully and convincingly argue how the science of AIDS has consistently and criminally ignored, mistreated, and denied the needs of HIV-infected women. Several women interviewed explain why direct action is necessary to make bureaucrats and researchers aware that while women actively suffer the pain of crippling diseases which do not qualify as "AIDS," they will not passively accept their invisibility in the eyes of AIDS science. Other women argue for legislative and educational action. A decidedly politicized, informed, aggressive, and activist vision of the political realities of science is envisioned in this tape's portrayal of women's relationship to AIDS. No posture of "balanced" journalism is present, because it is implied that one side of this struggle is corrupt and demands no respect. The tape insists that women have been held in the gridlock of red tape, sexism, and mistreatment by the scientific establishment. Although the interviewees detail the many ways that women have been victimized by "science," the tape ends with a victory. The CDC does at last change the definition of AIDS to include cervical cancer and pelvic inflammatory disease. Women can and must fight the enormous, faceless powers which have control over what is and is not AIDS and AIDS science. In this video, women are envisioned to have control—superheroines winning battles against their own AIDS monsters.

Permitted Looking

In the PBS science documentaries which chronicle and make visible the accumulation of knowledge about AIDS, one final system allowing the acquisition of pleasure is set in place: the delightful activity of watching and monitoring those who are objects of scientific study. Throughout the programs the audience is given permission, like the scientist, to watch the strange and curious lives of all kinds of social "perverts." In *NOVA,* scientists delve into the lives of prostitutes, Africans, homosexual men, and individuals with AIDS dementia. In *The AIDS Quarterly,* although the content is handled much more gracefully by allowing the "objects" of the study to speak for themselves, the camera pries into several private moments. For instance, when Belloo, who is suffering the side effects of AIDS dementia from his use of Compound Q, is confused, cannot form sentences, and is ultimately brought to tears, the camera continues to record him, and this footage is included in the final program.

Denying privacy is only one example of the gratuitous but condoned probing into the lives and bodies of others typical of the science documentary but not typical of work which documents from a position of sympathy, similarity, or sorrow. The particular power and pleasure of detached scrutiny is that the viewer of scientific activity is a *permitted* voyeur—the voyeur who gave himself permission to look. Unlike the conventional Freudian voyeur, whose pleasure is in seeing without being seen, knowing without being known (even if he may ultimately "accidentally" reveal himself), the scientist, the documentary camera, and the home viewer (who is offered identification with both of these sites) authorize their illicit act in the names of Science, Knowledge, and Truth. Metz speaks of a more complicated series of authorizations in the voyeurism of the fiction film. "The film knows that it is being watched, and yet does not know." He explains that the *institution* of cinema knows about and depends upon spectatorship, while the film itself is structured around the denial of an audience. In the case of the narrative film text, he explains that " 'seeing' is no longer a matter of sending something back, but of catching something unawares." [22]

In Metz's terms, each science documentary is similar to the institution of the cinema; it knows it is being watched and takes illicit pleasure in its control over vision. For example, at the end of "Can AIDS Be Stopped?" a sequence reporting upon a gay male PWA is presented. The man, identified not by name but by sexual preference, is participating in an unspecified study. But the narrator does say some things with great precision, for example, every year "he" arrives at "Ward 86" at "San Francisco General" for his part of the study. He gets a medical exam ("stick your tongue way out," instructs the doctor, as we are privy to this less-than-dignified moment of the patient's visit). The narrator concludes, "The medical exam is only the beginning. Volunteers are also asked to reveal the history of their sexual lives. What they did, with whom, how often, and with what protection." The real need to understand the relationship between sexual behavior and HIV infection seems somehow lost in this sordid inclusion of the study's demands about private sexual practice without including the study's purpose or results.

Then, in reporting a study on heterosexual transmission, NOVA's camera lingers on the spaces and bodies of the sex industry. Although the study considers three groups of women, NOVA covers only one aspect of the study. The narrator says, "the project's field workers go into the streets recruiting from those groups of women." The simple use of the loaded statement "in the streets" is enough to identify NOVA's interest in only one of "those groups" of women. But to make it crystal clear, his voice is accompanied by a lurid montage of images of the red light district: "LIVE!" "LIVE!" "LIVE!" "Erotic Nude Show!" Lights blink. Seedy men enter shaded doors. Only one short segment of an interview with a prostitute is covered. She is asked to calculate how many partners she had in a year. When she cannot work out the math, the narrator thoughtfully does it for her.

The way that NOVA reports the work of science and doctors—the knowledge and concomitant sexual pleasure gained from an authorized scrutiny of other's problems and life-styles—has a long tradition. "Science is a masculine viewer, who is anticipating full knowledge of nature, which is represented as the naked female body," writes Ludmilla Jordanova in her study of scientific imagery. [23] This metaphoric description of the work of science has a literal basis. The acquisition of knowledge has often been obtained by the sexualized scrutiny of women's bodies. In her book on primatology, Donna Haraway explains that even when the scientist is a woman, which is often the case in this field, she is constructed and understood as "female male."[24] And in his book on postmodern theories of televisual culture, Gregory Ulmer explains how knowing, in general, is similarly codified: "Knowing, in the modern paradigm is scopophilic. Regardless of gender, sex, class, race, or orientation of the knower, the one who knows, the subject of knowledge in the mind of science, is in the position of the voyeur."[25] And, I would add, is in the position of a man, just as the object of the gaze of knowledge is in a passive position, a position codified as female.

It is useful here to return to the workings of the horror film. For, as I mentioned, the monster in horror stories is always a "projection of unacceptable parts of the self."[26] The monster is the "locus of the most primitive":[27] sexuality, impurity, irrationality, and, most importantly for this analysis, femininity. Feminist theorists of the horror film have maintained that the monster stands in for "that area over which the narrative has lost control."[28] This is the "space of the feminine." Women and gay men transgress into the "space of the feminine"—those places unknown, uncharted, irrational. The AIDS virus, a fantastic biology cum monster that also transgresses boundaries and makes things impure, easily resides in this feminized position in a horror narrative like "Can AIDS Be Stopped?" But then, too easily, these feelings as the show presents them are displaced onto the literal bodies that are infected (or thought to be infected). "The virus is lost and, metaphorically speaking, the homosexual/prostitute/African/injecting-drug-user/hemophiliac body *becomes* AIDS," writes Patton about the ways that the body with HIV is pathologized by diagnostic medicine.[29] What is true in medicine is true in documentaries covering medicine. The women, gay men, prostitutes, and PWAs in the program—individuals who have often inhabited this "space of the feminine" in the rhetoric of dominant white male society—are themselves made into the AIDS monster against whom voyeurism and other forms of sexual control are easily condoned. It is an easy slip to allow those infected by the monster AIDS to *become* the monster themselves.

Yet it is equally easy and necessary to avoid such slips and to see PWAs not as monsters but as the heroes they really are. Such an image is created in *Amsterdam Treatment Report* (DIVA TV, 1992), which documents several male and female AIDS activists reporting back to the floor of ACT UP about the scientific information presented at the 1992 International AIDS Conference in Amsterdam. In this tape, AIDS activists are pictured as *the* experts on AIDS, both because they live it, and because they have as much medical and science expertise as the doctors and researchers whose work they follow. Nothing like spectacles, freaks, or helpless victims, the speakers in the tape are instead the articulate presenters of lengthy, uncut, talking-head interviews in which their authority over AIDS science is evidenced in their language, clarity, and control over complex information as well as the camera's legitimizing focus. The tape makes it clear that now that these AIDS activists have fully assumed the roles of experts, not monsters, scientists, not subjects, the responsibilities of power are theirs as well. One AIDS activist in the tape explains:

> Most of the leading researchers and the scientists realize that there are AIDS activists who know as much as they do about the disease, drug development, and pathogenesis. You name it, we have the knowledge base, and can dialogue with them on this in a productive way. . . . We have an influence on almost every area of drug development now, and a great knowledge of it. The trick is to come up with the right recommendations now that we are being listened to. The decisions are complex and affect a lot of lives. It is a heavy responsibility that treatment activists have to take seriously.

Conclusions: Alternative Pleasures

Sex here is the perfect metaphor for a particular admixture of power and pleasure. —Ludmilla Jordanova [30]

Power and pleasure are invoked by the sexually charged conflation of vision and authority. The science documentary confirms its privilege to see and learn at the expense of others—the bodies it "objectively" views and then objectifies. Clearly, the two science documentaries I have analyzed, both produced for public television, handle the reporting of the science of AIDS in different ways. Yet the two programs are also based upon similar paradigms which have real and lasting impact, whether this is the long-standing systematic control of women or the recent social controls enacted over people with AIDS.

What are the effects of representations which are based upon a sexualized and gendered gaze? How does pleasure transfigure itself into power? Putting AIDS into the gendered female position has easily translated, throughout the history of the crisis, into legislative and economic policy which treats PWAs in the same way our culture presently treats those who are culturally disenfranchised in other ways—punishing the victim by cutting funds, care, services.[31] Making AIDS and its bodies the monster has contributed to and perpetuated a culture where PWAs are actively discriminated against in all aspects of their existence from access to health insurance, burial services, and hospital beds to the less blatant forms of discrimination which occur in the neighborhood, workplace, and home.[32]

But other systems of pleasure can be used to make a documentary, or to study science. Rather than a system of distance and control, difference and power, structures of similarity and reciprocity are possible. Feminist science is based upon entirely different founding principles than the three truisms with which I began this chapter. Elizabeth Fee explains that in the practice of feminist science, "No rigid boundaries separate the subject of knowledge (the knower) and the natural object of knowledge; the subject/object split is not used to legitimate the dominance of nature; nature itself is conceptualized as active rather than passive."[33]

Alternative AIDS media differentiates itself from work like *NOVA* because it actively situates itself *within* the object of study, speaks *from* and *to* a position of infection and difference. Such work identifies with, instead of gapes at, the subject of study. Such work identifies with, rather than intensifies, the struggles of PWAs. In alternative AIDS media, to look is to see and know *yourself,* not the other—an entirely different route to pleasure and power. *HIV: The Other Side* (Anderson, Wendt, Flythe, Latz, 1993) is an excellent example of a documentary about AIDS science which comes from and is addressed to PWAs. This hour-long video of interviews is conceived of and produced by long-term survivors who discuss the alternative therapies which they think have made the difference in their life spans with HIV. Also interviewed are the health practitioners who these PWAs depend upon— Western M.D.s, chiropractors, acupuncturists, massage therapists, herbologists. The program speaks to HIV-positive people, insisting that long-term survivors and their health advisers are the most qualified experts on AIDS medicine, AIDS health care, AIDS science, AIDS treatment, and the creation of long, productive lives with AIDS. The immense *pleasure* articulated in this tape is that of living, the pleasure of self and community empowerment, the vital importance of loving oneself and maintaining a positive attitude, and taking control over systems which would otherwise control you. Power is actualized through study and knowledge of self, not of the other.

Finally, pleasure is not the only emotion upon which representation can be based. Much alternative AIDS media has been rooted in anger, the motivating power of political action.

5 CONTAINING AND UNLEASHING THE THREAT: WOMEN'S SEXUALITY IN THE AIDS DOCUMENTARY

The female population is, of course, a subject of anxious attention to (presumably) heterosexual journalists, since it is from this direction that they evidently think themselves to be at increasing risk [for AIDS]. . . .—Simon Watney[1]

An anxious male heterosexual journalist is at no greater risk for AIDS from women than he is from men or from an unsterilized needle. He is at risk for the transmission of HIV when the bodily fluids of another individual come into contact with his own bodily fluids. He can protect himself from such contact in many ways: with barriers like condoms and dental dams, safe sexual interaction that does not involve the interchange of bodily fluids, or a clean and personal set of drugworks.[2] However, these facts are not what is most typically represented in the AIDS documentaries of the broadcast media that are dedicated to heterosexual risk (which until of late has meant women's threat to men). In such programs the "realities" of transmission and protection are not what is mimetically represented. Instead, we see male anxiety about female sexuality, and then we see that anxiety contained through representation. I am curious about the anxiety of male heterosexual journalists over the female population. How does their ambivalence and anger seep into the images of women created in AIDS reportage? How is the attempt to assert control over anxiety about AIDS in broadcast documentary similar to other recent social controls over women? And then, how do female video producers respond to this male anxiety? How do feminists make work that unleashes the previously contained threat?

The disregard by heterosexual male journalists (and others) of women's lived and epidemiological experience in favor of constructing representations more ideologically beneficial to their creators underwrites the entire history of women and AIDS, not merely that found in TV documentary.

Gena Corea in *The Invisible Epidemic: The Story of Women and AIDS* focuses upon how consistently the medical establishment has misinterpreted "the story of women and AIDS." From the lack of a specific category for documenting women's epidemiology (other than "other") until 1985; to the exclusion of women from drug protocols because of their procreative capabilities; to the painstakingly slow acceptance of women's opportunistic infections like pelvic inflammatory disease and cervical cancer as legitimate indices of AIDS—the story of women and AIDS has largely been one of criminal indifference, sexist misassumptions, and racist disregard.[3] Paula Treichler explains that with more than enough scientific evidence to prove irrefutably that others besides gay men were at risk for AIDS, it was hard to let this "monolithic" picture go.

> The construction of AIDS as a "gay disease," for example, is not based on "material reality"—which challenges any stable division between male and female, gay and straight, "promiscuous" and monogamous, guilty and innocent. Yet the construction inscribed again and again throughout our cultural discourses radically contains and controls this diverse and contradictory data, producing monolithic identities of those "at risk" or not at risk, depending on their official classification.[4]

Similarly, according to Sunny Rumsey, the construction of AIDS as a gay disease long obscured the "material reality" that straight people of color were suffering. This kept funding, care, and education from communities of color until infection with the virus had reached epidemic, and no longer ignorable, proportions.[5]

In this chapter my interest is in charting the gap between some "material realities" (perhaps best understood for my purposes here as the unique but expressible lived and cognitive experiences of humans) and the reality represented in broadcast documentary. In some cases this misalignment of realities means the disregard of scientific data (i.e., the belief that heterosexuals are not at risk for AIDS), in others the perpetuation of reigning systems of values and representations (i.e., the belief that women's sexuality is only meant for procreation or men's pleasure). Given these vast disparities, it seems important to question how and why the maintenance of what Treichler calls "monolithic identities"—dependent upon secure and traditional understandings about the distinctions between men and women, whites and people of color, straights and gays—continues as one of the primary concerns, as well as structuring devices, of the broadcast media's representation of AIDS even in the face of an epidemic. I do not mean to suggest that mainstream representations of women's reality are themselves not diverse, or even true to the experiences and opinions of some Americans, and even of some women with AIDS. However, I will show how the material realities represented in broadcast documentaries rely upon cinematic and ideological structures which are themselves unrealistic to the needs of many women involved with AIDS. Thus, one of the definitive features of the alternative media is its commitment and ability to fill in this gap by attempting to represent the ideas and experiences of women which do not make it onto the nightly news.

A most important gap needing to be filled is the chasm created because the mainstream medical establishment and media refused for many years to acknowledge what had been verified scientifically as early as 1982, that AIDS affected women and could be spread heterosexually.[6] In 1986 and 1987, with the release of scientific studies establishing that HIV could be transmitted heterosexually and documenting the history of cases involving women,[7] the medical establishment and the media were forced to accept the existence of the female with AIDS. Before that time, when the reported cases of AIDS were predominantly from the classic "4-H risk groups" —homosexuals, heroin addicts, hemophiliacs, and Haitians—women were perceived to be virtually untouched by AIDS (even though all of these groups included women), and so they were left untouched by the television camera. But suddenly AIDS was no longer perceived as a disease of gay white men. The representation of AIDS altered accordingly.[8]

Now the bodies of (some) women could enter the screen. Consequently, their images served a time-honored role: to carry partial blame for physical and psychic contamination. Here was an image as familiar as patriarchy. Typhoid Mary, the prostitute dripping with disease, Eve. On the other hand, commercial television was as ever desperately trying to convince its fabricated general public—consumers who must never be so angered or alienated that they turn off the tube—that they were not at risk for the disease. What a conundrum. Acknowledging that women were at risk fed the familiar narrative of women's guilt, while it also meant that the female became the first potential "bridge" to the heterosexual male. How could women, in the terms of this particular crisis, be both culpable vector for the spread of disease, while at the same time *not* embodying a threat to the anxious white male maker and spectator of broadcast television who was desperately maintaining a position of unimplicated outsider?

Mainstream documentaries use "real" images of women and "real" images of AIDS to validate understandings of women's experiences with the epidemic that never "really" existed: heterosexual women (and thus heterosexual men) are not at risk; prostitutes are a great risk (to men) and need special containments; white middle-class women need special educational attention, *even though* their risk is supposed to be negligible. Although the "official" story of women and AIDS does change (broadcast television now acknowledges that women are at risk and that women experience AIDS differently from men), the effects of this slow and still incomplete change contribute to needless deaths and infection of large numbers of women.

Meanwhile, the video production of feminist activists attempts to express other interpretations of the same reality. Many alternative videos are grounded in a critique of patriarchal America. In this vision of reality AIDS exaggerates the cultural contraints which already keep women down— racism, sexism, lack of adequate health care, poverty, homophobia, the contestation of our control over our sexuality. Alternative videos about women and AIDS use a variety of approaches to reach and represent the many women in this society, each living a distinct and diverse "material reality."

By analyzing broadcast and alternative documentaries focusing upon women and AIDS, what becomes most clear are the conflicting ideologies about who women are, what they do, and how they are to be seen in an era that is rife with changes in the experiences and understandings of women. In 1986 and 1987, broadcast television responded to the "crisis" of heterosexual transmission with several AIDS documentaries geared specifically to alleviate the fears of the heterosexual "general public" and ostensibly produced to explain to them their potential risk. I analyze the representation of women's sexuality in four such productions: *Life, Death and AIDS*, a Special News Report produced by NBC; *AIDS Hits Home*, a CBS Special; *Donahue: AIDS Ward*, again for NBC; and *AIDS: Changing the Rules*, an independently produced documentary by AIDSFilms, aired on PBS.[9] I have chosen these productions because their shared goal—to inform the "general public" of possible heterosexual concerns about AIDS—means that these programs, unlike the majority of programming at that time which focused upon gay men, devoted time and energy to the representation of women. I will contrast these documentaries with work by feminist activist videomakers who have struggled to make video that contradicts the misinformation consistently produced by the broadcast media about women and AIDS. As one of these videomakers myself, I share a kind of frantic desperation to get the "real" story out. Competing visions of reality, or at least what is really important, distinguish the work of alternative and mainstream producers.

Yet, of course, these realities are constantly shifting as the cultural meanings of AIDS, sexuality, and women change. So I will conclude by analyzing two commercial productions about women and AIDS from 1992, *Something to Live For: The Alison Gertz Story* (an ABC "Sunday Night Movie") and *Playing It Safe: The Entertainment Video Program for Women of the Nineties* (an industrial produced by G. D. Searle & Co., the makers of the contraceptive pill Demulen 1/35). Like Arsenio Hall's *Time Out*, these 1990s' productions played a largely corrective role, attempting to convince the white, professional, straight women who were told only five years earlier *not* to worry about AIDS, that they must now "play it safe." Five years later, however, these programs continued to represent "good" and "bad" modes of transmission (and thus the "good" and "bad" people one should watch out for), which does not and never did protect people from HIV, although it may safeguard a system of values. Furthermore, by maintaining a white-bred vision of AIDS education (refusing to image or address lesbians, poor women, women of color, female IV drug users), these 1992 productions continued to maintain an unrealistic and downright endangering image of the AIDS crisis.

As in previous chapters, my analysis works through particular documentary texts and in no way attempts to be a systematic review of every interpretation of the AIDS crisis produced during a particular period. My purpose is specific in its scope: the close analysis of six commercial AIDS documentaries and several more alternative productions focusing upon the representation of women and the meanings of women's sexuality and AIDS constructed through such representation. The six mainstream programs under discussion themselves span a range of systems of finance and production. *AIDS: Changing the Rules* is an independent project aired on PBS but also distributed as an educational tape. *Donahue: AIDS Ward* is a vehicle for a particular media personality. *Life, Death and AIDS* and *AIDS Hits Home* are productions of network news departments. *The Alison Gertz Story* is a network made-for-TV movie, and *Playing It Safe* is a promotional freebie, given to gynecology patients in order to sell birth control pills.

Their different economic and formal conditions withstanding, the six programs I analyze share a similar outlook and response to their representation of women's sexuality vis-à-vis AIDS: great (and legitimate) fear about the changing demographics of HIV infection, as well as much less legitimate methods to curtail this fear. In the AIDS documentaries of 1986 and 1987, women were depicted as *contained* threats, an oxymoronic representation that allowed them to register simultaneously as iconographic site of danger and as easily controlled subject. In the late 1980s it was not merely in AIDS media that an anxiety about women's bodies was being resolved through the power of containment.[10] For it seemed that the *threat* that women posed was not just viral transmission, but the very gains of the women's liberation movement—economic, political, and sexual independence. The varied forms of *containment* (through AIDS documentary practice, U.S. Supreme Court decisions, and the mobilization of the Christian Right), were representations, suggestions, or even laws that tried to return women to the constraints in place before women's liberation, that is, monogamy, marriage, children, economic dependence.

The "cultural wars" which began during Ronald Reagan's and George Bush's administrations continue to this day. The nation is split on issues of morality, sexuality, and culture: abortion, the rights of gays and lesbians, the impact of sexual harassment and pornography, sexual liberation, feminism, the meanings of AIDS. To a great extent these wars continue to be waged through cultural production. The Far Right and the Left produce television and video in unprecedented volume, while the broadcast media pretends an unbiased middle ground. While it may be safe to say that the networks do not take up the agenda of the religious zealots on the Right, and it is equally clear that the networks refuse to represent the ideology of the "feminists" and others on the Left, it is unclear whose sexual reality they think they *are* representing in the ongoing coverage of women and AIDS as well as in other debates which center upon sexuality.

The ways in which women's sexuality is represented in these broadcast documentaries have very little to do with how most American women lead their sexual lives. Instead, a fabricated sexual reality is offered that is akin to what Raymond Williams has called *residual culture:* "experiences, meanings and values, which cannot be expressed in terms of the dominant culture, [but which] are nevertheless lived and practiced on the basis of the residue—cultural as well as social—of some previous social form."[11] What is seen in such documentaries is not the status quo, the present and ugly state of affairs of which I wrote about in *chapter 3.* Monogamy, marriage, and children may be the *desired* state of affairs according to those who represent women's lives for them, but they are not the conditions under which most women live their sexual or economic lives. We need think only of the furor raised over former U.S. Vice President Dan Quayle's condemnation of the network TV show *Murphy Brown* for us to understand the power of representation to muddy the boundaries between residual and dominant culture. Simon Watney argues that this attempt to hold on to residual culture "is precisely what the mass media were invented to do, since they have evidently never responded to the actual diversity of the societies which they purport to service."[12] Using this logic, the function of the alternative media can be understood as working to represent that diversity. In the case of women and AIDS, this means two kinds of diversity, sometimes, although not always, interconnected—women who are "diverse" because of class, ethnicity, or sexual preference, and those whose diversity is one of ideological beliefs as much as lived experiences.

Why does the mainstream media present the residue of traditional sexual and "family" values as if it is the sole reality? How is the representation of woman as contained sexual threat set into place in the AIDS documentary? Throughout mainstream representations of women and AIDS, distinctions are drawn *between* women. Sander Gilman explains that in the representation of AIDS, boundaries are drawn between different "types" of women. "A new group has now been labeled as the source of the disease: women, but not all women, only those considered to be outside the limits of social respectability. Even while acknowledging heterosexual transmission, the attempt is made to maintain clear and definite boundaries so as to limit the public's anxiety about their own potential risk."[13] Categories of safe and dangerous women are drawn, not surprisingly, along already established lines which couple assumptions about race, class, and age with expectations about women's sexuality. In the mainstream documentaries that I analyze here, I identify six distinct types of sexual women into which all the women represented in these programs neatly fit: the middle-class yuppie single; the unmarried, procreating, low-income woman of color; the teenager encouraged to say no; the procreating white wife; the promiscuous prostitute (and tossed into this category, the African/Haitian woman as well, because of her assumed promiscuity); and, lastly, the unseen, therefore unsexed, lesbian. When representing women and AIDS, separating women into these six distinct categories of blame-for-their-risk is the broadcast documentary's first order of business.

Safer Sex for the Single Straight Woman

Once a woman is labeled and identified by her sexual practice, the programs I look at here use a variety of representational strategies to perform the more complicated feat of containing and controlling each category by denying or limiting the very "type" of sexuality that has served to identify her. How is this done? An excellent example occurs during the segment called "The New Rules" in *Changing the Rules*. This segment is one of three which organize the tape. Ronald Reagan, Jr., narrates a segment on why "normal" (straight) Americans should now take the risk of AIDS seriously, actor Ruben Blades demonstrates how to use a condom on a banana, and super model Beverly Johnson gives safer-sex education for straight women. Other informational and documentary segments which the narrators introduce include a montage on "safer-sex" behavior, an interview with a straight couple in which the male partner has AIDS, and pseudo-documentary (scripted but shot as if spontaneous) statements by a variety of actors who explain that they have AIDS.

In "The New Rules" section another rule outside those of safer sex is laid in place: how the single woman, by cultural definition a woman looking for sex, can at once be defined as such, only then to have her sexual activity controlled. Beverly Johnson, a beautiful, tall, thin, black media celebrity, narrates the segment. To the program's credit, she precedes her lesson by explaining that not only are women at risk, but that women of color are disproportionately at higher risk than white women. However, this savvy, politicized talk becomes part of a more devastating setup to come, the setup where Johnson, a new kind of straight-talking, sexually free young woman becomes the voice and image of an old kind of sexual conservatism. Johnson begins by telling us that abstinence is the safest sex of all. However, her scripted narration is hip enough to know that the 1980s' gal is not going to "just say no." Instead, Johnson suggests "Rule #1," which is to use a condom, every time, because "there's AIDS virus in vaginal secretions and semen. You know"—pause . . . pause . . . pause—"cum." Here we begin to see how the all-new desexed single woman is created by the TV documentary. We have a beautiful, young, intelligent, articulate, polished, and even political black woman talking freely about sex in a respectful medium-shot. She looks directly into the camera and talks, as only a "sexually liberated" woman could, about premarital sex and vaginal secretion.

So why then the pause . . . pause . . . pause before the word "cum"? Why wasn't there a retake so that this sentence would flow as evenly and flawlessly as the rest of her lines?[14] Besides heightening the dramatic effect, her pause is the filmic equivalent of the apologetic quotes used for colloquial slang in written discourse. The power of the close camera framing and pseudospontaneous monologue format are what make the point. We are intimately aware of the subtleties of her narration. We are intimately assured that it is only natural for a young woman to be embarrassed over the word "cum." Perhaps Johnson felt that such an apology would endear her to the

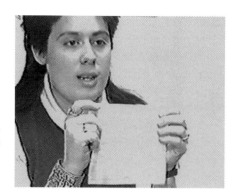

Figure 11   Denise Ribble, *Living with AIDS: Women and AIDS* (Alexandra Juhasz and Jean Carlomusto, 1988).

"general public" to whom she was speaking. But this is precisely how the falsely prudish residual sexual adult is produced and affirmed in culture, even as that person becomes harder to find. More importantly, such an apologetic device is antithetical to good AIDS education. AIDS educators need to demonstrate a comfort with sex and sexuality so that the people they educate can envision this sort of comfort for themselves. This is necessary to empower women to make the difficult changes required to negotiate safer sex with often resistant partners. In countless alternative AIDS educational tapes female AIDS educators speak all of the words necessary to educate viewers about safer sex without embarrassment.

Like *Changing the Rules,* alternative AIDS videos also feature beautiful, intelligent, cool, and sexually savvy women articulating safer-sex education to female spectators. Denise Ribble, a New York City AIDS educator who is featured in *Women and AIDS, Women and Children Last,* and *Testing the Limits,* discusses cum—and much, much more—without a flinch. She explains with clear and careful consideration how a condom or dental dam should be used when someone goes down on a man or a woman. She discusses the value of fantasy and nonpenetrative sex. Then she makes sure to tell women how to protect themselves when they *are* penetrated, by tongue, hand, or penis (figure 11). Her words are free of sexual orientation. She assumes her female audience is straight, lesbian, and bisexual, and so she educates accordingly. Robin Gorna writes about how difficult safer-sex education for women has been, not merely because of the concerted suppression of sexual information coming from the Right, but because of a more generalized uncertainty about and unfamiliarity with women's sexuality by men and women alike. In her discussion of the hard work that goes into eroticizing safer sex for women, she acknowledges that many women first have to eroticize *sex:* "there is a core of health promoters/educators seeking to prevent HIV sexual transmission within a holistic context of sexual health. This holism is rooted in the belief that sex is fundamentally good, and sexuality, sexual acts and sexual behavior form continua. . . . We cannot seek to prevent one sexual disease without addressing the roots of sexual dis-ease."[15]

A generation of safer-sex educators have learned from Ribble's calm, reasonable, inclusive promotion of holistic sexual health. This school of safer-sex educators offers judgment-free factual information about HIV transmission, and, more importantly, these educators do so with a performance of sexual ease. For example, Sarah Adams, the peer AIDS educator in *Safer and Sexier: A College Student's Guide to Safer Sex* (Lay-Techs Entertainment Group, 1993), stands alone in a room, her clothing speckled with latex condoms, dental dams, and gloves; she might as well be talking about going to the cafeteria for lunch, her attitude is so blasé as she demonstrates which latex item to use to have sex with another's penis, anus, or vagina. Until other college students can mimic this untroubled relationship to latex and sex, safer sex will continue to trouble them. You have to know what to use and how to use it if you are going to have sex and not contract the many sexually transmitted diseases which are epidemic on college campuses; but more importantly, you have to be able to talk about sex if you are going to negotiate safer sex.

The teen educators featured in *No Rewind* (Paula Mozen, 1992) evidence another necessary aspect of AIDS education beyond comfort, openness, and skill; the best education comes from individuals who are themselves members of the community being addressed. The AIDS educators in the tape, the majority of whom are teens of color, are taped as they conduct workshops at racially diverse schools. Meanwhile, unlike Beverly Johnson, they address with *words* rather than performance style how embarrassing, difficult, and scary safer sex is. This allows teenagers in the audience to address the implications of embarrassment and to begin to articulate how important it is to get beyond it, regardless of how feminine, or even "natural," it may seem. Denaturalizing the acceptable interpretations of sexual behavior must be one of the primary goals of safer-sex education for women.

But back to embarrassed Beverly. She has finished the first lesson about condom use for both vaginal and anal intercourse, which is then followed by this enormous pause. The camera continues to roll, but she stops and takes a big breath. She is upset. Finally, she spits it out, "Oral sex . . . ." Then she takes one big, long swallow—lips, mouth, neck—and clears her throat. "When a woman goes down on a man, the man must wear a condom every time." What is this all about? First, it assumes that oral sex is something that is exclusively performed on a man. A continuing problem in safer-sex education for women is that condoms are the only safer-sex device referred to—signifying that women have no genitals of their own to cover with latex so as to help protect their male *or female* partners. Second, reference to Freudian *convergence* seems unavoidable (he said Dora's throat irritation was a hysterical symptom which translated psychical excitation about the fantasy of a penis in her mouth into physical terms). Finally, it demonstrates that although Johnson is a little prissy about "cum," she is downright physically uncomfortable about talking about those practices, such as oral sex, deemed "kinky." Why? So that the video, like late-1980s' America, can create for the single woman the impression of sexual freedom while reassigning an archaic system of rules and regulations which purify and make small the reaches of her freedom. Oral sex gets Johnson no closer to the conjugal, child-producing bed. No wonder her throat hurts.[16] Although she never says *words* that limit her sexual possibilities, the way that she expresses her message suggests opinions about the liberated sexuality she describes. In this vein, Treichler warns of "an epidemic of signification" which uses AIDS as justification for monogamy. "Meanwhile on the home front monogamy is coming into its own, along with abstention, the safest sex of all. The virus in itself—by whatever name—has come to represent the moment of truth for the sexual revolution. . . ."[17]

The most crucial rebuttal to the AIDS-prevention-requires-monogamy camp is that safer sex has no necessary connection to numbers or practices. Effective use of barriers does not hinge upon quantity of partners or limitation of sexual activity, but rather upon the use of a condom or dental dam when appropriate.[18] Therefore, what is being suggested for single, straight women has nothing to do with safety. Rather, the advice that monogamy and prudery (not barriers) should be the single person's response to AIDS manipulates real fears to falsely legitimize the dismantling of what sexual liberation tries to encourage: the separation of sexual pleasure from reproduction, marriage, and traditional family life. It is also another example of the mainstream media's trade-off between much-needed information and the construction of the residual sexual reality of their making.

Many alternative tapes represent safer sex for women from a more educationally valid and sexually liberated position. For example, *Party Safe! With DiAna and Bambi* (Ellen Spiro, 1992) documents the AIDS educational work of DiAna DiAna and her partner, Dr. Bambi Sumpter (figure 12).

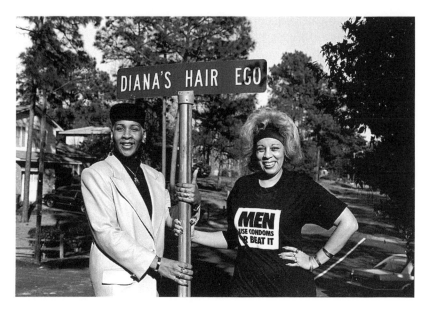

Figure 12   Dr. Bambi Sumpter and DiAna DiAna.

The tape begins with the explanation, "In addition to daily AIDS education within her beauty parlor, DiAna DiAna has taken her safer-sex gospel on the road. She and her partner Dr. Bambi Sumpter have hosted safer sex 'game shows' for artists, activists, homeless people, clergy, hairdressers and students among others." In this funny, sexually charged videotape we see scenes from several of these parties held across the United States and Canada. A diverse vision of sexual America emerges. We see single straight and lesbian women, we see lesbians and straights who claim they have lovers at home; there are rural southern African American women, and urban northern Asian-American women; the women are many ages, some are skinny and some are heavy, they are shy, they are turned on, and they espouse a variety of religious and moral values. "But they all want to be sexual or sensual in one way or another," says DiAna. As people loosen up by playing games, the safer-sex fantasies they articulate are as diverse as the participants' races, ages, and sexual preferences. A white man in drag says that he would like to take off his bra and shake "his massive yaboos" at his partner; in the meantime, he has taken out two prostheses from under his dress and is shaking them like rattles at DiAna. A shy and reserved black woman, wearing a sweatshirt which reads "Jesus" where "Pepsi" would be in the familiar logo, says that she would have safe sex with two men, one "licking her boobs," another having oral sex with her through safe-sex panties. DiAna and Bambi do not care what you do, or even what you want to do; they simply want to show you how to do it all safely. And yet, the message of the tape is even more far-reaching. Safer sex does not mean the closing down of sexual horizons, but the opening up of more and more sexual possibilities—by showing people sex toys, erotic games, and the fantasies and sexual practices of others; by teaching people to talk about sex; by allowing women to know it is okay to ask for, and get, what they want, as long as they do it safely. DiAna explains, "The game show first started back home in Columbia, South Carolina. I was working with students and they told me I was telling them all these things they couldn't do, and they wanted to know what they could do. I came up with some games I thought would be easy and interesting because that was the only way to get people to talk openly and honestly about sex."

How to Have a Sex Party (House O' Chicks, 1992) shows a group of young, urban dykes meeting at an apartment to have a sex party. A title card suggests that "It might be a good idea to start your party with a live demonstration." We then see a woman taping a dental dam onto another woman and performing oral sex as a third woman massages the second woman's ass while the other partygoers watch. "Ya'll getting the idea now? I am," someone says off camera. The tape opens with safer-sex information printed on the screen ("Be sure to have lots of lube. latex gloves. condoms. tulips. beverages. finger food"), and then the fun begins. For fifteen minutes we watch this group of women pleasure each other in a variety of configurations, positions, and rooms with a variety of tools (fingers, mouths, flower petals, dildoes), and it is all safe, hot, and nothing like monogamous. The tape suggests that HIV is not the reason to return to monogamous, heterosexual, missionary-position sexuality, it is the reason not to!

Of course, the reinscription of the monogamous, if not the married and procreative bed, is not the agenda of mainstream AIDS education alone. The New Right's vehement battle for the reinstatement of "the family" was under way before AIDS fueled the debate. However, AIDS became the rhetorical linch pin for the Right by providing a whole new vocabulary under which science, the threat of disease, and sexuality could be linked.[19] AIDS, in all its scientific glory, gave words for a hysterical conjoining of germ, desire, gender, race, and sexual preference. These words then legitimate a line of thinking which uses AIDS as proof that sexual and other liberations have proved themselves dangerous and flawed.[20] And, importantly, it is not just the Right that uses AIDS to endorse their sexual morality. Gorna reflects upon how the women's movement, or feminism, has been divided around issues of sexuality since the early 1970s. Many feminists maintain that sexuality is dangerous to women; AIDS intensifies this belief, thus endorsing a sex-negative position. Other women believe that penetrative sex is anti-woman, or that sex-without-love is antifemale. For these feminists, AIDS supports a position of monogamous sexuality (especially without penises). Gorna concludes her essay by asserting that "AIDS presents the possibility of a justification for the sex-negatives. . . . It offers opportunities for the 'politically correct sex mafia.' . . . Or it can offer us the potential to respect the complexity of human sexuality, to welcome and enjoy our erotic selves, to embrace and celebrate the diversity of sexual desire and, from such a position of strength, make the healthy choices we want."[21]

Clearly, broadcast media programs like *Changing the Rules* have fueled and contributed to an understanding of women's sexuality that does not allow us "the position of strength" from which to make whatever safe-sex choices we want. Rather, these images serve to return women to the embarrassment, prudery, and discomfort about sexuality which generations of feminists have fought against. For example, in *AIDS: Changing the Rules,* this occurs when restrictive images of sexuality are presented as if they are sexual—when *not having sex* is presented as a "sexual" option. (As Denise Ribble says in *Women and AIDS* [Carlomusto and Juhasz, 1988], "abstinence is an option, it's just not a *sexual* option.") Certainly, there is a great deal of debate about the value of abstinence in women's sexual lives. Yet in this program the power of representation makes it appear as if not having sex is the consensus about the new rules for women's sexuality. In the segment of the show called "Casual Contact," a most extreme message is offered about being single and sexual. The segment is a montage of perky images of men and women edited to a synthesizer soundtrack. The "safer sex" represented in this montage segment does not suggest the range of behavior that is sexual, not penetrative, or not involving the exchange of bodily fluids (masturbation, mutual masturbation, sex toys, role playing, etc.). In fact, imaged here is not low-risk *sexual* behavior, but low-risk *behavior*: businessmen shaking hands, three people eating Chinese takeout, a scientist looking at slides, a couple in a cool convertible drinking imported water. This is the soft sell—say no to sex; chum around instead.

Two ad campaigns by alternative media artists show how to do a soft sell that is still very sexual. *Kissing Doesn't Kill* (GranFury, 1990) and *SaferSister* (Maria Perez and Wellington Love, 1992) sexualize perfectly safe behavior like kissing, stroking, fondling, and pinching. In *Kissing Doesn't Kill* a series of beautiful men and women, in a variety of gendered couples and a range of races, kiss in this fast-edited, music-inflected, commercial. GranFury uses the style of perfume, high fashion, or cigarette ads to sell their politicized message as well as their vision of hot and entirely safe sex: "AIDS is a political crisis"; "Kissing Doesn't Kill . . . Greed and Indifference Do." In *SaferSister,* a series of four public service announcements in both English and Spanish, a highly stylized image of a female torso is traversed by a seeking hand. As the hand moves off screen toward the female torso's unpictured vagina, a quick cut is made to the hand grabbing and then putting on a latex glove. Deep and erotic breathing are the only sounds on the soundtrack, and we do not see, but are forced to fantasize, the safer penetration which is suggested. Instead, the title, "Please practice safer sex" or "Por favor cuando haga el amor use proteccion," emerges as the breathing continues. Safe sex is hot sex, not not sex.

The hard sell is pictured in the opening sequence of *AIDS Hits Home,* a conventional news documentary with an unpictured male narrator, which is organized around the themes imagined to be most relevant for the home audience. The narrator begins with "AIDS is what homosexuals got. But a scary reality is starting to hit home: that the AIDS virus is out there and it's not just gays who are catching it." The rooms of an aerobics salon/singles gym accompany this voice. Taut, spandexed women are bouncing. A timely sound cut is made so that the voice of the aerobics instructor, who was dancing and shaking to the ominous threat of the narrator's voice, chimes in with "Here we go" to the aerobics tape's backbeat. Here we go into the world of sex and AIDS. Sexuality is to be transferred, displaced, and sweated out. Straight singles may lightly press flesh while exchanging exercise bikes or may rub against each other while spotting for squats. But the show insists that the *real* thing will kill you. A cut to an unidentified blond who tells a reporter that she does not date any more. "It's like Russian Roulette, one mistake and you die." That is not true. But it is framed as if it is truth, and so it becomes the show's truth, because it is left stated but unrefuted.

The Procreating and Promiscuous Woman of Color

Left unpictured in commercial television's representation of AIDS and the single woman's sexuality are images of single, low-income women of color (Beverly Johnson, though black, is rich and famous). The unmarried woman of color, unlike her white counterpart, is always depicted as a mother of children, establishing and confirming her historically assumed insatiability, irresponsibility, and uncontrollability.[22] When the single woman of color is represented in AIDS documentaries, it is as an unwed "welfare mother" whose children signify her lack of sexual and economic control. Such images are indebted to a long history of misinformed notions about the sexuality of women (and men) of color. Historian Elizabeth Fee notes in her discussion of the battle against venereal diseases that "blacks were popularly perceived as highly sexual, uninhibited, and promiscuous . . . white doctors saw blacks as 'diseased, debilitated and debauched,' the victims of their own uncontrolled or uncontrollable sexual instincts and impulses."[23]

Whereas the single white woman is contained through representation, the low-income, single, and childless woman of color is controlled through invisibility, absence, *lack* of representation. The low-income woman of color hoping to negotiate both safer and nonprocreative sex sees no model of herself in mainstream AIDS documentary. This negligence is especially disturbing on two counts besides racism. For one, black and Latina women are disproportionately affected by AIDS and need appropriate risk-reduction information and education targeted toward them;[24] two, the specific cultural and religious significance of sexuality, gender roles, and birth control in various ethnic and religious communities makes the issues surrounding safer sex that much more complex, requiring open and frank confrontation, not avoidance.[25] Correcting significant gaps in information, the alternative AIDS media has paid a great deal of attention to the culturally specific safer-sex education of women of color. Four narrative tapes, *Vida* (Lourdes Portillo, 1989), *Are You With Me?* (M. Neema Barnette, 1989), *Reunion* (Jamal Joseph and Laverne Berry, 1993), and *Se Met Ko* (Patricia Benoit, 1989), were made to address the particular needs of urban Latinas, African American women and men, and Haitians, respectively. Although these tapes cover information useful to many women regardless of race (i.e., negotiating condom use with resistant male partners), this information is also inflected by racial, ethnic, class, and gender specificity.

Thus, *Vida* has its lead character, a working-class, single mother who lives with her single mother, make the difficult decision to ask her boyfriend to use a condom, acknowledging the contradiction between his machismo, which is threatened by her attempt to control the sexual interaction, and her desire for affection and sex as a single woman. She is encouraged to put first her own psychic and sexual needs by her support network of female friends and family (figure 13). *Are You With Me?* pictures a middle-class black single mother and her daughter, both in the process of thinking through

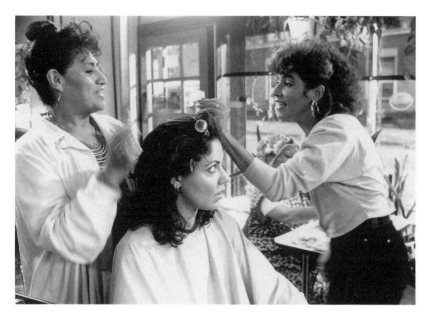

Figure 13   *Vida* (Lourdes Portillo; AIDSFilms, 1989).

safer sex with their boyfriends. In both tapes the protagonists know people in their neighborhood who died of AIDS; this brings the importance of safer sex home to communities (the barrio and the middle-class black neighborhood) rarely considered as home by broadcast television. For this reason, all of these tapes go into great detail to visualize the unique environmental feel of underrepresented communities by including a highly specific mise-en-scène: food, apartment decor, slang, dress, and social spaces (the barbershop, Central Park, the beauty shop). In *Are You With Me?* the specificity of age is also crucial. The mother (a nurse) initially believes her advanced age is her protection against HIV, even as she lectures her daughter about using condoms, even as she knows the medical "facts" about HIV transmission. The daughter, in turn, educates the mother, reminding her that her adult and "monogamous" relationship is also one that has included fights and even short breakups with her long-term boyfriend. In both tapes we see single women of color who are mothers and who are also employed, emotionally together, and sexually mature make the difficult decision to negotiate for safer and nonprocreative sex, even if it may mean the end of a sexual relationship (it does in *Vida;* it is unclear in *Are You With Me?*).

   Reunion is about an African American upper-middle-class family with three sons and their respective lovers/wives and children. Here we see the diversity of class, ideology, age, and sexual experience that defines the African American experience in the United States. One of the brothers, a buppie (black yuppie), is married, upwardly mobile, and HIV-positive. The second brother espouses black nationalist sentiments, is a construction worker, and will not use a condom, even though he sleeps with many women besides his long-term girlfriend. The third brother is in college and doing well after a few rough years as a teenager, which eventually led to his incarceration. His intelligent and vocal girlfriend is working on a report about safer sex in the black community, and she and the brother are rethinking whether they should have safer sex. In this tape we see a range of black women (and men)—one married with children, one unmarried with children, one unmarried and childless—make a range of decisions about their safer-sex behavior. *Se Met Ko,* like all of these tapes, occurs within the context of an extended family where more than one generation lives with and cares for the others. The importance for women of taking care of children, husband, parents, and neighbors is part of the culturally specific mise-en-scène in these tapes. The focus on their responsibilities for others also implicitly voices an argument for women to take care of themselves so that they can best do their work of caring for others. In *Se Met Ko* a single woman, who lives with her parents and a child who is perhaps a niece, decides that she needs to negotiate safer sex with her boyfriend. Over the course of the narrative he learns that she is right, and they both learn that they need to continue to care for (not discriminate against) the members of their community who are already suffering from the effects of AIDS.

Don't Tackle a Teen

Like low-income single women of color, teenagers of all colors are dangerously denied imaging in the broadcast documentaries I analyze. Like women of color, teenagers are frequently believed by our society to be uncontrollable. Instead of tackling an uncontrollable woman, the mainstream media's early AIDS documentaries ignored this highly threatened population of women. (Teenage girls are actively experimenting with both sex and drugs and are even less prepared than adult women to break societally inscribed sex roles to take control of their safety. According to the video *No Rewind,* teenage infection can now be considered the third wave of HIV infection, after gay men and then drug users and their partners.) Teenage sexuality is left unaddressed in the programs I analyzed. Broadcast television, like the New Right, seems to insist that by avoiding the discussion (and education) of teenagers, this social "problem" will go away. This attitude prevails in the education of teenagers. In many public school districts AIDS educators are legally prohibited from condoning (discussing) homosexuality and are subtly coerced to refrain from promoting condom use, as this is perceived to condone intercourse.[26] In New York City a ban is in place on AIDS educational materials that do not privilege abstinence as a means of AIDS prevention. Instead of educating young women about negotiating safer sex, the state and television offer "saying no" in a scare campaign aimed at teenagers, complete with threats of babies, herpes, AIDS, and death. A disturbing poster campaign in the New York subways showed an image of a boy cornering a girl in a misty, darkly lit alley, with print copy suggesting violent sexuality: "AIDS. If you think you can't get it you're dead wrong." Douglas Crimp argues that a similar collapsing of sex, death, and AIDS occurs semantically in the ambiguous use of the word "it" in the title of another ad campaign targeting teenagers: "AIDS: Don't get it." He continues, "AIDS will not be prevented by psychic danger to teenagers caused by ads on TV. It will only be stopped by respecting and celebrating their pleasure in sex and by telling them exactly what they need to know in order to maintain that pleasure."[27] In broadcast documentaries, if young women do not say "no" as they are instructed to do, they will be punished with disease, children, or other social penalties. Former U.S. Surgeon General C. Everett Koop, seated in front of a class of eager students in an AIDS video for teenagers called *Don't Forget Sherrie* (American Red Cross, 1988), explains: "People get AIDS by doing things that most people do not do, and do not approve of other people doing. Now what am I talking about?" What he means is abundantly clear. Again, an as-if wish about who "we" are—a forceful campaign in representation to turn "us" into who others may wish us to be—results in AIDS education that provides moralistic scare tactics and threats instead of useful information.

Therefore, in many of the limited programs made specifically for teenagers, a moratorium is placed upon their sexuality; they are not afforded even the token freedoms allowed other single women. For example, the videotape *Sex, Drugs and AIDS* (1986)—changed to *AIDS: Just Say No* (1987)—made by O.D.N. Productions specifically for distribution to teenagers in the New York public schools, was prohibited distribution until a controversial sequence was altered to condone abstinence over condom use. In the original sequence three girls discuss sexuality in a world with AIDS. Two of the girls have sex with condoms, and they are convincing a friend that she can also discuss this option with her boyfriend. In the second version of the sequence the discussion focuses upon choosing abstinence. This version is certainly providing safe information, but it is entirely unrealistic in regard to the sexual lives of New York City teenagers. This is an example of how an "alternative" production, because of funding and other institutional constraints, is forced to function in a manner similar to that of broadcast television: constructing images of a residual culture that have little to do with the realities of teenager's lives, but have a lot to do with a prevailing ideology about what teenagers' lives should be like.

Many alternative producers are not so restrained when providing information for teenagers. They produce sexually explicit and culturally specific tapes working with teenagers and without institutional constraints. Videos like *What's Wrong with This Picture* (Second Look Community Arts, 1991), *No Rewind,* and *It Is What It Is* (Gregg Bordowitz, 1993) are all produced collaboratively with teenagers who work with the videomaker to express the issues important to them in words and images that come from, and are addressed to, their experiences and sense of the world. In an article about AIDS media education for high school students, Brian Goldfarb suggests that "you can't expect to educate students about how to avoid transmission if you don't explain how it occurs, and how to prevent it. Realistically, this means moving beyond a biologistic approach that names the danger of exchanging bodily fluids to one that names specific practices associated with desire." [28] In *What's Wrong with This Picture? More Than Just a Video About AIDS,* the importance of using up-to-date lingo while also acknowledging desire is addressed in a scripted scenario. The scene opens with an uptight female educator talking to a group of teenagers. She is clearly getting nowhere, and the kids are bored and inattentive. One of the teens stands up and joins her in front of the others, saying, "Look Jane, I appreciate what you're trying to do here, but 'injection drug needles?' 'unprotected sexual intercourse?' What is that? Watch this: If you shoot up and share needles you can get AIDS, so clean your works with bleach and water. If you have sex without a rubber you can get AIDS. So always use a rubber when you have sex. Got it?"

Goldfarb also explains that teenage sexuality, like all people's sexuality, is intimately connected to the "interrelationship of sexual and cultural identities." [29] This means that AIDS education for teens must acknowledge the reality of homosexuality, drug use, race, and class as well as the diverse ways in which teenagers express themselves sexually. This occurs in the tape *Kecia: Words to Live By* (Peter von Puttkamer, 1991), which documents the AIDS educational work of Kecia Larkin, an HIV-positive Native American teenager. In her moving, honest, and forthright presentations to other teen-agers, Kecia discusses how violence, drug and alcohol abuse, anger, sexual exploitation, and racism contributed to her running away from home and taking up a life on the streets with other kids who "were looking for love, a hearth, a fire, companionship." We see Kecia addressing an auditorium filled with Native American youths. They are quiet, attentive, upset. "I knew a lot of kids like me down there. A lot of them were Natives. Most of them ran away from home for the same reasons I did. A lot of them were ad-dicted to something: anger, drugs, alcohol, drug dealing. And I realized that I was comfortable there because that was what I grew up with at home." In a well-lit talking-head interview she explains that "I'm presently traveling to communities talking about AIDS. I tell them what it's like to be HIV-positive, and how to prevent it. They think that you have to be a homosexual, prosti-tute, or a needle user to catch AIDS. That's what they see on TV. No one's in there saying these are the ways you contract it." Well, Kecia is in there, and as long as a ban remains on explicit discussions within schools and on com-mercial television about what teenager's sexual and social lives are like, she understands how crucial her work is, and how crucial it is for videomakers to document her doing it.

Babies Standing in for Mothers

Another "type" of sexual woman in AIDS documentaries is the female who has sex that results in procreation. Women who have children are represented as being as desexed as their infantless sisters in mainstream documentaries. Two kinds of mother are depicted in such productions: the "minority," poor, and guilty single mother of sick babies (who were already mentioned in the single women-of-color category but who are included here because it is through images of their babies that they are allowed the privilege of representation), and the white, middle-class, married mother of innocent victims. How is women's sexuality regulated through the depictions of these two motherly scenarios? In *Life, Death and AIDS* the two different types of mother are given opposing representational strategies. We are exposed to the first kind of mother at the tail end of the segment of the show devoted to drug users. Two highly stylized images are all "she" gets: a close shot of two black baby girls dressed up in light blue, one holding a rattle, the other a bottle; and the image of a young, lonely Latino boy, alone in a hospital bed. A correspondent's voice accompanies these images, saying, "Almost all of the hundreds of children born with AIDS are *victims* of drug users: either drug-addicted mothers, or mothers who got the virus from an IV-infected husband or lover" (emphasis mine).

What is to be seen here? Certainly not victimizing mothers of color, those uncontrollable and immoral baby vessels. For this woman is erased in the public image immediately after the act of unprotected heterosexual intercourse. Instead, her metonymic representation comes as unchecked as does the Right's agenda which places the rights of the conceived above those of the woman who conceives. Since it was established that mothers had a real risk of passing the virus in utero to children,[30] images of sick but pretty babies have become the overplayed symbol of this manner of HIV transmission. Such pictures of helpless children have been overemphasized by the media because they depict the unblamable PWA—untainted by sex, drugs, and, at this young age, even rock 'n' roll—they have done nothing to bring on their predicament.

The image of an "innocent" sick child establishes the guilt of the unseen and displaced mother. The lost and hidden mothers inferred by images of sad children cannot be shown, the narrator's voice explains, because their crime is too horrible—"victimizing" their own offspring through the selfish act of procreation. Unlike other women, females with HIV are not supposed to propagate. It is difficult to separate the message not to have children, which is given to the mostly African American and Latina women who are infected, from the genocidal messages that they have received for generations.[31] Furthermore, in a society that does not condone abortion, especially for poor women who cannot afford it, these images suggest only two options: poor women of color must not, cannot, and will not procreate—they must abstain from sex; or they must agree to accept the only solution that many states *can* legally fund—hysterectomy (sterilization). The long history of sterilization abuse against women of color makes this horrific possibility a real and important concern during the AIDS crisis.[32]

The implicit support of sterilization abuse aside, it is sometimes argued that the sad, pretty images of sick children encourage the support, money donations, and pity of a "general public" which is unable to empathize with those considered "socially deviant." Tolerance gained by submission to the structural intolerance and biases of our culture cannot be considered a progressive solution. Instead, alternative media often considers and analyzes our society's history of blaming the victim. An example of this approach is seen in the tapes *Women and Children Last* and *The Heart of the Matter* (Amber Hollibaugh and Gini Retticker, 1990 and 1993) in which one black woman discusses why she blamed herself for her husband's HIV infection, and even his later infection of her, and then how she worked to understand and get past this self-blame. In *The Forgotten People: Latinas with AIDS* (Hector Galazan, 1990) several HIV-positive *men* articulate their own deeply felt self-blame for infecting their wives and thus their children. And in *Pediatric AIDS: A Time of Crisis* (Pierce Atkins, 1989) a mother's support group at Albert Einstein Hospital is recorded. Here, we see how mothers (who are often HIV-positive themselves with HIV-positive lovers) struggle with, and overcome, their self-blame so that they can contribute to the highest standard of living possible for their sick children and themselves. These women are courageous and strong, fighting the obstacles of discrimination, ostracism, poverty, illness, pain, and the extreme grief associated with caring for sick children. We hear their financial and practical as well as their moral concerns. Who will take care of their children if they die first? How will they afford the healthy foods that ill children need? One mother says, "If I would lose my daughter, my intention is to be a mother to those children that do not have, to try to make things a little easier for their parents. I won't give up." The inability of broadcast television to see beyond the oppressive structures on and through which it reports is precisely what distinguishes it from much alternative practice. In my analysis of commercial television I often appear to be blaming programs for that which, in effect, defines their mode of production and distribution—distance and the inability to change or challenge the operative cultural structures upon which they report. Rather than blame, however, my intention is to demonstrate that this defining feature can and should be contested.

Infrequently, as in *Donahue: AIDS Ward,* the low-income minority mother herself makes it onto the prime-time screen. This show, perhaps the most offensive of those under consideration, documents the host, Phil Donahue, as he "visits" an AIDS ward in a New York City hospital. A camera follows him as he walks down the hall of the ward and into a series of hospital rooms in which AIDS patients await his entrance. In the sequence in which he interviews a Latina mother who is quite ill, we watch our host enter her room in the ward. He is armed with his technically unnecessary but phallically useful microphone (such interviews are amply recorded by powerful microphones off-screen), which he sticks into the face of a scared woman on a bed. A handheld camera follows him, catching his entrance with bumpy integrity, and finally comes to rest upon the woman. "Hi Martha. I'm Phil Donahue," he says. "How are you? I guess it's okay if I sit on your bed." We have been prepped in hushed tones while Donahue was in the hallway that "Martha is a Hispanic IV drug user with two kids." Donahue questions her only about these two things, her drug use and her children. What else could there be to know about her? "You probably got it from the bad needle," he wheedles. "How did you explain this to your kids?" he leers.

After more of this questioning than Martha can take, she breaks down. The camera relentlessly holds on the tear-streaked face, the microphone the only indication of Donahue's presence in this shot. His voice returns: "Martha, I'm sorry. We have to leave. There's not really a graceful way to do this. [A graceful way to blame a woman for her illness, remind her that she is dying and leaving behind small children, push and prod her into tears?—no, I guess there isn't.] You're a courageous mother. And that's the best thing one can say about a woman, isn't it?"

No. There are many societal constraints which keep women from being "courageous mothers" and many of the other powerful things women can be. Courage is not always enough in a world where women (who are mothers and other things) are forced to confront poverty, drug addiction, lack of self-esteem, racism, physical and sexual abuse, and sexism. The video "I'm You, You're Me": Women Surviving Prison, Living With AIDS (Debra Levine and Catherine Saalfield, 1993) critically investigates, with female ex-prisoners, why this largely African American, Latina, and poor population has struggled with motherhood and many other facets of their lives, and how they have the courage to try to change. We are introduced to a group of women who have set up an HIV support group while incarcerated at Bedford Hills Maximum Security Prison for women in New York State, and who have then gone on to continue to run the group on the outside (figure 14). We learn about the many struggles these women face, from explaining to lovers that they are HIV-positive, to depression because their futures seem to be full of only grief and illness ("with the HIV, it's rough, what's going to happen tomorrow? How will I deal with this when it comes?"), to fear of idle time now that they are out of jail and not using drugs, and, finally, to their fears about raising their children. "Many of the girls are getting their children back and don't know how to deal with them. I don't know how to deal with them either, but we'll do it together," one explains. These are women who are willing to admit they can attempt to learn to live their lives in more constructive ways and that they are helped in this difficult task by sharing their struggles with other women. Several of the women from the group have gone on to be AIDS educators on the outside as well as continuing their work on the inside. One of these women, interviewed with her infant daughter, tells us that she has had three other children. Two were "lost to foster," and the third she willingly gave up to adoption because she did not feel fit as a parent at that time. Her youngest child is HIV-positive,

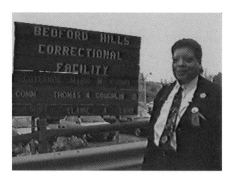

Figure 14   Linda Gang,
I'm You, You're Me:
Women Surviving
Prison, Living with AIDS
(Catherine Saalfield and
Debra Levine, 1992).

and she takes the baby with her when she goes to health centers to talk to women about living and staying on the outside. "I want you ladies to be able to make it like I am. I'm trying to show society that if us ex-convicts can do it, the ones that are already in society can do it without having to go to jail to learn how."

Another reason why the media may deign to include images of a mother along with her baby, besides the kind of drama invoked by Donahue, is to capitalize on the high sentimentality of a mother and baby presented sick and sad together. For example, in *Changing the Rules,* an actress with a sweet baby on her hip, faces the camera in the tightly framed, well-lit style of that production. The show uses the codes of documentary to make us believe that this is a real, spontaneous interview, not scripted, acted, and highly constructed. Tears are welling in her eyes. "I have AIDS, and my baby has AIDS. Every night I kneel and pray to be strong. I pray my baby won't die." And then she really breaks down, tears pouring, and the camera stays and stays. Interestingly, it was scenes like this one and the others I described from *AIDS: Changing the Rules* which brought about the production of the three excellent educational tapes I also have mentioned—*Vida, Reunion, Are You With Me?*—by AIDSFilms. As was detailed in the case study of AIDSFilms in chapter 2, the small nonprofit organization totally reorganized its mode of operation and production to better educate the communities of color which are disproportionately affected by AIDS. The changes in AIDSFilms' production strategies and projects (AIDS educators and filmmakers involved with and from targeted communities participate in every aspect of production) exemplify several important points about AIDS media. First of all, the biases and misrepresentations in *Changing the Rules* were not the result of the bad, mean, or wrong *intentions* of the individual producers who organized and financed the film, but they resulted from conditions of production that did not include the ideas, information, and attitudes of the very people being represented. Such a disparity, I would guess, is more often than not the case in mainstream AIDS reportage. Second, the very capability that AIDSFilms had to change its mode of production in relation to criticism (and the fact that the company sought out reactions, other than ratings, in the first place) demonstrates a flexibility that often defines the alternative media.

The Nonblameworthy Mom

In the imaging of procreating women there is a flip side to the guilty, weeping, or missing mother. Nonblameworthy infection is assigned to Amy in *Life, Death and AIDS.* Unlike the women of color who are displaced by images of babies, Amy, the white, Middle American mom, is allowed an entirely different representational strategy. First, an introduction by Tom Brokaw, the show's host, "And now, a victim of chance." Brokaw explains that this *chance* victim is a 24-year-old Indiana woman who received three blood transfusions for a bleeding ulcer in 1982. Other than babies who are cuter, and hemophiliacs who are already cursed with an unfortunate disease, blood transfusion recipients are the most holy of PWAs, again because their behavior and life-style is unconnected to contraction of the disease. Brokaw concludes his heartrending, melodramatic background information by saying, "She was married a year later, and in the same week, in 1984, she learned that she was pregnant on Wednesday and on Friday she was diagnosed with having AIDS."

My purpose here is not to condemn Amy for being a female PWA spokeswoman. Her work is important and valued. However, what is necessary to contest is that Amy is given respect by the camera and the narrator that is wholly denied the other mothers and PWAs represented in the program. She is allowed not only her own image, but her voice as well. She is given her name. She can tell her story. She is allowed the comfort of her own home, soft chair, and husband's hand for the understandably intimidating interview. Unquestionably, such respect should be the norm for all documentary interviewees, but only Amy, in this hour-long show, is so treated. Why? Brokaw and the camera tell us: she is from Indiana, she is blond, she wears blue eye shadow, and she cooks meals in her clean, spacious kitchen. She is the PWA acceptable. Not only does she look like a "normal American," she is married—as akin to the fictional heroines of prime time as any PWA could be. And on the sexual hierarchy, Amy is A–OK. Treatment by the TV camera becomes yet another social incentive for privileged forms of sexuality. For just as Amy is given every comfort and respect by the documentary camera (eye-level, steady medium shot, her own voice, her own home), those less privileged on the sexuality scale are punished by documentary form just as they are by society.

A large body of mainstream AIDS media tells the story of the middle-class, white, "innocent victim." The mainstream media has paid an inordinate amount of attention to the New York City doctor who was infected by a needle jab and is suing the hospital where she was employed. A *People* magazine cover dated July 30, 1990, appeared, along with countless other magazine and newspaper articles, talk-show appearances, and, finally, a made-for-TV movie (to be discussed later in this chapter) devoted to Alison Gertz, the young woman who first got a rose from the date who also exposed her to HIV: "Her date came with champagne, roses . . . and AIDS." The hours of talk-show appearances by the Glaser family–friends of Ronald Reagan and other Hollywood celebrities—work to confirm the guilt of those Others who do not conform to a public-relations-perfect family pattern and who therefore do not get represented.

All of the women and their families who have done the difficult and political work of "coming out" about their infection are not to blame. Neither are the reporters who tell and retell these women's sad and moving stories. Nevertheless, the special attention paid to them, as well as to the message that women who are doctors, well-to-do dates, or Hollywood wives are somehow "innocent" victims of this virus, is a sad testament to the structures upon which our society and its broadcast documentaries are built. Cindy Patton spells out the difficult terms of this problem:

> The goal is not to teach "compassion," because this still positions "the public" outside the reality of the AIDS episteme, positions them as a class with the privilege of being kind toward an "other," positions them as health imperialists nostalgically charting the story of continents wasting with the disease. Rather, we want them to understand their complicity in the systems of AIDS discrimination and their position relative to the highly fluid boundaries of the so-called risk groups, a complicity typically assuaged by altruistic "othering" in our culture.[33]

Acting Up for Prisoners (Eric Slade and Mic Sweeny, 1992) is an excellent example of an alternative AIDS tape that documents individuals attempting to evaluate their "complicity" in regards to AIDS discrimination. When people on the outside began to find out that the HIV-positive female prisoners at Frontera Prison for Women in California were being neglected and mistreated, the people on the outside responded with direct action—not pity—as well as an *analysis* of how discrimination against female HIV-positive prisoners was part of a larger system that ultimately endangered all women with AIDS. "Prison is the lowest level of how we treat PWAs. We need to set a standard below which the system will not fall," says an interviewee on the outside. Women from ACT UP/San Francisco and the ACLU staged several protests throughout California to raise consciousness about the situation of HIV-positive female prisoners, and they also directly confronted the California Department of Corrections, resulting in real changes in the treatment of female HIV-positive prisoners.

Punishing Otherness: Prostitutes and Africans Can't Speak

So, what about the woman who repudiates the confines of married, procreative sex? How is her documentary image controlled? In *Life, Death and AIDS,* prostitutes are represented for one fleeting moment as another visual point to be made during the segment on IV drug users. The camera, in voyeuristic and slightly blurred long shot, scouts women on the street as they lean over and look into cars to proposition the men inside them. The voice-over reminds us that "many of the street prostitutes are drug addicts." And that's it. Such imagery, stolen from a safe distance, merely reinscribes prostitutes into society's favorite pictures of them. First, the distance of the camera from the scenes depicted informs viewers that proximity spells danger. But second, the zoom lens ensures that even though the prostitutes are dirty, their hot pants and four-inch heels can be recorded from a safe distance with no danger. The camera in this scene, removed but curious, is certainly not interested in offering these women the respect and power of self-articulation in the more customary form of an interview.

The show's producer is uninterested in talking to street workers, perhaps scared to find out the "unimaginable," "outrageous" things they do. According to Priscilla Alexander in her article "Prostitutes Are Being Scapegoated for Heterosexual AIDS," this fear is based upon discriminatory misinformation. Most street prostitutes used condoms long before AIDS was ever a threat, and most street prostitutes perform *oral* sex, only a minimal risk to the man while being a real risk to the woman unless she takes precautions.[34] All kinds of erroneous deductions are drawn and perpetuated about prostitutes' risk (this meaning, of course, their risk *to* their straight male clients) when images are offered as index cards of historical misconceptions about who prostitutes are and what prostitutes do. Stereotypical images reaffirm stereotypical (and incomplete and inaccurate) assumptions.

What we can learn about prostitutes from such images is that these documentaries have the same agenda about these women that has been dominant in society, a desire to contain women who have always been targets of social control yet have never been entirely controlled. These images attempt to control prostitutes' sexuality by at once affirming sexuality to be their identifying feature (in the seductive, stolen, curious images taken of them), while denying them the ability to explain their sexuality by literally unplugging the microphone. The images hold these women captive in poses which confirm their guilt—seducing men, ready to let the germ-flow begin—while keeping in check any education or information about how to curb the spread of HIV from women to men, and much more easily, from men to women. Finally, such images reify criminal penalties which punish prostitutes—never their johns—regardless of what kind of sexual activity is being sold, so as to sweep these women off to jails and other places of quarantine where they cannot be heard (or educated).

My Body's My Business (Vivian Kleinman, 1992) and *Safe Sex Slut* (Carol Leigh, 1987) give us an entirely different image of prostitutes. *My Body's My Business* features direct interviews with prostitutes who are well aware of why they must protect themselves and their customers, and who have been doing so for a long time. One woman repeats the effective argument she makes: "I don't know what you do, and you don't know what I do. So, to be on the safe side for both of us, we'll just use the condom. They're just a part of my life-style now, I never leave home without them." We also see prostitutes educating other working women about how to put condoms on resistant johns so the customers will never know the condoms are there. Then, after a prostitute explains to an educator that she was offered $1,000 in cash to have sex without a condom, the educator shows her (and the viewer) how to make her hand feel like a vagina, by applying lots of lube and pulsating it, so that the man would never even know he has not come "inside." In *Safe Sex Slut*, Carol Leigh espouses with humor, camp, and sex appeal the importance of safer sex for all people, including "sluts," as she performs a tantalizing dance to the words of her own song: "I live just like a Mouseketeer, I don't mess up the atmosphere. The bedroom is the last frontier, condoms leave a souvenir. Safe sex." All of Leigh's videowork features articulate, knowledgeable, and angry female prostitutes who discuss the complicated social, political, criminal, and economic ramifications of AIDS for the lives of prostitutes and their johns.

The representation of African and Haitian women can best be understood as another example of the to-be-seen-blamed-and-not-heard system used for the imaging of prostitutes. Some worries have developed in the United States about statistics in Africa because African AIDS demographics, unlike U.S. statistics, show that the male/female ratio of the disease is virtually 50-50. Americans worry that Africa is a portent of things to come; that here, too, AIDS will eventually become a disease of heterosexuals (as if it isn't already). This concern is displayed in a typically U.S.-centric way in the mainstream documentaries I analyzed. Three of them ignore international demographics, as if the heterosexual nature of AIDS transmission in Africa is somehow insignificant to Americans, and the fourth, *Life, Death and AIDS,* searches for that one, furtive, distinguishing feature that will explain why heterosexual Africans are having this problem but why "we" never will.[35] The furtive feature, the program decides, is that well-known African character trait—their un-American and prolific sexual behavior. A 1987 *Cosmopolitan* article, "Reassuring News about AIDS: A Doctor Tells Why *You* May Not Be at Risk," by Robert Gould, explained that African statistics do not apply to American women because "men in Africa take their women in a brutal way." The media has used AIDS as an excuse to perpetrate inane and racist descriptions of Africans' sexual behavior, and *Life, Death and AIDS* proves no exception.

In the show's special sequence on Africa, we see from a low side angle, in an underlit shot, a woman in a hospital bed, while the commentator says, "In Africa, AIDS is spread not through insects. Cuts. Rats. Needles. But heterosexuality . . . ." (Can you hear the unspoken word "women" as you see her image?) The next cut is to a male African doctor who says, "A young single woman can't talk about it. Most women are hesitant to discuss their sexual lives. She might be having more partners than she's telling us." The image and the words confirm that AIDS (and more) are the fault of the unidentified "she" in the previous shot. Not only is she promiscuous, but she lives in a society where women are taught to keep silent about their sexuality. Yet if she does so, she then gets blamed for not telling how many partners she had. The camera, then, like the culture, denies her her voice and image by filming her from a bizarre angle and at a hygienic distance. At the same time, she is punished for *not* speaking because the voices of the male narrator and doctor get to dictate how she is to be understood.

Say No to Cosmo: Doctors, Liars and Women (Jean Carlomusto and Maria Maggenti, 1987) provides an important critique of the racist misreading of African statistics found in most mainstream media, as well as a great

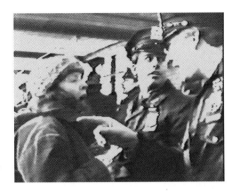

Figure 15   Maxine
Wolfe, *Doctors, Liars
and Women* (Jean
Carlomusto and Maria
Maggenti, 1989).

deal more. The tape is about the response of the then newly formed ACT
UP Women's Committee to the *Cosmopolitan* article by Dr. Robert Gould
(figure 15). We watch a small group of activists plan and then stage a demonstration to confront Dr. Gould, after which we see broadcast television's
manipulative and hysterical coverage of these events. Self-critical discussion
by the women involved (including Carlomusto and Maggenti) highlights the
power and importance of self-representation. When the women are alone
with Dr. Gould, they are in control. They ask direct, informed questions
which prove how unqualified he is to speak about women and AIDS and
how highly qualified they are. "You say in your article: 'Then, too, many men
from Africa take their women in a brutal way.' " "This I got from nurses from
many countries in Africa who describe this sort of sexual activity." "That
implies that men in the United States don't do that. One-third of women will
be raped in their lifetime, and we don't know what happens to the other two-
thirds." However, when the mainstream media takes up and frames these
debates, a great deal of power is taken from the female activists. Carlomusto
explains in an interview in the tape: "When we were in control, things went
well. When we lost control was afterward, when the media got control of the
event. We lost our representation. I was in on the organizing, I was documenting it. We had control of our image." We then see clips from several local
and national talk and news shows where the female activists are not even
allowed the power of rebuttal. Meanwhile, Dr. Gould continues to express
his misinformation on the air—women will not contract HIV through "normal heterosexual intercourse." Carlomusto ends the tape with a call to video
arms. "I hope women will feel comfortable taking the camera and bringing
it to places where things are happening. . . . documenting their own lives.
I want these women to be in the editing room; to restructure and represent

their own history." Only when the people misrepresented by the media or medical establishment (women, Africans, prostitutes, lesbians) record their own history, can we hope to see other agendas served. Video provides a powerful tool to organize direct criticism against the ongoing and dangerous misinformation reported on broadcast television.

The Unseen and Unsexed Lesbian

Finally, these AIDS documentaries make no mention of those women whose "unspeakable" sexuality is so alien to the media that it is offered up as nonexistent. In the media's pictured world, lesbians should not, and therefore do not, lead sexual lives. They are desexed through non-imagery. Zoe Leonard writes, "Lesbians have been absent from most discussion of HIV-infection. The most common attitude seems to be that AIDS is not a lesbian problem."[36] Of course, this denial has real ramifications. Here, the media once again perpetuates the highly prejudiced "risk-group" versus "risk-behavior" fallacy—i.e., the attitude that knowing someone is gay or Haitian means that they are at risk, as opposed to knowing what sort of behavior a particular gay or Haitian person participates in so as to determine his or her potential risk. In "Lesbian Safety and AIDS," Lee Chiaramonte debunks the "fairy tale" of lesbian nonrisk. She writes that to believe that lesbians are entirely safe "I would have to believe we are either sexless or olympically monogamous; that we are not intravenous drug users; that we do not sleep with men; that we do not engage in sexual activities that could prove as dangerous as they are titillating. I would also have to believe that lesbians, unlike straight women, can get seven years' worth of honest answers from their lovers about forgotten past lives."[37]

Furthermore, as in their handling of prostitutes, the media's unwillingness to ask lesbians what their lives (sexual and otherwise) are like ensures that an exotic, unnatural, unimaginable picture remains grooved in the imagination of most Americans. The most dangerous consequence of such uninformed fantasy is that there has been little or no scientific research conducted on the transmission possibilities of lesbian sexual behavior.[38] Chiaramonte confirms the dangerous consequences of this particular threat in an interview with Dr. Charles Schable of the AIDS Diagnostic Laboratories at the Centers for Disease Control. "To my question about any correlation between lesbian sexual behavior and AIDS exposure, he replied, 'What sexual behavior? I thought lesbians didn't have much sex.'"[39] Gorna writes about how this invisibility of lesbian sexuality to the society at large makes safer-sex education difficult. "What has become evident is how little information exists, even within the lesbian community, about the types of sexual activities women are engaging in with one another. . . . Without information about the practices, there can be no possibility for health education initiatives assessing their risk and promoting safer sex." [40]

(An) Other Love Story (Gabrielle Micallef and Debbie Douglas, 1990) demonstrates that lesbians do have much sex, and their attempts to practice this sex safely is made extra-hard by their exclusion from almost all AIDS educational materials. The tape begins in the bedroom of a lesbian couple cuddling in bed as they watch a news program reporting on AIDS. This self-referential device serves the specific purpose of pointing a finger at the culpability of TV journalism. The narrative occurs within an interracial, urban lesbian community where AIDS is still not considered to be a lesbian issue. At a bar the tape's protagonist, Adrianna, admits to another woman that she has become worried about AIDS. "But you're a dyke." Adrianna insists, "We don't cancel out because we're lesbian or monogamous. AIDS is a big issue for women." But her friend is having none of it. "Dykes don't get AIDS." The video then charts Adrianna's and her lover Veronica's slow realization of the reality of AIDS within their lesbian community as they learn that a close friend is HIV-positive and as they discuss their own need to consider safer sex in their relationship. The tape ends with the couple hosting a safer-sex party for their friends. And in the final scene Veronica arrives with a gift for Adrianna—a bag of dental dams. The two play with the pieces of latex and begin to kiss. These lesbians have sex, and the implication is that it will be safe sex from now on.

Women's Invisibility in Mainstream AIDS Documentaries

Invisibility, certainly most severe for lesbians in mainstream documentaries, seems to be a most common choice that the broadcast media makes to cope with their anxiety and ambivalence about women's role in the AIDS crisis and about women's sexuality in general. What seems most surprising about the representation of women's sexuality in these AIDS documentaries, is in fact the immense lack of it. For, although I have devoted this chapter to the representation of women's sexuality in early AIDS documentaries focusing on heterosexual risk, surprisingly few images of women were available from which to draw my analysis. Rather, in these AIDS documentaries most of the airtime is filled with male narrators, male patients, male doctors, male health administrators, male scientists. This interests me because it challenges some very basic tenets of feminist film theory. AIDS documentaries contradict the idea that film, unlike other aspects of patriarchal society, has historically been too attentive to women, at least in terms of imagery. The work of feminist film critics in the early 1970s focused upon this surfeit of visibility in fiction films. Later, feminist film theory attempted to explain how the filmic apparatus uses these overabundant images of women to help construct our lived sense of ourselves as female or male.

Yet here are mass-produced and mass-received texts that are simply not operating under this structure. Feminist theories of women's representation in fiction film do not seem entirely useful for analyses of other uses of film and video which are not organized around women, or, for that matter, narrative (i.e., most documentaries or television sports.)[41] Nevertheless, the tradition of feminist film theory engendered the kinds of questions I have been asking in this chapter. How is the representation of women related to the lived experiences of women? How does the media express current attitudes toward women and women's sexuality through form as well as content?

Yet, more specific theories about women's representation which consider the representation of illness, or the representation of authoritative knowledge, allow for a more nuanced approach to AIDS documentaries in which we see men talking about, analyzing, and knowing women. Although feminist film theory helps us understand the pleasures evoked by viewing women's bodies, other routes to spectatorial pleasure are left unaddressed in these accounts of the underlying structures of narrative film. "Voyeurism, fetishism and narcissism are present but seldom occupy the central position that they have in classic narrative," writes Bill Nichols about the documentary. "The difference in this regard between fiction and documentary is akin to the difference between erotics and ethics."[42] Nichols's theorization of documentary holds true in these broadcast AIDS programs, for even though they are highly concerned with women's sexuality, men's control is not accomplished through voyeuristic and erotic mastery over women's bodies but through cognitive and ethical control over the meanings of women's experience. Mary Ann Doane describes a similar erotics of knowledge in discussing medical melodramas in her book about the woman's film of the 1940s: "Medicine introduces a detour in the male's relation to the female body through an eroticization of the very process of knowing the female subject. Thus, while the female body is despecularized, the doctor-patient relation is, somewhat paradoxically, eroticized."[43]

In 1940s' woman's films and AIDS documentaries alike, the pleasure of gazing at a woman's body is displaced by the erotics of watching science see her. Therefore, in many AIDS documentaries instead of seeing women, we see men gaining cognitive control over women. In a world with AIDS, the surface or image of a woman's body is not all that a man needs to know of her. If she is not only symbolically but potentially diseased (and, more importantly, the cause of men's disease), then patriarchal society is less concerned with sexual fascination over the surface of her body than with scientific control over what is going on inside her body and societal control over what she can do with her potentially contagious body. Nichols explains how the "desire to know" is the structuring pleasure of the documentary. "Documentary realism aligns itself with epistephilia, so to speak, a pleasure in knowing, that marks out a distinctive form of social engagement. . . . In igniting our interest, a documentary has a less incendiary effect on our erotic fantasies and sense of sexual identity but a stronger effect on our social imagination and sense of cultural identity."[44] Thus, the viewing of these broadcast documentaries concerned with AIDS and heterosexuality invokes the pleasures of doing and viewing science—the pleasure in systematic knowing, control, and permitted spectatorship discussed in *chapter 4.*

Late 1980s' broadcast documentaries about heterosexual transmission displayed a primarily white, heterosexual, male anxiety toward knowing that AIDS was not their problem. Maintaining a sense of control over stable sexual and social boundaries for women defined a great deal of the agenda of these programs about AIDS and heterosexuality. Images of women's bodies and sexuality, or the lack thereof, were used to secure a hold upon a residual sexual reality that was in fact nearly obsolete because of feminism, sexually transmitted diseases, divorce, and women's economic hardship. Yet by the early 1990s, even if the desire to uphold residual family values through the control of women's sexuality remained, there was no way that the kind of blindness about HIV transmission necessary to fabricate this sense of stability concerning AIDS could be maintained. It became impossible to ignore that women had AIDS, that people contracted AIDS heterosexually (heterosexual sex is much more dangerous for females than for males), and that all Americans needed to consider AIDS a part of their sexual and social reality. Some commercial programs at last shifted their focus entirely to women's experience. In the two 1990s' tapes I am about to analyze, the programs work overtime to insure that the "normal" female protagonists shown can and do get AIDS. Although this means that women's bodies are highly visible (they are all that we see), it should come as no surprise that all we see as well are the bodies of straight, white, professional women. As these tapes work to discredit the messages of earlier broadcast programming by insisting that all women are at risk for AIDS because women do have sex and AIDS is transmitted sexually (drug use by women is not considered), they reaffirm many of the biases about what kind of sex and what kind of women are worthy of media consideration and concern.

A New Visibility in Mainstream AIDS Documentaries

Both *Playing It Safe* and *Something to Live For: The Alison Gertz Story* use conventional realist narrative to give national, big-budget attention to the little-told story of women and AIDS. These two programs are devoted entirely to the difficult task of educating a previously placated audience of women that they too are truly at risk for HIV infection and that their sexual practices will have to change so that they can protect themselves from transmission. Unlike the 1980s' documentaries I analyzed above, these 1990s' products are not invested in alleviating the anxiety of straight white men. Instead, the nineties brings us women's stories, told from a woman's point of view with the generic codes of the woman's film, meant to acknowledge the need for (some) *female* anxiety about women and HIV. Yet these tapes make their newly visible females into the most conventional of postfeminist gals—professional and powerful, sexual and spunky, but white-bred as hell. The consequence of this approach is the valid enlightenment of a group of women about their proximity to HIV, while also maintaining the familiar and erroneous concept of female risk groups (or types of sexual women) and the prevailing hierarchies of guilt, innocence, blame, and fear which may promote and alleviate panic but which do not protect anyone from HIV (even the white heterosexual professionals who are the tapes' intended audience).

Playing It Safe tells the tale of a woman who is a radio talk-show host on a popular program called "The Working Woman." She answers call-in questions about taxes, office etiquette, getting raises, what to wear on business trips, how to avoid harassment in the workplace. But calls keep coming in about AIDS and other STDS, and she does not know what to say; this is not her area of expertise, what does this have to do with the working woman? She finally decides to air two programs interviewing an expert, a female AIDS doctor, who can answer these questions. In the meantime, she is beginning a new relationship with a coworker and is trying to practice what she preaches: to discuss sexuality with the guy before they have sex, to ask him to wear a condom. *The Alison Gertz Story* tells the real-life story of the young, upper-class Manhattan designer who, while in her teens, was infected with HIV after having intercourse once with a date. The program is structured by a narrative frame which depicts her telling her story to an auditorium of rapt high school students in her current role as straight, white, rich AIDS spokesmodel (if I can get it, if I have it and you can't see it, anyone can). Her narration follows her too slow diagnosis (since she was white, straight, and rich none of her doctors tested her for HIV) and her gradual transition into acceptance of her HIV status. We watch her unsuccessfully attempt to negotiate safer sex in two relationships, and we at last see her take up her new calling, not as married mother and professional as she had always dreamed, but as AIDS educator and foundation head.

The agenda of these two tapes is a new one—to convince "normal" American women that normal American womanhood now encompasses AIDS. Refusing to participate in the construction of another residual sexual reality for women, these tapes show a "new" reality of postfeminist women who use the same balls they have in their professional lives to organize their sexual lives. These girls want sex and will take the initiative to get it. Yet what empowers the women in these remarkably similar tales is eventually what also traps them (and the tapes which present their brave stories) in much of the same old muck that has organized stories of women and AIDS from the start. In their attempt to reach "normal" women the tapes conventionalize the protagonists' race, class, sexual orientation, and life-styles, so that the narratives reinforce the dangerous myth that there are good and bad modes of transmission (meaning good and bad people who transmit HIV) and that good (normal) women do not ever participate in bad activities (lesbian, bisexual, kinky, nonmonogamous sex, drug use or sex with drug users), so these behaviors need never be addressed. Education which has been carefully prepared so as to avoid alienating its intended audience is based on naive assumptions about who that audience is, and in the meantime such assumptions serve to provide incomplete information.

In *Playing It Safe* the doctor tells women who call the radio program a number of extremely important "facts" about HIV transmission as well as other STDS. She knows statistics, rates of infection, and she knows how hard it is for women to ask men to use condoms. For these reasons, she frames her detailed information with the advice "to choose your partners carefully." But she never says what this advice means because she is relying upon what "we" already know. The tape condones the implicit suggestion to do exactly what many women already do, which does not protect us one stitch: find out a guy's salary, where he grew up and went to college, and make assumptions about his safety from clues which have nothing to do with risk for HIV.

Choose your partner carefully. And, although *The Alison Gertz Story*'s central message is precisely the dismissal of the common belief that "choosing your partners carefully" is a protection against AIDS, it ends up confirming similar kinds of misinformation through the film's extended quest for the "cause" of Alison's infection. One of the clumsiest and most cliché-ridden sections of the program is dedicated to this search. Alison starts having flashbacks about a night of hot sex in the glory days of disco. She meets a blond, feathery-haired bartender at a club, and he arrives at her uptown apartment a day later with roses and wine. A soft fade finds the two making love before a warming fireplace. All of this romance, the innocence and candlelight of the encounter, made even more excruciating by our knowledge that Alison is usually monogamous and this is her one youthful fling, points to the fact that she is an *undeserving* PWA, an *innocent* victim. She had sex on a date with a nice white boy. The film ferrets out the route of her transmission—this one slip from innocence, one night of youthful lust—to validate Gertz's claim to AIDS superstardom. If, instead, Alison had flashed back to five years of living on the street of the Lower East Side as a junkie, no film would have been made to tell her story. Her innocence gives her her voice. If only she had followed the adage "choose your partners carefully." . . . As an AIDS educator, Alison is explicit that it is her whiteness, her wealth, her heterosexuality, her one-shot infection that allows her to speak to and reach teens who wrongly feel protected by their own privilege. Yet this undermines, and in fact silences, important information (use condoms and dental dams since outward signs are never an indication of HIV), even as it serves to reach people.

Nothing is wrong with educating straight, white, heterosexual, professional females about their real risk for AIDS, but it is worthy of note that these large-budget, mass-release programs do not address the female audiences whose needs are proportionately much, much greater at this stage in the epidemic (the urban poor and working poor, who are largely women of color, who may be drug users themselves and are even more often the partner of a drug user, who have inadequate access to health care, who cannot easily adopt safer-sex practices because safer sex is birth control and often religiously and/or culturally taboo). When will these women get to see their story in such a culturally legitimate form? When will such mass-release projects, such large budgets, be turned toward this deserving female population? And until then, what else should be done? Although I have emphasized the importance of targeting educational approaches to specific audiences by tailoring images to replicate the specificity of mise-en-scène and cultural codes—language, clothes, values, locales, and sexual practices—of the intended audience, I have also stressed that to understand the story of women and AIDS we need to know about the *many* stories which make up this crisis. Programming made for white-bred America may serve this legitimate audience, but it does not begin to reflect the multiple ways that even straight, white, middle-class Americans live their sexual lives, nor does it pretend to acknowledge the manner in which most American women live. To educate about safer sex, one has to make room for the variety of ways that women are sexual, not rely upon assumptions, judgments, or stereotypes.

The surreal and ironic capping off to my initial viewing of *The Alison Gertz Story* demonstrates why creating narrative structures dependent on innocent and guilty PWAs and good and bad routes of transmission endangers us all. Immediately following the film's airing on ABC's "Sunday Night Movie," there was a promotional ad for a Philadelphia station's "Action News," which was to air next. We were informed that the top story would be about Edward Savitz, Philadelphia's "AIDS/sex offender," and then we also would get the bonus of seeing Alison Gertz in person. Savitz's story had, in the previous few days, become one of those national AIDS megastories we get every year or so (the house bombing in Arcadia, Ryan White, Magic Johnson, Kimberly Bergalis, the Florida dentist, Arthur Ashe), and many Philadelphians were following it with greedy attention. Days earlier, Savitz had been the victim of a highly publicized police porn bust. After months of spying, taping, tapping, and photographing him, he was arrested for paying young men for sex (it turned out that he had supported generations of Philadelphia high schoolers). As the story unfolded, it became unclear whether his greatest crime was being gay, having sexual interaction with minors, paying for it, buying their underwear—or having AIDS. Lost in the citywide panic which followed (an increase in calls to AIDS hot lines by the hundreds, free counseling for any boy who had "known" Savitz and that boy's friends and family), and never would be retrieved, was that Savitz's sexual behavior with these boys was perfectly *safe* as far as transmission of HIV was concerned. His fetish behavior (an interest in socks, underwear, and maybe even feces) kept him from participating in unsafe sexual interactions with the boys; they rarely even touched and never had intercourse. I do not want to go into the horrific and criminal details of this case, but "Fast Eddy" or "Uncle Eddy," as he was called, was repeatedly harassed in jail, was set an egregiously high bail so that he had to stay in jail even though it was known that he was attacked and harassed there, and ultimately was released to an AIDS hospice only in the very last days of his life.

Edward Savitz was treated like a monster, a lunatic, a murderer, a criminal, in part because of a social and representational system that on the same evening could use this same AIDS logic to treat Alison Gertz like a helpless victim, an innocent, pure princess, an AIDS darling. Savitz died a miserable death, and one of America's largest cities was allowed to let its prurient interests get the better of its ability to think clearly about sex, safety, and AIDS. Whatever may or may not have been wrong with Savitz's smelling boys' undergarments, it kept him from infecting anyone with HIV. The creation of heroes and villains, of good guys and bad, of risky people and safe people, endangers all of us as it permits already operating biases, that themselves have nothing to do with protection from HIV, to structure AIDS representation, AIDS education, and AIDS legislation.

Introduction: The Words, Art, and Theory of WAVE

In this chapter the Women's AIDS Video Enterprise (WAVE) takes the form of words. Here, I will focus upon my own video project—from preproduction through distribution of the videotape, *We Care*—to describe making activist video—at least for me. I will use words to explain our video exercises and late-night phone calls, the quirky and diverse women who were the project's participants, and my large doubts and small triumphs. I will call this process of writing letters, asking for funds, eating dinner at group members' homes, choosing to include a particular image in our tape *We Care,* and taking the completed video to a homeless shelter in the Bronx, "art." I will call my subjective descriptions of these many activities "theory." I may sound defensive. I guess I am worried. These are important words to be used for things as seemingly inconsequential as the particular, personal, everyday feelings of an individual engaged in activist video production.

But I hope that the idea of the alternative AIDS media which has accumulated incrementally to this point in the book leads us inevitably to the conclusion that to best understand what the alternative media is and what it does—to best understand the tapes we make, our art—personal knowledge about the processes of funding, distribution, production, and viewing is essential. My words detailing a project I know from the inside out are the best example of a theory of this kind of art—not because they are the most true, or accurate, thorough, or systematic, but because they attempt to enact as closely as possible, without being there yourself, what making this work feels like to an individual who undertakes it. If the most precise definition of alternative media depends upon its unique capacity to allow individual makers and viewers to construct themselves as marginal subjects through a dominant form, then the closest thing I can imagine to a theory of alternative AIDS media is to scrutinize and even reenact this function with words.

The following words about WAVE are best understood by mobilizing three varied but often intersecting theoretical traditions about art, writing, and the relationship between theory and practice. The first could be called a Marxist sociological study of art or, as Terry Eagleton explains, theory that assumes that "art is first of all a social practice rather than an object to be academically dissected. . . ."[1] My "academic dissection" of the videotape *We Care* will be framed with a discussion of the social practice of the group of women who produced it, the "pressures, hierarchies and power relations"[2] that structured the project and the lives of the individual women involved. To understand our video, our lives, needs, problems, and relationships need to be understood too. Janet Woolf maintains that "in the production of art, social institutions affect, amongst other things, *who* becomes an artist, *how* they become an artist, how they are then able to *practice* their art, and how they can ensure that their work is produced, performed, and *made available* to a public."[3]

Whereas a certain kind of art production—that by professional "artists"—may rely upon a somewhat standardized account of who an artist is, how she is able to produce, and how her work is made available to consumers, for activist art production by nonprofessionals this is never the case. The kind of "artist" who might not call herself an artist, who makes her work when she is not really at work, the kind of artist who has neither a degree nor training nor the personal and institutional support and validation these things allow, this kind of "artist" may understand art production as a kind of unaccustomed and rare privilege. This kind of artist might lack the confidence, or time, or money to produce, yet she produces nevertheless. Therefore, to think about alternative media production by this kind of artist, I must also talk about the real difficulties of real people's lives. That is, why it is harder to work on and complete an art project when one is poor because so many other responsibilities interfere (taking the baby to the hospital, cleaning the house, going to work, taking care of husbands and parents and nieces). And why it is harder to work on and complete an art project when you are a Latina who has been taught that your words are not important, when you are a lesbian who has been taught that you are not creative or smart, or when, as a woman, you are instructed that this is not your realm. The underlying motivation for WAVE's organization as a support group is this understanding of art. The production of art cannot be separated from the other tensions, anxieties, and problems that women encounter during their daily lives and in their sense of themselves.

Here, the second theoretical tradition—that of feminist theory—

comes into my analysis. I will be describing the personal interaction and growth of the female participants in WAVE, including myself, and to do so my tone will be necessarily descriptive and anecdotal. To understand what alternative media is, we must first understand the local effects of media production and spectatorship on real people. How little is a tape like *We Care* understood if it is not known how Aida took the tape to a community college and led a class there, thus becoming a college teacher for an afternoon? Or how Carmen showed it to her mother and finally began talking about her husband Willy's HIV infection? Or about how my relationships with these women profoundly affected the way I know AIDS and myself? None of that is made visible in our tape. It can only be written about here, because I know, because I was there. Needless to say, this extratextual information is central to a full understanding of our work of art.

Which brings me to the third theoretical tradition which shapes this chapter—the Birmingham Centre's "ethnographic approach" toward media studies, founded upon the belief that talking to real people about their relationship to the media will alter what theory says about the ideological functions of this institution.[4] So I am going to talk with myself—write—what my relationship was to the media, and to the other women in WAVE, as we made and showed *We Care*. My understanding of "theory" recognizes that chicken and rice at Carmen's house is not simply a part of putting theory into practice but is part of theory itself. Knowing about the details and difficulties of her life alters my *ideas* about her, and my *ideas* about her relationship to the WAVE project and video production. Cross-cultural, cross-class, cross-town friendship—the sharing of a meal, the enjoying of wedding photos, the pleasures of hospitality—organizes our abilities to produce video together, organizes the videotape we produce, explains its content and form as much as any abstract idea about education, representation, or AIDS. Aida's self-empowerment—that she was afforded the opportunity to be an expert, a teacher, an artist—*is* academic. My expanded knowledge of AIDS, through the experience of people who live with AIDS in households other than my own, facing different obstacles, *is* theoretical. The day when nobody came to our weekly meeting because babies were sick, friends had died, people could not deal with the long subway ride on a snowy day *is* deeply about how lived experience affects production and, therefore, production's theory. Although academic theory structured this project (detailed below), the making into practice of that theory altered, contradicted, and transformed it into something else. What came out on the other end were not generalized statements about the meanings of media, but specific and sometimes uncertain words about the everyday processes of video production with and for real and diverse people.

The WAVE project was a group of seven women who met and discussed AIDS' impact upon our lives, while learning how to make video, munching on doughnuts, and drinking coffee. Aida, Carmen, Glenda, Juanita, Marcia, Sharon, and I met weekly for six months. Words can only mimic, shadow, stencil the twenty-two long and hard Saturday meetings we shared.

> For six months, a video-support group for women will meet weekly with a social worker and videomaker at the Brooklyn AIDS Task Force (BATF) to participate in an innovative education. The members of the group will discuss the impact and toll of AIDS on their lives, while at the same time analyzing how the media has covered (or ignored) the crisis, particularly as it impacts their community. Basic education in video production and media criticism will coincide with the group's progress. As they decide what is most lacking in the AIDS education offered to their community, they will respond by producing their own video, to be actively distributed. (Excerpt from funding letter)

The videotape we shot shows what we looked like and the words we said during those twenty-two weeks. But even with these reminders, it is hard to recall how it felt each week: the fear, the humor, the sadness, the challenges. Funny, how even the most self-consciously recorded, documented, preserved activities like this project nevertheless come back to words. How else to describe the cold Sunday wait for Juanita at the AIDS Walk, or the hot summer subway ride to Sharon's at the Far Rockaways? The video documents of these days are more selective than my memories—incomplete, fragile, dated; they tip off my recollections. On videotape are recorded the people we were in 1990. Today some of those people have died; we are thankful but wary of their video images, records of a time when we still hoped for their long life, their healing, the happy days we would share. And today the women of WAVE are changed. When we see our video images from 1990 we notice that we have put on and lost weight, we have grown out our hair, we have married, changed jobs, moved; our ideas and hopes have changed. When we watch who we were in 1990, we feel nostalgic and we also feel connected to the past, our work, and to each other. Video initiated this connection; it still feeds it, but now we are also friends outside video. *We Care* is effective AIDS education, and WAVE was a successful video project, because each took into account the specific needs and lives of individuals. I hope to capture and convey that concern in the words that follow.

Preproduction: January 1988–February 1990

The WAVE project started as words in my head, words discussed with my friends and professors, words which eventually were typed into my computer, printed out, and sent to seemingly countless offices of nonprofit organizations as funding requests.

> WAVE intends to produce AIDS prevention education that is hitherto lacking and greatly needed: community-specific information made by and for the low-income, minority women who are at great risk for this disease. WAVE proposes to shift the hand on the video camera from the distanced and punitive control of the mainstream media to the women who come from the communities most affected by this crisis. The women participants in WAVE will be enabled to articulate and then respond to their concerns about the present state of HIV education and treatment by producing their own educational videotape for their community. (Opening paragraph from a funding request letter)

After almost two years those words became money, $20,500, minus 5 percent to my nonprofit funding sponsor, plus in-kind donations of editing time, and later a $5,000 distribution grant. After that, the money became "art": the three videos produced by the WAVE project, *We Care: A Video for Care Providers of People Affected by AIDS, A WAVE Taster,* and *WAVE: Self-Portraits.* So said, it sounds easy. Immediate. But a great deal of word processing, mailing, and rejection letters occurred between my requests and the cold, hard cash. My words now will never evoke the disappointment, the uncertainty, the massive expense of energy, time, and passion which was the funding process of one political art project during the Reagan eighties. It has been difficult to remuster that level of dedication, commitment, and faith in my project which was the minimal requirement for getting WAVE funded. So, as with many other experienced, enthusiastic, and capable artists, the daunting prospect of facing the humiliating and draining work of fund-raising keeps me from making tapes like *We Care* more frequently.

I am not the only WAVE producer so blocked. Several women involved in WAVE who hoped to continue to produce on their own have been unable to break through the highly professionalized requirements of arts funding. Juanita has been hoping to make a tape about lesbians of color and AIDS. Sharon speaks of a video project about anger. But without a professional fund-raiser's command of written English and film jargon, knowledge of receptive organizations and the ability to network, or even the ownership of useful computer programs and laser printers, the women who come to art production with a great deal of passion but without the privilege of an art school degree, a B.A., or a summer internship with the right gallery are virtually excluded before they begin.

It is not simply my determination, but my education, my contacts, my knowledge of what was "in" conceptually, theoretically, and politically, and my access to and power over words, that eventually allowed WAVE to be funded so that our video could be produced. Art funding is hard to explain or predict—a complex system of favor-trading, of people you know, of where you have shown, where you went to school, what is "in," who is "in." A key to the funding of WAVE was that during my two years of fund-raising I was an active participant in the New York City art scene through my involvement in the Whitney Independent Studio Program and NYU's Department of Cinema Studies. The gulf between the motivation to produce, an excellent concept of what will be produced, and the acquisition of even minimal funding needed to do camcorder production is not typically bridged by talent and enthusiasm alone.

Thus, a complete reading of any work of video needs to be aware of how and why it was funded and all that *was not* funded as that particular work received backing. During the grant cycle in which the WAVE project got significant funds from our primary funder, the New York Council on the Humanities, Amber Hollibaugh and Gini Retticker were also attempting to get funds for *The Heart of the Matter* (1993). My request marked the second time I had applied there. After my first unsuccessful attempt I was invited to apply for a "minigrant" from the agency for what was admittedly unnecessary "research"; this process actually represented the hoop I had to jump through to make my application properly fit the category of "humanities." On this second time around, Amber and I knew that the agency would not grant two projects on women and AIDS in one cycle. What were we to do? Stagger our funding requests to this agency, meanwhile upsetting one project's funding rhythm? Compete against each other when we were friends and colleagues who entirely supported each other's extremely different projects? We decided to each include a letter in our applications supporting the other project. Yet this did not safeguard us from what we already knew would occur. I received funding that year, while *The Heart of the Matter* had to go through more rounds before being granted NYCH money.

For two years I attempted to raise funds for a project that empowered people to educate themselves and, in the process, made them stronger, more articulate participants in their own lives and communities. For practical as well as theoretical reasons I chose media production for this project. A tremendous amount of AIDS education has been produced in video. Such videos are easily integrated into the kinds of educational outreach being deployed against the crisis. AIDS tapes easily play in the places where PWAs meet and are treated. Although pamphlets have been produced in great number, printed literature in English is not effective in educating people who are either illiterate or non-English speakers. Furthermore, as is often argued by proponents of media literacy, people are already highly educated consumers of television.

But even though those involved in AIDS education have known about the importance and feasibility of localized education for a long time, it took several years to fund WAVE into action. The project fell through the cracks of funding compartmentalization; it was neither strictly art nor strictly therapy, neither entirely activism nor entirely education. Ultimately, WAVE was funded by arts and humanities (not health or social service) organizations because arts support sources were the ones that I knew to turn to, and my skills, connections, and resources could most effectively be used among them. Admittedly, too, AIDS was a trendy funding issue during the late 1980s and early 1990s. Even as arts support became defunded, timid, and censored, some of the most effective and powerful responses to the AIDS crisis came from "cultural" producers.

Yet Douglas Crimp emphasizes that an "idealist conception of art" is often what is behind a celebration (and funding and showing) of AIDS work as either commodity or act of redemption.[5] He argues that although many of the producers of AIDS activist art receive funding and art world acceptance for their AIDS art, they remain "wary of their own success. Such success can ensure visibility, but visibility to *whom?*"[6] I remain wary of our art world funding and our art world successes, even as I also understand how vital they were and are to the production and dissemination of this video project. Certainly, in the case of WAVE and *We Care,* the success and visibility of our work as "AIDS art," rather than AIDS education, served to further the progress of our AIDS education. Art world screenings mean money and dominant cultural affirmation in a way that homeless shelter screenings never can, even as homeless shelter screenings are the primary intended use of the tapes. An art world screening gets a review in a magazine, which then gets clipped and included in a grant request for distribution. You get the grant because you have received validation where it counts. This kind of dominant cultural affirmation leads directly to the "real" or desired affirmations of educational and political art. In the case of WAVE, the "success" of the project in the dominant art scene allowed for the raising of funds which let us distribute the tape for free.

It is a testament to the courage and experimentation of small or adventurous funding agencies (NYCH pushed all of its boundaries about "humanities documentaries" to fund this never-for-PBS project) that projects like WAVE get money. But it is equally a testament to the way in which most highly endowed agencies *cannot* fund such projects that projects like WAVE must operate on minuscule budgets in relation to less political, less experimental, and more expensive work. For example, the reasons that WAVE was *not* funded by the NEH are very revealing. After sending off a boxload of application materials to the NEH (the massive application requirements of such agencies, which cost a great deal in copying and mailing alone, keep many poorly funded agencies from applying in the first place), I received a terse and immediate response. My project could not even reach the stage of project evaluation, because it did not qualify for an NEH grant on several counts. One, NEH-sponsored media must be in a "professional format" (¾" or 1" videotape) because all NEH-sponsored projects must be eligible to be considered for PBS airing. This was a highly suspect position on their part, for media technology now allows any format to become "broadcast quality," for example, the playing of home video footage on the nightly news. Interestingly enough, after *We Care* was selected to be screened on New York City's WNET's "Independent Focus," it was later determined by the technicians there that the tape was not "broadcast quality," and they did not air it. This occurred even after I had returned to my editors who carefully remonitored what the editors insisted was a perfectly broadcastable signal. Broadcast, then, is no technical standard but an ideological one, which means politics, not professionalism. The policy that material produced on ½" video cannot be funded for or aired on PBS is political, because it keeps low-budget, community-specific work from arenas of mass distribution. Secondly, WAVE did not qualify for NEH funding because such grants were designed specifically to join "media professionals" with humanities scholars. I was hiring no media professionals; therefore, I did not qualify for an NEH grant. The very point of my project—to challenge the notion of who a professional could be—did not, in the eyes of NEH administrators warrant breaking their needlessly prohibitive, exclusionary protocol.

Another telling example of missed funding involves a New York City Department of Health grant, which would have been perfect for this project, but for which I did not apply, again for illuminating reasons. The grant, which involved considerable funds for community-based AIDS service organizations doing risk-reduction education, required an application form that was quite literally a book. The process of getting DOH money, appropriate for hospitals and other large health organizations with fund-raising staffs and the necessary equipment, machinery, resources, and time to fill out a book, makes no sense for the very cash-hungry, resourceless organizations that DOH was trying to target.

Yet an industry defined by such funding hypocrisies has not kept alternative AIDS media from being produced. In fact, great quantities of work get funded despite such hurdles, for many of the same reasons that WAVE eventually got funded: alternative producers participate in labor-intensive, dedicated funding drives, or they work with shockingly small budgets. For the most part, I received small grants from small, politically identified funders: ArtMatters, Women Make Movies, the Astraea Fund. My two "large" grants ($19,500 and $5,000, respectively) from New York State's Humanities and Arts Councils allowed for the tape's production and distribution.[7]

Because of the money I finally did raise, BATF took me seriously enough to consider sponsoring my labor-intensive project. It was my money, more than my ideas, that convinced this beleaguered and often broke community service agency to take on yet another project. I had decided to approach them to sponsor WAVE because of their close connection to the communities they serve. While, again, I cannot devote words here to the years of BATF's social service work that built the level of trust necessary to encourage community participation in a project of this sort, this is another vitally important extratextual condition which allowed for the project's successful outcome. With my grant money and this AIDS service agency's backing, resources, staff, and, most significantly, its connection to Brooklyn communities of color, WAVE at last began its life beyond words on paper. Needless to say, a great deal of thinking, soul-searching, planning, and theorizing had been expended before I finally wrote a successful grant application and raised the money which allowed us to begin work one cold Saturday in January 1990.

Three years earlier, during the summer of 1987, after having lived in New York City for a little less than a year, I decided to volunteer for the Gay Men's Health Crisis (GMHC). At that time, like most of my fresh-from-college friends, I knew no one personally who was HIV-infected. Yet, like any politically aware person, I *knew* one thing, and *assumed* another. I *knew* that AIDS was becoming a hot spot in our society, where the political concerns which were most important to me churned, collapsed, and reverberated—politics of sexuality, health care, poverty, race, and gender. I *assumed* that soon I would know someone—many—who would be infected. I look back and see that my initial knowledge and assumptions, both political and personal, have with time been proven only too true.

I was assigned to GMHC's media department, which consisted at that time of one woman, Jean Carlomusto, who was single-handedly funding and producing a weekly cable television show, "Living With AIDS." After completing a few menial assignments for her, I asked if I could produce a half-hour show on women's issues and AIDS. As hard to believe as it may seem now, at that time there was very little being written or produced in video about women's relationship to the crisis. *Women and AIDS* (Carlomusto and Juhasz, 1987), the first tape I produced for GMHC in response to this lack of attention, broadly sketched the social and political context of women's relationship to the epidemic and thus helped to fill the enormous gap in available resources for and about women. Because of this lack of needed materials, the tape virtually distributed itself, being shown nationally and internationally at museums, at AIDS conferences, before AIDS support groups, and at colleges and universities, among other arts and service venues. After this tape, I produced two more shows for the "Living With AIDS" series. Each of them—*Prostitutes, Risk and AIDS: It's Not What You Do, But How You Do What You Do* (1988, with Carlomusto), and *Test for the Nation: Women, Children, Families, AIDS* (1988)—approached with more detail some of the issues raised in *Women and AIDS*.

My work on these video projects, in conjunction with my experience as an AIDS activist and my graduate education in cinema studies and ethnographic film, forced me to rethink my production strategies and intentions. For reasons academic, lived, and artistic, I needed to move beyond telling women's stories "for them." First, although by this time my relationship to AIDS had become personal as well as political, I found myself in my video work mostly documenting the lives, concerns, and political needs of *others,* specifically, low-income women of color, the female population earliest and hardest hit by the crisis. The media has never been kind or sensitive to such women, whatever their health, and alternative media practitioners like myself come to such communities with this legacy before us: abusive interviews, promises of anonymity unkept, words used out of context.

Even though my interviews for GMHC were different from the classic mainstream interaction, and even though I tried to include my own relationship to the crisis in the productions I made, I found it increasingly difficult to continue to produce this kind of work. I felt that—good intentions be damned—I was still enacting some version of the typical and highly suspect power dynamic of the filmic exchange: me taping/"them" speaking. Me white/they black. Me rich/they poor. Me outside the crisis/they inside.

For reasons theoretical and personal, these dichotomies made me uncomfortable. Feminist film theory speaks of an innately aggressive apparatus, a system of looks which are inscribed by patriarchal power relations. (I wondered if this remained true even when a woman, myself, held the camera.) The ethics of the documentary interview have long been a necessary area for academic and practical concern. (I wondered if even a consensual interview was not necessarily manipulative.) Even though I would meet with my "subjects" several times (unlike the more usual one-shot affairs of TV journalism), and even though I shared a personal and political agenda with them, and even though I did not *want* to abuse the power granted me by the video camera, I found that the structure of making media left me in an uncomfortable position. I was *taking* and *having* others' images to use again and again, to edit to my liking, to use in making my videos, which, in turn, would further my career, even if this was all primarily in the service of getting the word out about AIDS.

Finally, the legacy and inherent contradictions of anthropology and ethnographic film made me wary of my position as cultural, white outsider (with my own, personal relationship to the AIDS crisis nevertheless), asking women different from myself to illuminate devastating and personal experiences for my camera. Similarly, Frances Negrón-Muntaner, the producer of *AIDS in the Barrio* (1989), writes:

> When media professionals ask, "How can *we* awaken *them* (communities with little or no political power) to the potential of media?" we assume a patronizing position. As a Puerto Rican and lesbian film/videomaker, I am aware of the double bind of being both part of the power (as a professional) and marginalized by it (as a cultural and sexual Other), and the effects of these contradictions in the power relations one establishes with communities that we claim as our own. . . . It is important to ask these questions if mediamakers are to avoid reproducing the power structures we amply criticize in our work and our discourse as independents.[8]

I attempted to ask these questions and to respond to this double bind by organizing WAVE, a video project where I would cast myself as a teacher and a member of one small community, a long-term video AIDS support group. There, I would be revealing as much or as little as would my once subjects, now my fellow group members. There, I would be taking as much responsibility for speaking, holding the camera, deciding the questions, as would my peers. Of course, I was still the motivating force behind this "need to awaken them," but the participants in the group would actively choose to participate in this awakening; they would be told up front what they would get from (and give to) taking some control of the media.

I am certainly not suggesting that this project was a "solution" to the structural problems and contradictions in the power relations of filmic interaction. But I am suggesting that paralysis in the face of these difficulties is an even less effective approach. Independent videomaker Annie Goldson explains how working on the series of tapes she coproduced with international movements labeled "terrorist," *Counterterror* (1987–92), contributed to analysis, rather than concealment, of the structures of domination and oppression. "For whites not to address racism is to deny we are already implicated in its processes and institutions. To remain silent is to carry out the self-fulfilling prophecy that we will return to a position of liberal guilt, inactivity, and perhaps—depending on one's class—privilege. . . . The mute guilt "expressed" by many producers of European descent (although I reject the term "Eurocentric"—again it is universalizing, eliminating differences among whites) positions whiteness as superior." [9]

The point is not that as white, or middle-class, or college-educated, or HIV-negative producers we should not involve our work with issues of race, class, or sero-status, but that we *should*, responsibly. Videomaker Michelle Valladares writes that "white artists carry the burden of an historical legacy as 'observer.' No matter how well-intentioned their observations, they must be held responsible to this history." [10] Thus, I organized WAVE in an attempt to take responsibility for the legacy of white involvement with otherness and observation while also acknowleding my implication in the history of the AIDS crisis. I first acknowledged that altering my position as observer was not as simple as giving a camcorder to people who never had the opportunity to use one. Taking responsibility for these histories inspired my attempt to address power imbalances on all levels of the production process. In preproduction this meant a dialogue about our backgrounds, current life conditions, and our relations to each other—our similarities and differences. I wanted to think through with more fluidity the essentialist notions of identity which would keep me from working with this community (and them from working with me) because I am white and the other group members are black and Latina. Negrón-Muntaner discusses how her AIDS work led her to understand how the word *community* "falls short of describing the multiplicity of experience within these groups."[11] I believed that I could be part of a community with women of different class, ethnicity, sexual preference, and HIV status from myself. Part of the group's work would have to be defining what our particular "community" was. Making a video would help us (force us?) to raise these difficult questions.

Furthermore, WAVE seemed an appropriate response to some of the difficulties I was confronting in my video work because I was learning about the kinds of risks that women take when they speak about their HIV status publicly. Beyond the discrimination that anyone is likely to face after disclosing sero-positivity, women are highly likely to have children for whom their fear of discrimination is paramount. In addition, the ways in which many women who are infected lead their lives are illegal (because of their own drug use or that of their lovers, or because of the link between prostitution and drug use). Thus, to ask a woman to speak about AIDS before a camera is often a setup for discrimination or even prosecution. The process of making tapes for GMHC about prostitutes' or maternity issues was frustrating but illuminating about this aspect of AIDS educational video production. Even the designs and desires of an alternative media approach to these sensitive issues were not enough to empower women with personal experience to talk in front of a video camera and microphone, let alone to make their own videos about such issues. I knew only one prostitute—Carol Leigh, the AIDS, prostitute rights, and video activist—who was comfortable speaking on camera. For the tape on maternity, only one white female PWA would speak on camera with her image recorded.

This is another reason the project was organized around a "support group" model. Dr. Dooley Worth, who served as a project consultant, established the first peer group for high-risk women. She found that women, especially women of color, needed time and space to begin to trust AIDS education as well as to feel comfortable admitting and discussing their own relationships to the crisis. "The response of black women to personal risk for AIDS must be considered in the context of the risks associated with living with sexism, racism and socio-economic oppression on a daily basis, of constantly being reminded that one is distinct from and "inferior" to the majority, that one has limited access to addressing one's needs. Black women's wariness of self-disclosure is part of their larger survival strategy."[12]

Inefficient filmically (a video "about" these women could have been produced in two to three weeks), but efficient in more important ways, particularly in terms of the kinds of responsibility I needed to take as a producer/outsider, the joining of video production with the usual work of a support group expanded both of these activities. As our personal troubles and concerns regarding the impact of AIDS upon our lives were revealed to the group, we would think about how such issues could be expressed in the even more public forum of video. In fact, the structure of a video, with its necessary relationship to narrative, gave us a ready-made form which channeled our own narratives. Because a video was to be made, we needed to speak. Because a video needs to be coherent and organized, linear and structured, our words sought similar patterns.

Finally, WAVE was the outgrowth of one further difficulty I had found with my previous video projects: my knowledge that the most effective AIDS education comes from the specific communities to which it is targeted. Renee Sabatier explains that "AIDS prevention can only be effective if it changes people's sexual behavior. In the Third World, and among ethnic minorities in the North, this is unlikely to happen if AIDS education is perceived to emanate from a predominantly white, relatively privileged, outside establishment. Instead it must be made compatible with the aspirations and plans which those communities are drawing up for their own development."[13]

At present, the only precaution against AIDS is risk-reduction education, and one of the best responses to infection is sensitive, knowledgeable, culturally specific information. As the numbers of infected rise steadily, especially among poor urban women of color, it is clear that a crisis exists in such education. New educational tactics, which take into account the particular needs and values of the distinct communities suffering most from this epidemic, are sorely needed.

Yet knowing about the power of community-specific education and seeing it happen are not necessarily the same. For the very structures of oppression which made low-income women of color more susceptible to this disease (and others) denies them attention from the powerful institutions which make and fund media, and more significantly, these oppressive structures rid their communities of the resources necessary to make their own media. Catherine Saalfield and Ray Navarro in their article about activist AIDS media by and for people of color explain that "to issue demands for culturally sensitive materials without taking into account the economic, cultural, and racial obstacles that exist in the independent sector of film and video assumes that people of color will be able to easily overcome such well-entrenched barriers. . . . When asking, 'Where are the videotapes from minority communities?' one may as well be asking, 'Where are the Black physicians, the Latino dentists?'"[14] The programs that have successfully brought media production to disenfranchised communities (i.e., Challenge for Change, Worth and Adair's Navajo Film Themselves Project, the Inuit Broadcasting Corporation, the Walpiri Media Association) depended heavily upon outside funding, which was never stable or fixed and came and went with the political tides.

Even when the political or cultural tide is in one's favor, the differing effects of dominant cultural affirmation upon various members of our group provides a telling reminder of the discrepancies in power and privilege that divided and divide us. Surely, when *We Care* does "well" in dominant cultural settings it affects all of us in positive ways, yet only some members of the group have résumés upon which the information that the tape played at the Whitney Museum matter, and even fewer of us have résumés upon which such information is relevant. When a reporter from the *Village Voice* attended one of our meetings and interviewed everyone afterward for a story on the WAVE project, we were all excited, proud, nervous—even those of us who did not read or care about the *Voice*. Great, we thought, this is just what we need—public attention, affirmation in a dominant form; we can show the article to our friends; we can show it to potential funders. When the story took weeks and then months to be written and rewritten, and then never ran because of conflict between the writer and her editor, we were reminded of the underside of "real-world" attention: you don't control it. But more so, it became clear to me that the *Voice* was indifferent to the specific functions of this manner of art production. The *Voice* did not recognize or respect the tenuous relationship to authority, vulnerability, and expertise felt by these artists. To run the piece would build up authority, to pull the piece was to confirm vulnerability. For the women in WAVE—unlike other "artists" who may have experience with attention, reviews, coverage by the mass media—it was a painful, and distrustful experience to open up to someone from the mass media. When the article did not run, everything that we suspected about the dominant culture being uninterested in our story, being manipulative, tricking us, was proven true. The women of WAVE were both hurt and scornful. We gained nothing but pain from this attention which came from outside where we worked, who we were, what we made. Nevertheless, the experience did not keep us from producing; it simply further entrenched our sense of why our project was unique and deeply important.

Production: February 1990–August 1990

"Tell me about your mother/sister/daughter," Sharon's voice queries.

Images of her daughters, sisters, mother answer back, their black faces etched with familial similarities: "If you want my opinion, I'm very proud of her," says her daughter.

"But what about AIDS?" Sharon wants to know. *"Does she devote too much of herself to AIDS, and doesn't this make you angry at her?"*

"Sure it makes me mad when she's gone so much. But maybe she doesn't know that, even so, I understand. . . ."

In her self-portrait, these interviews with her family are intercut with Sharon speaking on the beach. I videotaped her one afternoon as she stood on the rocks looking at the ocean. The crashing waves forced me to stand directly in front of her with the Camcorder. In tight close-up the microphone mixed her words harmoniously with the ocean's steady beat.

She speaks of the way the ocean purifies her, washes her clean. AIDS' toll has been enormous on her, bringing the death of countless friends, and the illness and death of more family members than I often have the will to contemplate. She goes to the beach at the Far Rockaways "to get lost:" to lose herself in the breeze, waves, and the roar of airplanes taking off; to momentarily lose her memories, her duties; to get the strength to pick up and do it again (figure 16).

The first meeting of the Women's AIDS Video Enterprise was a nervous encounter. Suddenly, all of these real women were sitting around the table with me. I had to make them like me. I had to make them want to come back next week. I didn't know how carefully I needed to trod the AIDS territory. Could I say the word?

The participants had been recruited by BATF, specifically by Glenda (their employee who was to be an administrative liaison between the group and the agency, while also participating as a group member). All I knew about the women sitting expectantly (reservedly?) around the table was that they were concerned enough about AIDS to have both tapped into BATF and to have found the idea of a group like this one appealing. They each had signed a contract accepting the terms of the project: a $15 weekly payment, carfare, child care, and a six-month commitment. "Things were better than I could've imagined—because they were real, real women—with their uniqueness, their own intelligence, their own stories, their own limitations.

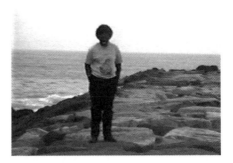

Figure 16   Sharon
Penceal, *Self-Portraits*
(WAVE, 1990).

They *all* were dynamic, committed, for real and personal reasons. Proud. So different from my usual crowd—some parts so similar to me" (excerpt from my journal, March 24, 1990).

We went around the table and explained why we were there. This process was rewarding, but not easy, for our backgrounds were both challengingly dissimilar and surprisingly the same. I said I was hoping to make a new, useful, effective AIDS video. I hoped we would get to know each other, learn about AIDS, discuss AIDS' impact on our lives and our communities, learn how to think critically about media, and learn how to use the camera, microphones, and lights so that we could make an important contribution to the limited body of AIDS media. Aida spoke of family members she had lost as well as of discrimination and fear in her neighborhood. Glenda wanted to learn how to make tapes. Sharon's brother had died the week before, and she was both angry and depressed. Carmen started to cry when she explained that her husband was HIV-infected. Juanita, a volunteer for BATF, once had aspirations to be a filmmaker. She said this project joined two of her greatest interests. People were tense, wary, not sure if they should give. The room felt cold. Everyone was jittery. Yet only with hindsight do I know how truly distrustful the participants were—of each other, but mostly of white, professional, nervous me.

After a bagel and coffee break we watched two videos, BATF's *Mildred Pearson* (1988) and AIDSFilm's *Are You With Me?* (1989). "Had to make people see and talk about media other than as content or as jumping off point for personal history. Should one want to? Is this enough?" I wrote in my journal that day. As the weeks went by, people got better at looking "my way"—beyond content, at why something was made the way it was, not just at what it said. Basically, though, we were always drawn to tapes that created or recorded the power of a personal connection to AIDS, the power of real passion, commitment or grief, regardless of the form. Thus, we talked a lot about the different effectivities of documentary or scripted work. Which form best allowed for this power? Which would we choose? We discussed what it meant to make something "community-specific." Did videos made for specific communities actually encourage and exaggerate cultural stereotypes? Juanita commented that in *Vida* by AIDSFilms, all the Latino characters wear crosses around their necks, the man is macho and irresponsible, the woman is a single mother and lives with her single mother. She said this confirmed racist assumptions about families of people of color. Aida said it looked like her house. I said, it looked nothing like where I grew up, but that issues which the characters were confronting made sense to me—how to negotiate using a condom with a resistant lover, for instance.

After the first week I returned home (as I found I would do for the following twenty-one weeks) extraordinarily spent. So much responsibility, too much coffee. I was responsible for everything going well, but I was also responsible for not using too controlling a hand. I was responsible for this thing to work—for a video, a good video, to come out of this hodgepodge of faces, this jumble of stories. I was responsible for the grant money, and for buying breakfast. After our second meeting I wrote, "And I feel my own prejudices fall into place as I doubt my desire to be *friends* with these women outside the project. Is this okay? I wonder about my own lack of sensitivity when I thought I could enter this world, ask to know their problems, and then not give on a larger level than my weekly meetings. *Is* this my responsibility as filmmaker, human, friend?" But after even that first meeting, I realized one other thing: they were responsible, too. Responsible enough to have devoted most of a Saturday to AIDS education, personal empowerment, and contributing to altering the course of the epidemic by leaving kids and lovers, warm beds, and late breakfasts. *They* would take up some of the responsibilities for the project's success because it was their project, too.

Glenda has piles of snapshots of herself and her loved ones which she shuffled and organized endlessly, preparing to shoot: five pastel baby faces smiling, she and a friend posing at the beach, her mother dressed to party. She put the camera right up to those photographs, and, after finally making sense of the macro-lens, her chosen images filled the frame.

Then, she interviewed her coworkers at the Brooklyn AIDS Task Force. "How do you see me?" she asks. "Skinny. Funny. Smart. Moody. Into music. Into your church," they say.

Glenda and I met one afternoon and edited together her self-portrait.

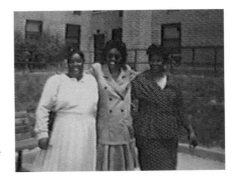

Figure 17   Glenda
Smith-Hasty and
family, *Self-Portraits*
(WAVE, 1990).

We edited their comments about her in succession. But she frames these interviews with a musical and pictorial montage.

Her portrait begins with the song "Lean on Me," illustrated by her many images in photographs. At its end, quite artistically I assure her, the self-portrait closes with the end of the song, accompanied by the blurred and lilting images taken of her by her mother, after she received a brief lesson in Camcorder operations from Glenda. Glenda mugs to the camera, smiles at her mother, and is lost from view as the camera wiggles, swings down, and finally pans the room to find Glenda again as she sticks out her tongue (figure 17).

The first hour of our weekly session was usually devoted to the support group. Marcia, a social worker, led this part of the meeting, although she was a member of the group as well. However, on some weeks (our second meeting, for example), conversation filled the full three hours. "We talked and talked—a lot—too much," I said in my journal entry of that week. "Filled the time allotment. But I figured, especially early on, getting to know each other, to loosen up, is more important than the 'real work.'"

The function and importance of the support group facet of the project cannot be stressed enough. Here, we found a comfortable and comforting place from which to speak about and face the private and difficult issues which are raised for us as women, people of color, people affected by AIDS. The kinds of issues we articulated in our final videotape are not easy to speak about in public; they are private and painful. It took comfort with the camera and talking aloud about these things to equip us for the deeply intimate interviews we gave. Furthermore, it was here, in our long and dangerous meetings, that we began to understand something much more than our individual problems. We also started to discern who we were as a group,

in relation to each other. We talked about what our "community" could be—
the WAVE community, the seven women we were. The power relations of
this project were complicated—who speaks for whom? But the response to
this realization, if at first fear, subsequently led to discussion. For when we
talked, we learned things about our similarities and differences and about
the numerous deployments of "power" throughout the group. For some of
the members of the group had (and still have) more money than I did, and
some less; many of the group had suffered the losses of AIDS more than I
had, while others had lost less. And if I had more words to contribute about
critical theory or media production, the others as quickly responded with
ideas and expertise of their own. Only by talking could we begin to explore
our similarities. Only by talking could we get to the more complicated place
of comprehending the differences *within* our similarities.

For example, we spent one session discussing sexism in the workplace for the full three hours. After we had shared experiences ranging from
practical jokes (a bucket of water poured from a doortop onto a shirt, making
it see-through), to more angry symbols of distrust (a tampon on a desk: you
must be on the rag), we agreed that as much as feminism had allowed us these
possibilities for work, it had not altered many of the conditions which define
interactions between men and women. We also began to understand that
some working environments are more sexist than others. Another session
was devoted to a discussion of racism. We moved again during the course
of this discussion from the experiential details which mar all of our daily
lives to larger conclusions about the society we live in. We discussed how
few opportunities we have had to spend time with women who are of different ethnicities from ours, let alone to become friends, to become intimate.
And a great deal of pleasure was taken in talking about stereotypes about
whiteness—how I proved them untrue, and often, just to tease or "read" me,
how I confirmed them. Few opportunities in my life have offered me the opportunity to reflect upon the impact of racism within a space that was both
interracial and safe, where there was room to tease, to push, to question, to
hear. At our reunions, the girls continue to poke at me lovingly about my
white, skinny body wearing outrageous clothes and standing out in group
photographs. So much is worked out in these remarks; I remain an outsider
as I am drawn right in.

In the WAVE group we were all vulnerable, we were all safe. What
endangered us, what we were scared of, what hurt, what we could make fun
of, was different for each one of us. During our second meeting we spoke

about disease, illness, death, how to go on. Sharon, after talking about her brother, her many other infected family members, and the thirty or so friends she had lost, asked, "What's it all for?" This was simply my first taste of the high pitch of catastrophe and crisis from which my own class privilege had sheltered me. Sabatier comments on class issues and crisis in her book on worldwide AIDS. "AIDS is in reality the latest crisis to emerge besides all these other epidemics—of infant mortality and malnutrition, of stds and other infectious diseases, of heart disease, stroke and diabetes, of alcohol and drug misuse or psychological distress and social disruption—which disproportionately affect the globally disadvantaged." [15] Over the course of six months together, the seven of us faced more personal tragedies than my family and friends will confront in twenty years. Babies falling out of highrises and dying. Child and wife battering. Teenagers hit by cars, AIDS deaths, unwanted miscarriages, fathers with heart ailments, brain tumors. What I also saw, however, was, if not an ease, then an acceptance of crisis and death as a part of life also unmatched in "my community." If class privilege allows most of my family and friends to lead long, relatively healthy lives, it also allows us to avoid mortality and the incorporation of disease and death into the normal cycles of life. First for middle-class gay white men, and then for others of privilege, AIDS has thrown a wrench into our tidy expectations about life. However, for society's less privileged, AIDS is just one more insult, just one more catastrophe, illness, upset among a life already full of them. "How to answer the question of Sharon: what's it all for? She didn't have an answer—and mine, to get out your heart, soul, knowledge, love into the world, was superficial and bourgeois in her world of death and disease. Who am I, with my privileged relationship to life, to communicate my world vision to her? I have no answers, and can frankly not even hear what she says about her own pain—I've had so little of it" (March 31, 1990). Of course, AIDS brings crisis into my life. I used the group to learn to gear up for my own AIDS pain. I taught the women how to use the camera; they taught me how to confront the disease and possible death of loved ones.

At the end of the second session I asked everyone to take a turn recording someone else's brief "hello." It was unclear what was scarier—to say something, unrehearsed, before the others and the camera or to pick up the camera and make it work right. Humor, silliness, and uproarious laughter were the responses. Juanita pretended to do a commercial, Glenda spoke "street," I jumped onto a table and begged permission to come down, Sharon admitted that "she loved the camera, the camera was hers." However, after our six months of taping, people relaxed on both sides of the camera. Practice, familiarity, and noticeable improvement grant technical confidence to those who initially resist.

For her self-portrait, I shot Aida lounging on a white sofa in her two-bedroom apartment in Bensonhurst. She wore no makeup, had not done her hair, and chose on a hot July evening to be taped in a loose T-shirt. Although she called attention to this several times before shooting, and then again when we were editing, she felt no urge to formalize our interaction.

For a good forty-five minutes—interrupted only by a quick check of her dinner simmering on the stove—Aida spoke candidly and articulately about her past, her goals, the changes she's gone through, her beliefs. She credits her seven-year-old son, Miguel, with giving her purpose and strength, even when things were at their worst. A single and young mother who left home at sixteen, Aida has gone through a lot. And it's only recently, she informs me, that she's turned into the responsible, giving person I now know. "I give a lot of love," she explains. "Even if I don't get any back."

In her edited self-portrait, after she refers to Miguel, Aida cuts to footage she shot of him sitting on the stoop.

"What does your Mommy like to do?" she asks him.

"Well, she likes to listen to music. Spanish music sometimes. And she likes to sit outside. . . . And drink."

"Mikey!" She stops the camera. "Answer again. You can't say that."

But later, when we are all watching the footage, helping each other edit our self-portraits, everyone agrees that that interaction must be left in its entirety (figure 18).

The last two hours of our meetings, under my supervision, were dedicated to video education, both how to use our camera, microphone, and lights, and how to think about AIDS media critically. We watched many tapes about AIDS and videotaped ourselves discussing these tapes' values, shortcomings, assumptions, targeted audiences, stereotypes, formal strategies. One week we compared my *Women and AIDS* (1988) to an NBC News Special *Life, Death and AIDS* (1986). As usual, the group criticized the broadcast media. Although they were quick to condemn the News Special ("Tom Brokaw's not talking from knowledge, just off a piece of paper," said Sharon), I also encouraged people to critique my work. Too many issues covered, too many concerns, it left you confused, a little daunted, they said. Perhaps this is one of the reasons why our tape, *We Care*, is so clearly focused, so specific

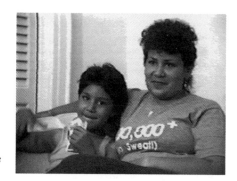

Figure 18   Aida Matta
and Miguel, *Self-Portraits*
(WAVE, 1990).

in its intended use and purpose. As we watched AIDS tapes, preparing to make our own, I was always pounding two questions into everyone's head. Who's it for? What's it for?

We also had visitors who discussed theories of representation, their own alternative AIDS media, or the factual information we needed to know about AIDS. We taped these presentations, constantly increasing the pool of images available for our final videotape. Also, in preparation for our final project we did a series of short exercises to familiarize ourselves with the equipment as well as with a range of possible formal strategies. Our self-portraits were the last of these exercises. We also taped role-plays (a lesbian couple learns that one partner is HIV-positive), scripted scenarios (two children argue about how HIV is transmitted, and their mother corrects them), our own conversations, the building where we were meeting and its surroundings, interviews on the street, public presentations by our members, the Gay Men's Health Crisis' AIDS Walk. These weekly exercises were extremely important, making us delve deeply into a small project, enjoying the pride of completion, learning from self-critique.[16]

However, on the third week nothing like these things occurred, because nobody came. It was snowing. It was gray and cold. I knew I had blown it. Scared them off. Bored them. Things were too heavy too fast.

> The problem. Oh the problem. No one came. No one. Aida and Carmen called, and finally we called Sharon and Juanita. People are sick, babies are sick. Sharon seems to be depressed. I'm not sure if I should take it personally (I failed/the project failed) or work this all into the reality of this project which involves women who have *a lot* of other worries and responsibilities—and to also remember

that this feeling unsure about the group is a natural (not necessarily bad) part of the whole deal. I'll call everyone this week. As long as they come back, this may be good for us. A break. (April 7, 1990)

After this week, I broke down a lot of my resistance and ambivalence about communicating with the members of the group outside our Saturday meetings. They needed to know I was their friend. I needed to know the same. On April 14 I wrote, "I called people over the week, and that seemed to make a big difference. *My* initiative to break down that line. There is an answer to that responsibility question: I do have a responsibility to follow through." These calls began a still continuing relay of phone conversations that goes on between all of us to this day. For a lot of fear was raised by the project. Fear that during the "support" part of the group we were exposing too much. Fear about our abilities to succeed in this important undertaking. Fear about making the tape, and ending the group. The calls were to confirm our abilities, to remind us about the others' friendship, to buoy worried spirits, to support in times of duress.

Finally, the calls brought about the event which settled my qualms about the group's viability more or less for good. During Week Thirteen a small coup occurred on the phone in regard to the proper role of Marcia, the social worker. "There's a little discontent brewing (and articulated) among the masses (Juanita, Aida, Carmen). No more psychoanalyzing they say! We came to learn about AIDS. After more talk, it seems that several have been hurt by Marcia's straight (personal, opinionated) advice/analysis" (June 16, 1990). This was all expressed to Marcia, and she pulled back. Things had gotten too heavy, which was not what people wanted. If it was upsetting that people were bothered by aspects of the group, I also saw this interaction as a claim on group ownership. My leadership, Marcia's leadership, had been challenged and overturned. This was *our* group. Its shape and definition were the concerns of every one of us.

Juanita went to sva *(School of Visual Arts) in New York City for a year, many years ago. That touch of filmmaking has never left her, and it is one motivation behind her participation in our group. Her self-portrait documents many aspects of herself, including her long love of film, poetry, and other literature. As her voice reads one of her poems ("Misery Dane," the poem's title, is also her pen name), images of herself, her home, family, political concerns, and favorite books pop in and out with her use of stop-action technology. Piles of books grow and shrink on her bureau.*

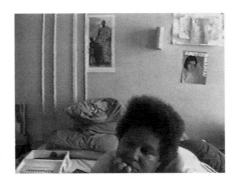

Figure 19   Juanita Mo-
hammed, *Self-Portraits*
(WAVE, 1990).

"Books are the things I crave. Books give me lives, new and old."

Then, it's her family we see, jumping rhythmically to her stop-action recording. Husband, daughter, and son, posed on a colorful couch, shift position, form new pairs at her whim. "Things appear, things disappear," she says.

At one point her two-year old son, Shah, appears, hugging a book entitled AIDS in the Mind of America. *Juanita's voice-over says, "My life's ambition, to help people understand AIDS."*

But mostly her self-portrait concentrates on her image as she changes, quickly and repeatedly, using costumes, glasses, wigs, and other props. Momentary glimpses of her lying on her bed, eating a sandwich, reading a book, wrapped in a sari, are replaced with a mocking pose as she reclines on a couch. "I'm weird. I guess you're not," says her voice, which concludes, "Misery Dane, that's my name" (figure 19).

The camera gave all of us, if Juanita especially, the power to organize and control the small details of the bedroom, bookshelf, and family—something that is often difficult for women in "real life." Books and self-image rearranged, children on the fly, the camcorder gave Juanita an opportunity to express herself as a strong black woman, activist and worker, mother and wife, reader and writer. And this capability of expressing herself has continued beyond the time span of the project for everyone, if for Juanita most of all—she bought her own camcorder, then volunteered at AIDSFilms, and is now producing segments for GMHC's "Living With AIDS Show." She and her daughter, Jahanara, have formed the production company Mother/Daughter Productions and have completed several tapes together.

A camcorder is not difficult to operate. With practice, the images become stable, the framing centered. Carmen uses her father's camera to record family gatherings, her daughter's kindergarten graduation. Willy, her husband, told me she had learned a lot. She knows words and does things with the camera he had never heard or thought of. "You know, she could take a media arts course," he said in the interview I shot of the two of them for our final tape. "She has ideas." Carmen blushed, but looked pleased. After Juanita acquired her camera, she began scheduling and shooting countless interviews. Her city councilman, her neighbors, her colleagues. She has tape after tape of interviews, and she ended up supplying nearly half the final footage for *We Care.*

WAVE was about a series of empowerments. Feeling better about oneself as an individual among a community of women with similar concerns. Feeling good about oneself for making an important, valuable, and professional videotape, which others use and like. Feeling good about oneself for having a skill that can be applied as often as one wishes outside the organized group, even after the project is completed. Walk down any street, go to any event, even turn on the TV, and see "real" people shooting small, lightweight consumer cameras. And, after watching *Our Favorite Home Videos* (showing viewers yet another tripping mailman or baby tipping over), remember that all "the people" need is a real project to work on, a real purpose for their work, to make something like *We Care,* as well as their goofy home videos.

Marcia's self-portrait raises questions of aesthetics and politics. Days before we shot, she made a collage of magazine images, handprinted words, a pair of earrings, the cutout names of black female authors, the initials of her loved ones. These items are glued or printed upon a rectangle of white tagboard. Glenda panned the camera over the particulars of Marcia's life made small and neat on one sheet of paper. Later, we taped, then edited in, Marcia's voice as she explained how she composed her self-portrait.

She says how hard it was for her to think about her own life in this objective way. Ultimately, she decided to split her life into three significant pieces: her friends and family, her work, her interests outside work. For all of her initial trepidation, she comes off as the incredibly motivated, together, and independent woman she is, dictating with confidence her ambitions, her qualifications, her desires (figure 20).

The documentation of the life of one black woman—"MSW" tells her degree, "JR" identifies her boyfriend, her name in big, black letters "MARCIA," holds the center of the white field—is both beautifully personal

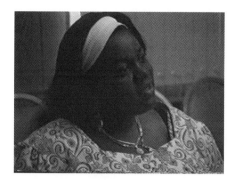

Figure 20   Marcia
Edwards, *Self-Portraits*
(WAVE, 1990).

and desperately political. In a culture where the privilege of self-expression
and its public articulation depends upon financial and social privilege, the
voice of each black woman describing herself, her life, her work, her needs,
especially in media, is political.

This is not to say that all of the women in the group define what we
are doing as "political." In many ways, at least on initial discussion, these
women would define themselves as defiantly apolitical, uninterested in the
disruption and anger of politics, seeking instead a stable comfort and local
improvement. If anything, the political dis-ease of the postmodern condition
hits the already culturally disenfranchised hardest. For they best understand
the overwhelming distance that separates individuals from political and economic power. The women in WAVE may not want to picket or march about
an issue, but we still have much to say. We watch TV, and we read news-
papers and magazines, and we know that our stories are not being told. We
note bias and distortion, prejudice and stereotyping, even as we take note
of the news that is being reported or the TV soap opera that endlessly plays
on. We know that a black woman is thirteen times more likely to have AIDS
than her white counterpart, and that a Latina is nine times more likely.[17] We
know that AIDS is political. Give us a camcorder, and this is what we say,
call it what you will.

Carmen did not have the chance to produce her self-portrait. Her
husband had not been feeling well, and she decided that her Saturdays were
better spent with him and her daughters.
We told her to come back when things became easier at home.

Neither was Carmen with us for our editing sessions, but everyone
else made it. Until this point (Weeks 14–15), we had shot everything in long

take or edited within the camera. But, the self-portraits were different. We were to conceive of these projects on our own, with the promise of editing defining their conception. Some people shot their tapes during the Saturday meetings, others took the camera home. I shot Aida at her apartment, Juanita shot me at BATF. Then I bullied over and over, "Log your tapes, it'll make editing so much easier."

If there is any part of video production which I obsess over, it is editing. I love to edit. Sitting in that artificially lit room for unclockable hours, scrutinizing and moving with the most minute technical precision little moments of once real time. I am precise in my imprecision in the editing room, and I usually cannot deal with intrusions from realtime, be they in the form of people, phone calls, or breaks. And yet, there I was, with six women crammed into a room, all of us editing our self-portraits, often with no real plan about what shot would follow another. I worked the machines, but the ideas came from the group. Theirs was a highly literate grasp of the power of editing; people used the cut not simply as a mark of progression, but of opposition, expansion, comparison. The self-portrait maker would turn to the others and ask their opinion. Should I make this cut here, or should the take run longer?

During the editing of *We Care* my blind dedication to editing as a private affair was shattered for good. Although, in this case, I arrived in the editing room with typed lists, game plans for organization, ideas about the shape of the final tape, I learned the most simple lesson about other strategies of editing. For, obviously enough, the ideas and brainstorms of a group of people are ever more expansive than the plans of one individual. We made up things as a group in the editing room that I could not have thought up on my own. Of course, this slowed the process (again, the reason why this kind of work is inconceivable with mainstream media deadlines), but it expanded the process at the same time. The idea for using the poem "We Care" was that of our intern, Kimberly Everett, who came to the project from Women Make Movies. We needed something to pull our diverse ideas together. We needed a different kind of footage from the talking heads which made up the bulk of the tape. The definitive mark of our tape—its title, and the reading of the poem which inspires it—was conceived after the fact of production, during editing.

And for me? In my self-portrait, the camera allowed me to obsess over my body. Funnily enough, most of my fellow self-portraitists cast themselves out of the picture—as voice-over, photograph, other's description. But

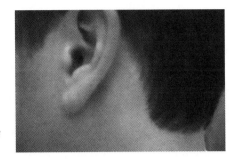

Figure 21   Alex
Juhasz, *Self-Portraits*
(WAVE, 1990).

*if this would have suited me in earlier times, during the WAVE project I could
not help but be obsessed with images of my own body, what with this virus
ever on the peripheries of my vision — in my work, in my friends, potentially
in me. In my self-portrait, images of my old body, from photographs, are
juxtaposed against too-close and very ugly images of my skin, my knee, my
hand. I used to want this body to hold the shape of me, but now I'm not
quite so sure. If that body holds antibodies that are not me, then I scream
to denounce its form. This is what I say in the poem I read over my images
(figure 21).*

I was uncertain about the reaction to my words, my AIDS, as I recorded my poem and my skin on a Saturday, I wondered if my ideas, my
feminism, were useful for the other participants in the group. As much as
I say in these pages that we were honest and open with each other, that
WAVE was safe, I also need to emphasize how closed and calculated this
honesty could be. There were many things about myself which I tried to
keep hidden — aspects of my life-style, aspects of my politics. Perhaps they
seeped through. Who knows? My hesitancy to expose myself came as much
from my understandings of who the other women in WAVE were (rightly or
wrongly) as they did from my understanding of myself (rightly or wrongly).
I crafted the personality which was Alex-at-WAVE in response to the personalities who were Juanita-at-WAVE and Glenda-at-WAVE. My self-portrait
made me feel vulnerable because I spoke in a different voice when I made
it: Alex-at-home, Alex-afraid, Alex-the-academic, Alex-the-AIDS-activist.

The complex power relations which occur when the filmmaker, the
teacher, that person who is typically *outside* the group, is also an *insider*,
even as she retains her status as outsider, is the focus of much experimental ethnographic film, embodied especially in the work of Trinh T. Minh-ha,
who has stated, "Undercutting the insider/outsider opposition, her interven-

tion is necessarily that of both deceptive insider and deceptive outsider. She is the inappropriate Other/Same who moves about with always at least 2/4 questions: that of affirming 'I am like you,' while protecting her difference, and that of remaining herself: 'I am different,' while unsettling every difference of otherness."[18] I would never want to deny that I was the teacher, the director; I had certain knowledge that I wanted to share. I had real skills that I contributed (my ability to raise funds, my knowledge about equipment and the media). But in so many ways I was the learner, and in so many ways I was willing and hoping to disperse the power typically offered to me in the position of director. My hope was not to get outside the dynamics of power created by ethnicity or race, access to knowledge or equipment, but to multiply and feed the complex weavings of power that define any interaction. I wanted to begin to take account of a videomaking process where *all* of the participants, not only the white director, are deceptive insiders and outsiders. I know that it is too easy for the onus of responsibility for this project to be placed on my shoulders or to be taken up by me (because I am white, because I initially raised the funds, because I directed the project), even as it would be too easy to say that I was "an equal" participant in the making of this project (because I am white, because I initially raised the funds, because I directed the project). The making of identity and community, across difference, through video production, acknowledges the impact of binaries of power, even as it collapses them. How else to work together?

Because I make WAVE into words here, because I have that privilege, or desire, or skill, we invariably hear my concerns, my viewpoint, my issues. I am well aware of this control, how this control mirrors other controls I had during the production process. Yet in the video production process, control was much more dispersed than it could ever be in writing. This, obviously, is another reason why committed artists choose to make their work in video.

We Care: A Video for Care Providers of People Affected by AIDS

We Care begins with a poem of the same name by our in-house poet, Misery Dane. She wrote it for an AIDS awareness day sponsored by BATF, which the group documented. When we were all sitting in the editing room deciding if we wanted music in our tape, and what kind, Kimberly (our intern from Women Make Movies) remembered the poem. We rerecorded it, and it is now the central, organizing force of the tape. All of our voices say the refrain, "We Care." Sharon's deep, resonant voice reads the poem's stanzas, "We care for people, people with AIDS. Why do we care you might ask? We care because people with AIDS are people like us. . . ." This poem is repeated twice more in the tape, playing under titles like a song with a familiar refrain.

The reading and meaning of the poem also make up the most literal site within the text that embodies and formalizes the collective production of the project. The tape has no narrator, no narrative voice, but the power that organizes it is the poem, and the poem brings the sounds of the many voices of the group into unison. Viewers have said that this harmonious voice then affects the way they see the tape's images, because these images are also then understood as a collective vision; no one hand selects what and how we see. This is a fair interpretation of a tape that was shot over six months by seven sets of hands. Its collective nature is a definitive feature in both the content and form of our video.

We decided to make a tape for care providers for two reasons which illuminate how the production of community media makes good education while also serving as a vehicle for the reproduction of community and personal identity. Having seen many alternative AIDS videos, we knew that virtually nothing had been produced for the ever-expanding population of people who are care providers. And we knew that the most effective media we had seen had a very specific and explicit agenda as media that announced its use value, that made explicit its address and intended audience. Secondly, as a group of seven diverse women, each profoundly affected by AIDS, the one thing that we held in common, which made us a community from which to shoot video, was that we were all care providers ourselves. This common place from, and to, which we spoke cut across the class, ethnic, and educational backgrounds that "split" us, and instead it bound us together in what we knew and in the concerns and experiences we had in common.

We sat down one afternoon and wrote down all the things we thought a person would need to know when just finding out that someone was HIV-positive or had AIDS. Those suggestions organized the tape. We distributed these sequences to teams of two to tape. Juanita giving advice to volunteers. Glenda and Sharon explaining available services. Marcia discussing issues around death and dying. A doctor giving her opinions. Sharon's lover, Marie, a fifty-year-old, HIV-positive black woman, giving a guided tour of her apartment. On-the-street interviews. A group discussion. The tape is organized into informative sections that focus on the advice of care providers themselves. Typically, a section's speaker will introduce herself to the camera and to the anticipated audience of AIDS care providers before speaking. The group used video as a method to record dialogue for an anticipated and acknowledged audience. The form of the tape reflects the concept of explicit, local address. "Hi, I'm Glenda, and this is Sharon. We're going to tell you about some of the services available to you if someone you know is newly diagnosed with AIDS." In the outtakes of this sequence, which are included in *A WAVE Taster,* we see Glenda and Sharon debating this atypical sort of media presence. "Am I supposed to know her?" "Who are we supposed to be?" asks Sharon. "Yeah, you know me," answers Glenda. "We are ourselves." This is our highly recognizable style: speaking to the audience members as if they are part of our group, speaking ourselves as if we are a member of this group, as if we are ourselves.

A most powerful example of this "as-if-ourselves" direct address is the sequence called "Being at Home with HIV." A direct cut from this title opens to an image of a beautiful and strong middle-aged black woman who looks into the camera and says, "Hi. I'm Marie, and I'm HIV-positive. I'd like to take you on a tour of my apartment and show you what has and has not changed, now that I'm positive." In a society where, because of discrimination and misinformation, it is almost impossible to be "out" with HIV as a middle-aged woman, Marie's comfort with the project is evident in her willing address and tour of her home. The camera is intimate, the eight-minute tour virtually uncut as she takes us through her living room, bathroom, and bedroom. The long take validates her knowledge and her emotions. We respect her work, we respect her words, we leave them unedited. In fact, all of the major sections of the tape are left almost entirely uncut. A person has something to say, and the camera records her saying it. "This is my living room. It's the same as it's always been. I need a new carpet, but that's another story."

The intimacy of the encounter makes evident a relationship between camera person and interviewee rarely seen in mainstream media. In fact, mainstream interviews typically take only one of two tactics. The interviewee speaks directly into the camera as if there is no camera, or the interviewee speaks to an interviewer, also included in the image. *We Care* uses neither of these conventions in its many talking-head interviews. Spectators of the tape have commented on the unusual "looks" in this section and others. Often the speaker does not look into the camera but at another person in the room. This constructs a pro-filmic reality that includes both the presence of the camera (and the audience-to-be it stands in for) and the other people participating in the taping event. In the case of Marie's interview, Sharon and I stood in the room and behind the camera. Marie spoke to her lover, as much as to the camera. Again, the group dynamic which organized the making of the tape organizes its form as well. We construct a shot which records a group, which *is* a group that itself brings the spectator into this collective, safe space.

To counter the rhythm and seriousness of the informative segments, we constructed six "Myth" breaks, which work to dispel dangerous myths about AIDS while adding a lighter, faster, and more "high-tech" look to the tape. These segments are highly edited with fancy effects (wipes, dissolves, freezes, an image that "blows up"). They begin with an image of my hand opening a book entitled *The Book of AIDS Myths.* The misinformed words of on-the-street interviews (or us, speaking the words we heard during interviews) are what you see and hear on the book's "first page." The footage which records people imparting incorrect information is continuously identified as *myth* by graphic effects like a big red "X" or a flashing "myth" sign. Then the incorrect statement—"You can get AIDS by drinking out of the same glass as them . . ."—is wiped off the screen. The page is turned. Another response wipes on, spoken by other on-the-street interviewees or by members of the group. An interview with Carmen and her husband, Willy, is often highlighted in these sections. "Sure, everyone's afraid of AIDS. I'd be lying if I said I wasn't. But I know how you get it, see?" Then the book slams shut, but it is now called *The Book of AIDS Facts.*

Criticism from some spectators of the tape about our presentation of "AIDS facts" reveals both the nature of the AIDS "industry" and the difficulties of cross-community education.[19] There is understandable contention in the AIDS community about what AIDS "facts" are (i.e., many believe that AIDS is not caused by HIV; some say that Saran wrap is not safe for oral sex). But, beyond these disagreements, the different politics of AIDS education, as people try to reach different communities, has created many different "languages" with which to talk to people. For instance, when Carmen says that she knows how people are infected, she explains that this is through "sex" or "using drugs." Many AIDS educators would insist upon using the terms "*unprotected* sex" or "*shared* needles" to make sure not to feed hysteria. But Carmen knows that people can have sex and can use drugs safely (she has lived with someone who is HIV-positive and is not HIV-infected herself), and this is what she says when she calmly articulates *her* education with *her* words. To challenge the way that Carmen offers the knowledge she has about HIV and AIDS would be to challenge the very expertise that is established by allowing her to speak on-camera. It is clear from community screenings of the tape that one of the reasons spectators hear these facts and insights in a new and powerful way is precisely because the speakers in the tape are *not* speaking like AIDS educators.

Another example occurs when Marie says that she does not let her three-year-old granddaughter use her towels. Many AIDS educators would insist that this statement perpetuates the incorrect information that HIV could be spread in this way. However, I believe (as did the several AIDS educators in the group) that her larger message (that you do not need to uproot your life to account for living with a person who is HIV-positive) overrides the "incorrect" information she provides about how she chooses to live—quite comfortably—with HIV-negative relatives as someone who is HIV-positive. To cut out this statement or other statements she made would be to radically question the very "expertise" that is constructed by allowing her to explain what she knows as she says it and knows it.

When watching other AIDS tapes (particularly those of the mainstream media), the women in the group were constantly explaining that the people in them were not "real." "Real" means many things, and one of them has to do with proximity to information. "Experts" are not real because they know about things from a distance—from reading or studying, but not from living or experiencing. Marie is real because she knows about "Being at Home with HIV" from doing it herself. A white male doctor reading all of the precautions one needs or does not need to know would provide an entirely different manner of education from Marie's tour. It might be "true," but it would not be real. The power of Carmen as educator is her real relationship to the virus. This realness is made evident in her uncorrected speech, her evident nervousness and her clear commitment to the ideas she espouses, all marked by the courage it took for her and her husband to talk about HIV on-camera. This is particularly important in light of this book's earlier discussion of distance, realism, and reality. In *We Care,* knowledge is closeness; reality is the *lack* of authority.

The tape speaks the voices of people who are living with this crisis: calm if sad, but also strong, loving, unafraid. For people who are not yet living with this disease, these voices testify to both AIDS' centrality in the lives of many communities and, sadly but importantly, to its normalcy. For people who are living with the epidemic, the voices are reassuring and stable; they identify a community. Thus, a binding together took place across boundaries of difference in our construction of the tape as well as in our conception of our audience. We made a tape assuming that the majority of our spectators, like the producers of the tape, would be urban women of color affected by AIDS. We assumed that they would be people wanting to know more, and people who would also benefit (as we had done) from a sense of community. We assumed our audience would share experiences with us, share our concerns. That is why the audience would choose to watch a tape with this title.

When I watch the tape, I know to whom it *will* speak, and I wonder for whom it will not speak. On its own terms, WAVE succeeded. *We Care* is community-produced, community-specific video that speaks loudly and lovingly to people who are similar to those who made it—a tape *I* could *never* have made on my own. All of the participants in the tape are people of color, except for me and the counselor who models deep breathing to relieve stress. Are people outside this community equally moved, educated, entertained by *We Care?* Are artists and mediamakers as interested in the process as I am? Are cultural outsiders intrigued by this access to a community other than their own? These are the kinds of questions that audiences answer. Addressing and learning from the actual needs of real viewers is what alternative distribution and exhibition is all about.

Distribution and Exhibition: September 1990–Present

But if we think about art in relation to the AIDS epidemic—in relation, that is, to the communities most drastically affected by AIDS, especially the poor and minority communities where AIDS is spreading much faster than elsewhere—we will realize that no work made within the confines of the art world as it is currently constituted will reach the people. Activist art therefore involves questions not only of the nature of cultural production, but also of the location, or the means of distribution, of that production.—Douglas Crimp [20]

WAVE, as an example of "AIDS activist art," challenges conventional notions about the nature, function, and production of ART, because it displaces—or traces—the meaning of art from production to exhibition. *We Care* was made to be needed by its makers *and* its spectators. And *We Care* most wants to be seen by the very people who are left unaddressed by the art market, the art world, the art museum. Thus, in its self-selection of audience—care providers of people affected by AIDS—our project must challenge the traditional mechanisms and economics of distribution. Our tape, *We Care,* not only wants to be seen, it intends to contribute to change. WAVE's videotape is one in a history of what Thomas Waugh calls "the committed documentary," because a self-aware focus on the possible political effects of distribution plays a major role in the nature of the project: "They are all works of art, but they are not merely works of art (although some have been reduced to this role); they must be seen also as films made by activists speaking to specific publics to bring about specific political goals." [21]

The history of film includes many such projects that emphasize distribution and exhibition because of a commitment to the process of change. Dziga Vertov writes of "film-cars" on trains and "film-wagons" to get films to the isolated peoples of the Soviet Union in the 1920s. [22] Producers of the Third Cinema like Octavio Solanas and Fernando Getino emphasize the revolutionary potential of the screening itself which "provokes with each showing, as in a revolutionary military incursion, a liberated space, a *decolonized territory.* The showing can be turned into a kind of political event." [23] And John Downing argues that Newsreel became increasingly attentive to screenings: "The basic concept, however, was a vital one and clearly defined Newsreel's commitment to the political *use* of film. . . . Newsreel began to argue that the film should never stand alone and the structure of the screening has as much priority as the structure of the film . . . the viewing event itself (became) a vital part of the politics of filmmaking." [24]

To understand art as a means toward social change is to understand "art as a verb": [25] to plan for art's *use,* not only its funding and production. Understanding art as a process and not an object profoundly affects the nature of artistic production and theory. For example, the making of *We Care,* its look and structure, was organized by our intention to speak certain things to a certain kind of person—to communicate to "specific publics" about "specific political goals." "Progressive art, more than any other, has got to communicate," says Lucy Lippard. [26] Thus, to make or make sense of progressive art—art of communication—is to take seriously the work that occurs *after* the object is made. We would ask: "Will a person who just learned a friend is HIV-positive want to know this?" "Will people in our neighborhoods be comfortable with this?" Items were cut and added during editing because of what we assumed the impact of a sentence or a scene would be on our conjectured audience. Many clips were included in the final video which came from a particularly beat-up tape of interviews that Juanita had shot. The impact of the words transcended the technical imperfections of the footage. Meanwhile, the imperfections of the tape quality formally signified our commitment to saying this particular thing to our intended audience.

Projects like WAVE challenge traditional understandings of art not so much because of an oppositional formal composition or aesthetics, but more because they foster a link between the work of making and the work of viewing. I am not implying that WAVE does not have an aesthetic—our tapes look and are constructed differently from mainstream media—but this aesthetic is one of purpose, of expressiveness. Writing about the Third Cinema, Teshome Gabriel explains that "we are talking here of 'activist aesthetics' and 'critical spectatorship.' The relationship between the two has a distinctive form which accounts for the character of the aesthetics of third cinema. These aesthetics are, therefore, as much in the after-effect of the film as in the creative process itself. This is what makes the work memorable, by virtue of its everyday relevance."[27] The scratched-up look of some of the interviews we included in the tape *signifies* to an audience that the content of these interviews mattered most, that its "everyday relevance" was its art. We included them *even though* they were not perfectly clean, perfectly recorded, perfectly framed. These "unaesthetic" interviews said things that we thought people needed to hear. Their aesthetic was their relevance, as much as it was the realness signified by their lack of "professionalism" or "broadcast standards." For, when you think about it, what exactly is "wrong" with a video image with a little dropout, those lines which lack resolution and look like scratches in the image?

Furthermore, if art is a verb, this explains how, for WAVE, our art did not conclude with the final edit session, but only began anew. The process of artistic production was clearly rewarding to the participants in the group. However, the process of artistic distribution is proving to be so as well. We have proudly taken the tape around to agencies and organizations in our neighborhoods. We have shown it to our families, coworkers, and AIDS professionals. Artistic *expression* here means the tracing from production through distribution: How has the tape been watched? By whom? In what contexts? How does it feel to show it?

Not surprisingly then, nearly one half of WAVE's total budget was devoted to distribution and exhibition. Besides the twenty-plus screenings for our neighbors, coworkers, churches, and agencies which serve the populations we are trying to reach, we have made more than seven hundred dubs of the tape which we have distributed free or at low cost ($30). We have sent out flyers, put ads in AIDS service publications, and entered contests. The tape has played in film festivals, on cable and on broadcast television, in church basements and hospital waiting rooms.[28] Our project is first and foremost about communication: first among ourselves, then to our local community, and, finally, to anyone else who will listen. "Where the dominant cinema prioritized exchange value, oppositional filmmakers have emphasized use value," writes Julianna Burton.[29]

One of the reasons so few producers take up this relationship to their production is that it is no easy task, especially with video. A sort of schizophrenic impasse seems to exist in the educational video industry. Low-budget technology means that more and more tapes are being produced by more and more people; it also means that more and more organizations and individuals are using video in educational efforts. Staff meetings and in-services inevitably use video at some point in the program. But, not surprisingly, since the costs of video production (and purchase) are much lower than that of film, the distribution of video is much less lucrative than film distribution, and so much less developed as an industry. The tapes are there, but it is not so easy to find or sell them.

When factoring an AIDS video into the already small network of alternative distribution companies willing to distribute low-budget, progressive, educational video, things become even more difficult. Nonprofit or progressive distribution companies streamline their work by distributing tapes about, and to, particular communities: women, health care professionals, African Americans, Latinos, Asian-Americans, unions, museums, and galleries. An AIDS tape can be useful to all of these communities. Most alternative AIDS tapes require some complex interweaving of these particularized distribution networks—and this mechanism for distribution is not already in place.

Furthermore, the people who most need to see AIDS tapes like *We Care* are the disenfranchised members of our society who are not going to be reached by even the methods of progressive distribution which still channel the work they handle through institutions and organizations. Effective distribution of educational materials to the people most affected by AIDS means nothing less than grassroots distribution, which means nothing more than labor-intensive, pro-active strategies that take the tape to the people who need it. Which means, in reality, that most of the work must be done outside the well-worked grooves of professional distribution: the maker becomes distributor (but rarely gets paid for the job). The "Seeing Through AIDS" program is a novel response to these dilemmas. Created through the unheard-of union of a media organization, Media Network, and a city health agency, the New York City Department of Health, the program sponsors AIDS video workshops for the people who most need to get their hands on alternative AIDS video. Facilitators bring to their audiences of AIDS educators, health care workers, or PWAs a range of hard-to-find tapes that will prove useful for the audience and their clientele.

"Seeing Through AIDS" notwithstanding, almost every really successful (useful and used, not merely screened at preeminent cultural institutions) alternative AIDS tape I know is distributed primarily by the people who made it. This means phone calls, follow-up, letter campaigns, follow-up, then long train rides to hard-to-find agencies, a small audience, and then, finally, few of the institutionally accepted markers of success. ("Send us reviews, PR, brochures," say curators, funders. Would a Xeroxed flyer from a church bulletin board count?) There is a flip side. A video in a well-known gallery that gets a *Voice* review will, almost guaranteed, play in a backroom where people waft in and out, catching the middle five minutes of a tape without any context. A *successful* screening finds a tape playing to fifteen members of an HIV support group or women's club, the tape introduced by the makers and then discussed afterward.

Therefore, for all these reasons (to get the tape where it needs to go, to feed the makers with active, responsive audiences, to allow the tape to have its utmost educational effect) WAVE's participants were paid $50 to screen the tape wherever they chose: homeless shelters, museums, drug rehabilitation centers, graduate school classrooms, the Queen's Department of Health. The economic incentive was important: allowing the WAVE project to continue to give. But, the self-empowerment found in media production is matched by the tremendous power and pride felt by the members of the group as we take our work to our churches, schools, jobs, and families. The viewing sites are endless, and reflect our different communities. I had enough funding for twenty-five such screenings, although we could easily have done fifty, and people have continued to organize and run screenings without pay.

There is a lot to be gained by running a screening: affirmation, critique, varied responses, which feed back into the meaning of the tape since it means different things to different people. The object changes in relation to the contexts of exhibition. Furthermore, these self-selected "community screenings" are precisely the sort most fruitful for alternative media, because the audience already shares some claim to an identity which joins them together and the presenter already has some relationship to this already-constituted group. Thus, Juanita showed the tape at her union clubhouse; Aida showed it at a community college where her sister is a teacher; I showed it to graduate school classes at NYU. "This means that the result of each projection act will depend on those who organize it, on those who participate in it, and on the time and place," write Solanas and Getino.[30]

"Where's the chicken?" Glenda asked, joking but serious, at the large screening we did at the Downtown Community Television Center.

Among the hundred or so viewers there, only a small number were people of color. It was my screening, on my turf, with my "community" out in force. The bagels, cream cheese, olives, and dried fruit I had picked up at the deli near my house was not what would be served at other WAVE screenings, would not be served at Glenda's screening. At the screening Juanita and I led at a homeless women's shelter in her neighborhood, grape soda and cookies were the appropriate fare. And, instead of big-screen projection, the tape played on the recreation room's TV screen, halting for thirty-two minutes the flow of soap operas that women were sitting in front of—and tuning out.

The audience at DCTV was attentive, communicative, supportive. The viewers at the shelter were less trusting, more divided in attention; some sat glued to the screen, nodding, responding, while others either watched with removed curiosity, slept, came in and out, or loudly opened bags of potato chips. But in all cases questions were asked after the screening, praise given, highlights and concerns discussed. The makers who attended these screenings led the conversations, answered questions, posed questions of our own.

At the DCTV screening a tremendous amount of interest was shown in the process: who did what, how did we edit, how did we come up with the structure. In fact, in this arena, another one of our tapes, *A WAVE Taster*, was the more popular. "The first tape isn't really for me," said one friend, an AIDS activist, who was implying that she did not need to hear AIDS 101 information, but was also referring, I think, to the fact that the players in *We Care* are not people like her. More to her liking, *A WAVE Taster* shows the process of the group, our interaction, the discussions, my role as educator, my relationship to the participants, their relationship to the issues and the camera. My friends with a less immediate relationship to AIDS than myself were more interested in the working of the group, its success (and difficulties) as theory made into practice. *A WAVE Taster* most typically shows at screenings where education about AIDS is supplanted by education about media production. At the shelter, the questions and responses were about AIDS transmission, AIDS facts, AIDS experiences. The video served as starting point for conversation about safer sex practice: what condoms to use, how to use a dental dam. Women wanted to talk about their friends and family who had died, about discrimination and the toll this had taken on them. After we talked, Juanita handed out free condoms. Was this why they had stayed to talk? And does this make the interaction any less valid?

If one thing seems to hold true across the varied communities which view our tape, *We Care* establishes a sense of ease and a lack of embarrassment about discussing HIV in public. Perhaps this is because the "experts" are real people who have really experienced what they talk about, or because the experts look and act like the real people who live and work with many of the spectators of our tape. I have developed many of my ideas about the reception of community-specific media by watching varied audiences watch *We Care:* women in the homeless shelter in Brooklyn, AIDS educators at GMHC, white, highly privileged prep school students in Southern California, academics at documentary conferences. The kinds of identification allowed by alternative media that I raised earlier—both within a self-defined community, and between communities—are evidenced in the many receptions of *We Care.* In some places, people watch the tape for the vital information it provides about services. For people less directly affected by AIDS, they speak of identifying as women who know the weight of many kinds of care provision, or as individuals who have experienced the totalizing effect of other illnesses or personal crises. Some audiences focus on their shared concern about strategies of video production.

Yet, all audiences speak of the sense of comfort, ease, and community, which is produced by the tape, and which invites them in, regardless of their class, ethnicity, gender, or HIV-status. This is hard for me to describe, but I know it is there too. I recognize this sensation to be an integral facet of successful alternative media, just as it marked successful "feminist documentaries" of the seventies, according to Barbara Halpern Martineau, "the relationship of commitment between filmmaker and subject, and between these two and the audience, provides a little-discussed dimension to the issues of how women are 'represented' in (feminist) documentaries."[31] This chapter has been an attempt to address this dearth of discussion. I have tried to show that the relationships among myself, the participants in WAVE, and our audience are definitive of our alternative video practice.

WAVE: A Coda for the First Group

The first WAVE group has been disbanded since 1990. Juanita told me not long ago how far apart we have all grown. Whereas we used to talk at least weekly on the phone, the calls are now much fewer and farther between. Much has changed in people's lives since we met: Willy died of AIDS in 1992, and Carmen is beginning to date again; Aida has moved to Chicago and is thinking of having another child with her new boyfriend; Juanita lost her job and landed another as a videomaker; Glenda got a raise, got married, and is getting her master's degree; Marcia also changed jobs and is thinking of working on her Ph.D.; Sharon's daughter had a baby, and Marie, her lover, has also died of AIDS; my friend Jim died, and I got and lost my first academic job and then found another. Such things now happen to individuals in the group, and others find out later. Our direct influence on each other's lives has ended. The group concluded, but people's lives go on.

Nevertheless, a scandal which occurred in the summer of 1991 got us all yacking on the phone again. We had been awaiting an article written about the group in *New York Woman.* A journalist from the magazine, having heard me give a presentation about the project, decided to write an article about us. She interviewed all of the women in the group and followed Juanita to some community presentations of the tape. Later, we received calls from a "fact-checker." My impression of the article was that it was responsible and interesting. The fact-checker assured me (as had the journalist previously) that no one's name would be included who felt uncomfortable about it, and every quote would be checked for its accuracy. I knew, for instance, that Carmen did not want her name published in this context. She and Willy were "out" about his infection only among a limited number of people.

Before I received my copy of the magazine in the mail, I got a call from Juanita. "Have you seen the article? Marie is really mad! She's trying to sue everyone in sight. Her family doesn't know she's HIV-positive." It turned out that the magazine had illustrated the article with stills taken from the video: one of these of Marie was accompanied, erroneously, with the words "Woman with AIDS."

Many problems stemming from this mistake demonstrate the innate sensitivity and difficulties of alternative media production. The most obvious lesson is known by anyone involved with journalists: although it is nice to get press, no one can handle your story with the sensitivity that you can. Although the magazine had carefully checked the facts printed in the article, this same care had not been exacted regarding the photographs. Marie would not have wanted her picture in the magazine in the first place, and she was particularly angered by the misinformation printed beside it. She believed that the picture could have very real consequences if someone who knew her, but did not know she was HIV-positive, learned about her infection in this way.

But further, Marie was upset with the WAVE project. She had agreed to participate in an AIDS educational video that would be seen by people involved in the "AIDS community." But she had not agreed to be in a video that would receive attention from the "general population." Yet the project had grown bigger than the group's good intentions. People see it and use it in places where we no longer have the same kind of direct control that we have when we are the ones who screen it. After all, there are nearly a thousand copies of the tape in circulation, many of them probably dubbed copies themselves. Marie's image is locked on to those thousand tapes. Although I felt assured that for the most part her image would be seen and used in ways that she had initially agreed upon, I could not have guaranteed her that her image would not show up again in a place or situation in which she was uncomfortable.

The lesson seems clear. The very reasons that Marie's testimony was so valuable are the reasons that she remained vulnerable. She agreed to the courageous act of being imaged in this public format. She understood how much good her interview does. She was proud of the tape and used it herself when she took part in AIDS education at conferences and groups. Yet her life had to go on in a world where she had real things to fear for being identified as an HIV-positive woman by the wrong people or in the wrong contexts. Although her interview does contribute to the lessening of discrimination against PWAs, she went on to live for several years in a world where discrimination also continued.

The Second Video-Support Group

In November and December 1990 I ran a second video support group for HIV-positive men and women at Woodhull Hospital in the Williamsburg section of Brooklyn. After the success of the WAVE group, I hoped that similar projects could be organized to be produced by and narrowcast to other underrepresented communities confronting HIV. AIDS educators at BATF who had helped conceive of the first project and had followed WAVE's progress were eager to try it again. A short while earlier, the agency had received a grant from the New York City Department of Health to run small support groups in underserved neighborhoods in Brooklyn. Nancy Warren, who administered this grant, thought it would be interesting to make one of these groups into another video support group.

A number of circumstances coincided to help us decide where, and for whom, we were to run the group. Sharon (from the first WAVE project) was facilitating a highly successful support group for HIV-positive men and women at Woodhull Hospital. Sharon's group had already gone through two eleven-week DOH contracts, and she was starting on a third because the group's participants refused to let it conclude. The group members were devoted to Sharon and highly committed to each other. For many of them, it not only was the first place where they had an opportunity to learn about HIV and discuss their feelings concerning it, but it was the only place where they felt a sense of community, where they could acknowledge their infection publicly without stigma. This seemed a good place from which to draw the new video support group—HIV-positive people already motivated and empowered about AIDS, people already involved with each other. Sharon chose four group members capable of taking on the extra commitment to join the second group. We would meet at Woodhull, and Sharon would lead the group.

For five weeks Sharon and I met two times a week for an hour and a half with Junior, Alvin, José, and Kathy. These meetings differed almost entirely from those with the first group, even though I attempted to follow the same model. Perhaps the reason was these participants were very different people from the women who made up WAVE. The four participants in the second group—three New Yorican men and an African American woman—were more economically disenfranchised than the women in the first group, and all of them were HIV-positive. Only one of them worked regularly, and this job was sponsored by a government program for PWAs that provided job training and employment in television repair. One group member was supported by family and was in the process of applying for public assistance (encouraged by Sharon's support group). Another, also living at home, was about to start a job as a home attendant (inspired by the HIV-support group). The fourth group member lived at Woodhull Hospital, a situation preferable to homelessness, but little more. All of the group participants had been or still were intravenous drug users; several of them had prostituted for drugs or money, and one had spent time in jail.

Another reason why the second video group differed from WAVE, however, was that we decided to conduct the group with little money. For the first project I had come to BATF with New York Council on the Humanities funds in hand, while in this case I was using only the funds available to BATF. To have stopped the ball rolling to raise funds would have diminished our energy and enthusiasm. But BATF's grant from the DOH covered only Sharon's salary. I already had video equipment, bought with WAVE's budget. All the other necessary expenses of the WAVE project (food, transportation, video stock, editing, payment for the participants) would have to be dropped, or covered by juggling the small reserves of BATF's budget. We figured out that VHS videotape could be donated by BATF's education department. My cab fare to and from the hospital—necessary because I was bringing video equipment—would be covered by BATF. I would try to find an organization that would donate editing time. All other perks (except for participants' subway fare to the meetings) would have to go. We decided that the positive effects of running such a group (the personal empowerment of the participants, the acquisition of a skill, the making of a video project) were more important than doing so in the relatively luxurious and ideal fashion of the first group. It did not make sense to wait the two years it would take to possibly get a grant to run another group. People were ready and waiting to make a video about AIDS; an agency and staff were ready to support the project. Had I been working with an organization that was not desperately staying afloat with a limited budget, the small amount of money needed to run this second project more effectively would have been easily available. Yet if I had been working with a wealthy and stable corporation, we would not have reached the very people and communities that the project aspired to involve. This is, of course, only one of the numerous catch-22s of low-budget community video work.

Choosing to run the group with almost no money was, then, my first mistake. For even though we advocates of camcorder activism delight in its relatively low cost, money is still the bottom line for media production. The WAVE project with its measly $30,000 budget ran upon a fraction of the usual cost of video production; but $30,000 is still $30,000. Low-end video is more expensive than other forms of artistic production (even if it is less expensive than film and professional format video), and it takes longer to produce and longer to learn. Yes, owning a camcorder allows individuals and groups the possibility of making a video for almost nothing, but other expenses that give integrity to a project and its participants must also be taken into account. People who are denied power and attention in most aspects of their lives need particular attention and care if they are to accomplish the difficult work of self-expression. This is a hard pill to swallow because the people who most need to produce media at minimal cost are those most in need of funding for "the extras."

Time was the second element in short supply. The DOH grants funded groups that met eleven times (WAVE had met twenty-two times). In halving the number of meetings, we needed to reduce the project's scope. Instead of viewing and discussing ten television shows and videos about AIDS, this group would see only two or three. Instead of participating in many preparatory projects before producing a final tape, this group would do only a few. And while the first group understood that it would be producing an important tape in response to the present body of AIDS media, the second group's aspirations were not as high. The members never believed they would produce a tape which would be watched by people they did not know. Instead, the participants would have a compilation of the work we produced to take home and show to their friends and family; the time commitment would be short, the editing costs minimal.

These decisions were important. We never could have asked for a six-month commitment from this group, as I had received from the first. These were people who had no idea where they would be in six months, if they would be healthy, let alone if they would be making the biweekly meetings of their video group. The short-term nature of the project fit the realities of their lives. Still, it was the long-term nature of the first project that allowed us to define our needs and concerns—and our voice—as a group. It was incredibly taxing to maintain six months of energy and commitment for the first project, but it allowed us to take ourselves seriously and to make a tape that would be taken seriously by others.

The second project raises the seemingly contradictory issue of how to produce artwork that is taken seriously by its makers and spectators when the conditions of people's lives make it difficult for them to do so. The space, time, and energy necessary to concentrate on something as consuming as a video project are precisely the luxuries that many of the underrepresented communities in our society do not have. Does this mean, again, that only the privileged can produce in the form of video? Or does it imply that our standards of what is "effective" and "serious" must alter as the range of media production expands?

The atmosphere at Woodhull was certainly not conducive to making people feel empowered or committed. Often our meeting room was locked because someone had forgotten to open it (everything at the hospital—toilets, elevators—was locked or guarded). Each time this happened, we had to ask busy, distracted security guards to let us in, and they would then need to call some other bureaucrat to get permission to do so. Our meetings were often interrupted by unapologetic doctors wanting to use a Xerox machine stored in our meeting room. If we wanted to watch footage, we had to sit in a locked section of the hospital where an outside agency was running a separate study. A woman who worked in these offices was so hostile toward the group that we often chose not to screen material at all. On the other hand, some members were extremely aggressive toward all of these figures of authority, which was an understandable but often undermining attitude. The contradictions here are similar to those I have already discussed. It was generous of the hospital to let us use its space, but with generosity like that, who needs opposition?

The positive effects that the project did have on its participants should not be undervalued. The members of the second group were extremely excited about the project and committed to it. They attended meetings religiously. Yet their understanding of the project, and my presentation of it, were very different from the way things had been for the WAVE project. For reasons both personal and organizational, video production for the second group was more a vehicle for personal introspection than community education. Lack of time and institutional support led me to present the project in more traditional terms than I had done before. The boundaries between me and the other group members stayed fixed. I was an outsider with money, skills, equipment, and a plan who came into their lives for a brief period (five weeks) and then took a cab back to Manhattan, which was exactly the kind of hierarchy I had attempted to challenge in the WAVE project. How could I transfer control of the project to the group when the group did not have the time, or the environment, within which to learn to express itself effectively through video production?

In this group it was, unfortunately, the most comfortable arrangement for me to be only the teacher, the giver, and for the participants to be the students, the takers. Members of this group were accustomed to people like me (social workers, clergy, medical professionals) coming into their lives, ostensibly to give them something for free. They are grateful but wary, all too aware of their loss of control and autonomy in this power dynamic. I also maintained a sense of wariness. I felt that the group members were extremely needy, that they would take as much from me as they could without giving much back. Since we had no time to get to know each other well, systems of social positioning already in operation were not challenged. I realize now that assuming the position of authority as I did was, in fact, a tacit form of taking. But the process of reevaluating and repositioning power relations among a group of people occurs over time and in relation to shared experiences that prove earlier assumptions to be invalid or incomplete. The lack of money and time reinforced more traditional power relations. I see this most clearly in my own writing about the two projects. When I discuss WAVE, it is always as "we," but when I discuss the second group, it most usually is "they" and "I."

Because of the largely unchallenged power relations structuring our interactions and because of the personal needs of the group members, the camera was used and understood in relatively straightforward terms as a vehicle for their self-articulation. For the WAVE group, on the other hand, concerns about the *process* of production were equally as important as its *possibility.* The second group recorded interviews, role-plays, poems, and scripted scenarios with a much less critical relationship to modes of representation. They had much to say, but they would say it in whatever form I suggested. Neither the time in group meetings nor the commitment outside them could be found to plan things in advance. The footage we shot was more loose, more raw, and often more powerful than that made by WAVE. The meetings had a similar feel. I learned early that this group did not respond well to preplanning. Sessions ran better when things felt slightly haphazard. I would come in, we would schmooze, I would suggest an exercise, we might get to it, we might do something else. I would ask people if they had worked on things since we last met. Sometimes they had, sometimes not.

These characteristics explain, in part, how we determined our final videotape. When we brainstormed, my ideas were given the greatest weight. I suggested that we pull together the footage already shot, using the concept of one evening of programming on a TV channel. This suggestion was unanimously accepted. Even though I said that the project was ours, it somehow remained either theirs or mine. Yes, they shot it and presented themselves, but since I remained the media professional in their eyes, as well as in my own self-presentation, my ideas came first. Then, although everyone was invited to come edit on a Saturday, I was the only one who made it. The editing facilities generously offered to me to use were in Manhattan, but the group participants were from Brooklyn. Thus, I edited our footage together in the loose pattern we had determined at the previous meeting. The role-plays became a "soap opera," scripted discussions about using condoms and dental dams became "commercials," the talk-show-style interviews we had shot became a program called "The Positive Hour."

The group's final tape, *HIV TV,* is somewhat difficult for me to watch. The interviews and role-plays reveal the pain and difficulty of the speakers' lives. At some moments their lack of command over English makes their attempts to communicate difficult, as, for example, when Kathy discusses the use of a dental dam with insight and honesty, but she trips over the words for dental dam and clitoris and must be prompted by those of us off-camera. At other moments, however, the speakers' ability to say something about AIDS or their own experiences is profound, exact, and powerful. For instance, Alvin talks about his experience of being HIV-positive while in jail. Kathy talks about her recovery from drug addiction. And the role-play that became the soap opera, "Living . . . ," chronicles two gay Latino men who meet in a hospital waiting room while both are waiting to hear the results of their HIV antibody tests. After each of them consults with a doctor, both of them learning they are HIV-positive, the two meet again in the waiting room and decide to go on a date. The usually censored messages that positive HIV status can be empowering and that HIV-positive people can be sexual are powerfully articulated through these scenarios.

HIV TV does not have the cohesive flow or tightness of *We Care,* in part because the group never really decided who or what the tape was for. While I strongly believe that a self-conscious and explicit understanding of audience and purpose is the key to building the foundation for alternative media production, in this case production served primarily as a first step toward a conscious and articulated political discourse. Clearly, if this group could have continued to meet and produce (if adequate funding were available, if their lives were easier), they would have "progressed" toward the manner of practice that I value. Is this what I should hope for? Are my ideals about self-consciously political and educational work fair expectations for all activist production? And what if this ideal cannot be reached by compromised, but critically important, production projects? *HIV TV* is a direct recording of the feelings, knowledge, and concerns of a significant community of people affected by AIDS. Clearly, making the video, and then owning it, was vitally empowering for the participants. It allowed them a forum to articulate for themselves, and to a larger audience, their ideas and knowledge about the AIDS crisis. And clearly, if that is all the tape can do, that is enough. *HIV TV* is useful to many people just as it is: people working with HIV-positive urban people, poor people, people of color.

The production of *HIV TV* demonstrates the complex play of elements that are required to do community-based media well. The initial WAVE project was successful because of a fortuitous and planned conjoining of talented, committed, intelligent producers, who had sufficient funds, time, and attention for them to feel empowered and educated enough to produce. These circumstances allowed both the goals and the process of video production to be clear to everyone. And WAVE's private funding allowed it autonomy from the chaos, poverty, and bureaucracy that exists even in many of the most well-intentioned community organizations.

It becomes clear why projects like WAVE are so rare and so difficult to repeat. It took years to get the money to do it properly. It took incredible amounts of energy and commitment to see it through. Although I have emphasized the seemingly utopian power of camcorder technology, the second project demonstrates the existence of blocks more significant to media production than limited access to equipment. Even if the positive effects of media empowerment through self- and community identification are real, the disempowering conditions under which individuals live their lives continue to be real as well. Furthermore, in a political climate of downsizing funding for social welfare, art, and education, it becomes even more difficult to raise adequate funding for this kind of political and educational community work.

I remain optimistic about the ways that video is being used by various communities in response to AIDS and other social crises, while I learn again and again to be cautious about the underlying conditions of oppression that do not change, even as media use expands. While I hope that I have shown just how important media empowerment can be in altering the understanding of AIDS for its producers and viewers, I believe I have also confirmed how vulnerable such already compromised individuals are. Yes, representations matter, but so do a multitude of other conditions. The politics of community-produced video extend beyond video's positive effects on individuals and communities. If we are to fully gain from the promise of the camcorder and other new video technologies, we must use a more conventional understanding of politics, one that moves beyond critiques of representation, to do the work needed to end the conditions that keep people down.

Conclusions

The many strengths and liabilities of the alternative media which have been discussed in this chapter point to what finally distinguishes this work from broadcast or mainstream media. The making and viewing of alternative media come from an urge to construct identity and community from the position of an endangered outsider. Working from the society's margins, the signifiers of "broadcast" video production are necessarily lacking—and good riddance. For alternative producers may lack professional training, massive funds, full-time attention to their artwork, or often even an adequate sense of self-worth. Yet these very weaknesses are the alternative media's strength. Speaking to specific publics about specific goals, the alternative media bridges the gaps between producer and spectator, viewer and viewed, addressing them not as a purchasing public but as an engaged and articulate community.

IDENTITY, COMMUNITY, AND ALTERNATIVE
AIDS VIDEO

Identity/Community/Video/1993: The First Conclusion to *AIDS TV*

It is the summer of 1993, and I am revising my doctoral dissertation into a book.

It is twelve years since the word AIDS was invented, and there have been so many videos produced independently about AIDS that I could never pretend to, nor would I want to, have seen them all, even if I must attempt some kind of comprehensive knowledge in these pages.

It is the summer of 1993, and my best friend and sometimes boyfriend of nine years died of AIDS on February 19. Can a gay man and a straight woman who have never had sexual intercourse be considered boyfriend and girlfriend? I think yes, and already the self-conscious and mobile sense of identity and community which will be the theme of this conclusion comes into focus.

I am living in a cluttered studio in the East Village with little cross-ventilation, and Jim's pictures are everywhere around me. On the bulletin board by my computer, magneted to my file cabinet, framed on the wall, propped up against shrines of Mardi Gras beads, candles, and perfumes. These things do not bring him back. But I tell my friends that I hope that when I'm least aware I'll catch one of these images of him out of the corner of my eye, and this will spark a fresh memory, a memory so fresh it will be real, and this will trigger a moment of return. No such luck. But I look at him now, smiling, posing, peeking at me in photographs as I work on the book, as I watch endless videos about AIDS; he was beautiful, I see love in his eyes, and he died of KS at the age of twenty-nine.

It is the summer of 1993, and I could say that at present I am a straight, white, HIV-negative, 29-year-old female professor and activist AIDS videomaker who is mourning my friend Jim as I spend a summer in New York revising a book about the alternative AIDS media.

But since this book, as I've discovered, is as much about identity as it is about AIDS or video—about how AIDS and identity conjoin in 1993, in video, and, in my life anyway, nearly everywhere else for that matter—I need to arrange my words more precisely so I can show who I am because of AIDS and video. I begin any day with who it is that I recognize myself to be—perhaps that white, 29-year-old professor I mentioned. Then, I settle down to watch, make, or write about alternative AIDS video because of my anger and despair, my whiteness and my youth, my mourning and my friend Jim's life and death. I can't deal with AIDS adequately as who I am alone. And then video works on me. Through video my anger and despair can be abated, my whiteness and youth may be contrasted with others' experiences, my mourning finds a productive release. My sense of my identity has been altered by AIDS and video. Because of Jim's death I must understand the "fact" of my age anew (twenty-nine! so young, a life to look forward to); because my friends and fellow videomakers from WAVE are women of color, I must try to take responsibility for the history of my whiteness; because I've had unsafe sex (even while knowing the risks, even while educating others), I must consider that at any time my hold on an HIV-negative identity could shift. I make and watch video to take some control back in the face of catastrophe.

I am fated to have an identity molded, in part, by video and by AIDS. As a straight (the majority of my friends are gay men and lesbians), white (three-fourths Jewish of German and Hungarian descent), HIV-negative (or so a piece of paper told me three years ago), twenty-nine years old (so young!), female (aggressive, controlling, strong), I could have chosen not to notice. Although as late into this history as 1993, I'm not so sure that even the distancing effects of all these safe labels could protect me from making AIDS a factor which determines who I understand myself to be. My identity continually shifts because AIDS affects me in ways both within and outside my control.

"Identity" is a much-contested word in the early nineties, at least for academics. We worry endlessly about its essential or strategic nature. We battle over whether its politics are self-serving and myopic, or liberating and diversifying. This book enters that fray from my particular vantage point, as something like a straight, white, HIV-negative, academic, activist, and artist overly invested in AIDS and video. From where I sit, I see hours worth of alternative AIDS video daily, I discuss new video projects with friends, I write funding applications for new video projects, and I see Jim out of the corner of my eye. AIDS, both as biological fact and cultural construction, alters my sense of myself, who I recognize myself to be each day.

So there you have it. I am not *essentially* anything. Today I am what AIDS and video make me to be! Yet I also know that the privileges of whiteness, sero-negativity, and a steady academic job make my sense of myself and my experience of AIDS different from those of the women with whom I made video in the WAVE project. AIDS and video can't deplete me of the variety of privilege and lack-of-privilege into which I was born. Essential or not, it's difficult to make some traits just disappear. Yet, video can change some aspects of one's sense of self. For all seven of us in the WAVE project, as diverse as we may be, the production of a video about our experiences allowed us to take some control back from AIDS, to make AIDS into what *we* wanted it to be, to make of our diverse experiences of AIDS and our lives something that we could agree upon. Of course, even the power of the video camera could not erase AIDS from our daily lives, from our friends, from our husbands. But it did allow us to show how our experiences—so rarely represented in our culture—mattered. It did allow us to show that our knowledge about AIDS—so rarely valued in our culture—was of great use to ourselves and others.

AIDS changes, videos change, and so do I; these three categories are never fixed because of both what I control and do not control. Through systems of representation, like the making or watching of video, I make desperate, hopeful, critical, angry statements about who I am in relation to AIDS. Through the viewing of video representations I learn, struggle, and join with others who communicate different experiences and worldviews. Then I return to who I had thought myself to be with something more—an identity touched and perhaps changed by the images of education, documentation, frustration, and celebration made by countless videomakers who are forced, like me, to confront and take a hack at AIDS again and again and again. I identify with these videomakers, even if I will never know them or the people recorded on their tapes, so as to forge an identity larger than my personal anguish and anger, so as to make and remake fighting communities. My identity, malleable and uncertain as it is, fixed and stable as it sometimes appears to be, means next to nothing in the face of a global pandemic. Yet my identity associated with others—those "like" me and those who are not—around the issues upon which we can agree (the difficulties of caring for a PWA, the anger at an unresponsive and unjust health-care system) feels as if it *could* matter. On good days we video activists believe we are making an educational, critical, or emotional intervention that will move many, that will contribute to change; on bad days it seems that AIDS rolls forward, blind to our cries and images. However, on all days these images serve to confirm a larger, politicized community—larger than any single AIDS identity—engaged in ongoing struggle.

In the summer of 1993, perhaps because of Jim's death, perhaps because I watch three or four hours of AIDS video a day, or perhaps because AIDS is nearly everywhere anyway, I know myself (partially) in relation to the representation of AIDS—the images I have made, watched, discussed, internalized, and hoped to forget—and I know, through video, that there are others like me. Therefore, alternative AIDS video is as much about forging community as it is about constructing identity, about how identities are turned into communities because of AIDS and through video.

By making AIDS into video, we make sense—not conclusively or irrevocably, but partially and transitionally—of our selves and our lives in the face of AIDS. Because of camcorders and cable, because AIDS changes daily, and because the broadcast media continues to represent this crisis using the limited and bigoted world vision which defines a great deal of their programming, many of us who are profoundly affected by AIDS use video—its making and watching—to respond, to rest, to scream, to educate, remember, contest, create—to communicate. Which is not to say that we do not communicate constantly about AIDS in other forms: on the telephone, in the hospital, over dinner, through writing. But communication through video allows for other levels of power: a larger audience, a mimetic hold on history, an accessible and familiar form. And because AIDS affects women, children, straights, bisexuals, whites, and Asians, when we use video to communicate, to reflect, the diverse experiences and issues of AIDS, when we use video to expand the reach of our words, we also inevitably show and see the multiple ways we experience AIDS and identity, and we often discover that we identify with aspects of others' experiences.

My careful invocation of identity after twenty years spent celebrating the loss or deconstruction of the subject is made obligatory because of the real needs and struggles around AIDS. Douglas Crimp believes that this contradictory relation to subjectivity is frequently found in the artwork produced by AIDS activists. "Identity is understood by them to be, among other things, coercively imposed by perceived sexual orientation or HIV status; it is, at the same time, willfully taken on, in defiant declaration of affinity with the 'others' of AIDS: queers, women, Blacks, Latinos, drug users and sex workers."[1] The formation of the particular and usually temporary communities of "others," like the women who made up WAVE, so as to produce and receive alternative AIDS media, demonstrates how individuals can and must declare affinity with others, must cross lines of ethnic, class, gender, and other differences, to form useful, if temporary, allegiances to alter the course of this crisis.

The women in WAVE found that our commitment to AIDS and to the production of an educational video provided a locus around which we decided to form community despite our other differences. We decided that the idea of "care provider" bound us together, and then it did, for a while, and within a particular context. We did not reveal all of ourselves, the parts that were not those of the care provider; we had other communities where we could be gay, or religious, or sexually explicit. Similarly, the temporary union of a group to watch our video provided a space where a minimal but operating sense of community was consolidated and defined, if temporarily, around people's lives and roles as "care providers." Since, ideally, AIDS videos are discussed after a screening, people can hear the ways that their reactions, identifications, and experiences are similar to those of others—in the process, consolidating a sense of community. Nevertheless, people also recognize how their other loci of identity must necessarily sever them from the other viewers in a room. A person who is poor, and caring for a PWA, will both share and differ in experience with a wealthy care provider.

Until PWAs (or people assumed to be infected with HIV) are not discriminated against in the workplace, in the hospital, in representation, or until women with AIDS are not discriminated against in clinical drug trials, there is every reason for them to call attention to the similarities of their oppression—to constitute a community around the work of combating these oppressions. It is in this sense that bell hooks wishes to claim "that there is a definitive distinction between that marginality that is imposed by oppressive structure and that marginality one chooses as site of resistance, as location of radical openness and possibility."[2] I suggest that the production of alternative AIDS media, which willingly speaks from and about a marginal and oppressed position and asks others to join one in this place "of radical openness and possibility," can be understood in hooks's terms as "that marginality one chooses as a site of resistance." Yet placing oneself into the "AIDS community," or even a community of care providers, does not necessarily establish that one knows precisely what that "means," or that there could ever be one meaning to this term or position. Even so, the moment when a maker or viewer agrees to identify himself or herself as the person specified by the title or content of an alternative work, and others who have done the same, is a moment of self- and community identification.

So, not surprisingly, many of the alternative AIDS videos help this process by specifying the contours of their making and viewing constituencies in their titles, if not in the body of the work—i.e., this is a video *by* PWAs, or AIDS activists, or the Latino community of Philadelphia; this is a video *for* care providers of people affected by AIDS, or black urban women, or workers.[3] Letting yourself be the subject hailed by a videotape contributes to a *process* of self-identification and self-construction, as opposed to a *fixing* of these states. For such self-identification, always inextricably linked to opinions, needs, demands, history, and videotapes, changes as the needs of individuals and communities change. But furthermore, such self-identification is only as stable as the videotape which holds it—impermanent, reeditable. Ideas change, then a new video needs to be made. Camcorder video production is cheap enough for such writerly revision to become economically feasible within the production of moving images.

I am suggesting that video—a form of mimetic representation which inherently attests to the reality of experiences that would otherwise be silenced and which is easy to use and easy to pass on—is so attractive to people involved in the struggle against AIDS because it enacts through its form an effect we strive for in the real world. Video and activists depend upon a sense of identity and community which is at once stable enough to fight with and malleable enough to change. Although many of these effects are temporary, in the case of the WAVE group our allegiances have become permanent. But such permanence need not be the case for the many communities which are organized in the struggle against AIDS. Thus, for example, Dennis Altman believes that the notion of the "gay community" has needed to expand in certain circumstances to include the many straight women doing AIDS work. "There are numbers of people who, without being homosexual in any sense, have committed themselves to working with gay community organizations, just as there are men who regard themselves as feminists."[4] In this case, "gay community" or "feminist" may have little to do with "identity" and much more to do with "identification."

Mark you, this is not the overriding or totalizing psychoanalytic "identification" which provides the foundation for feminist film theory and its critique of realist representation. Rather, I am speaking of a careful and conscious process of recognition across difference which occurs in real life and in representation for the understandable goals of interpersonal communication and political cooperation. Catherine Saalfield calls it "the enlightened self-interest of activism," a need to join with others who are not you so as to work toward your own, and most likely their own, empowerment.[5] Video facilitates this kind of identifying with others in the face of crisis, terror, anger, disease, political inaction, and death—a most productive, necessary, and empowering response. Forming allegiances through video production and reception is often easier than doing so in other forums. People live in isolated communities; people are closeted about HIV infection; people can carefully craft their identity and ideas in video, protecting themselves from some of the slips and stereotyping which often organize real-world interaction across difference. Needless to say, even as I celebrate the power of making identity and community through video, I am aware of the difficulties, problems, masks that are also part of this process. Forming allegiances through video is also dangerous, dangerous because of the pitfalls of misrecognition, misidentification, self-revelation, and the demands of difference which structure all social relations, even those that also occur through representation. Let me explain.

During the course of the WAVE project, Aida, Sharon, Carmen, Juanita, Marcia, Glenda, and I met for six months with the shared goals of video education, AIDS support, and video production. We had little else in common. Two women in the group are New Yoricans (New Yorkers of Puerto Rican descent). Four are black; two of the "black" women in the group have families in the South but were raised in New York, although one of these has a Latino father; another's family has lived in New York for several generations; the fourth is a first-generation American from Jamaica. I am white (three-fourths Jewish, but raised without religion; my first-generation Hungarian father had a Catholic mother and was raised a Catholic). The seven of us in the project ranged in age from twenty-five to thirty-five. Most of us are religious (fundamentalist Christian, Baptist, Pentecostal, Muslim). Four of us are married with children (one more has married since the end of the project). We all said we were straight. Our class backgrounds are complicated. Does class background mean how we were raised, how we now live, or how we *will* live after acquiring advanced degrees? In 1990 some in the group were out of school for good, some were attaining further degrees (A.A., B.A., M.A., Ph.D.), and we had a variety of professions: social worker, AIDS educator, hair designer, computer programmer, secretary, housing inspector, full-time graduate student. We had a range of relations to AIDS from actively caring for husbands, lovers, sisters, brothers, friends, and buddies, to being trained AIDS workers with no "personal" connection at all.

The seven of us held in common only two traits: our gender and our commitment to making a contribution toward abating the deadly effects of the AIDS crisis. From these similarities, and across all of our other differences, we formed a temporary community and collectively produced *We Care.* The tape has been shown in major art museums, at AIDS conferences, in churches, and in group members' living rooms. The effects of the group continue for the participants. In economic terms, the tape continues to make money. In activist terms, we continue to take the tape to people and organizations that can use it. In emotional terms, because we still are friends. I focus upon the success of this group—and our video project—because our success points to the most powerful and unique aspect of alternative AIDS media: the strategic and conscious claiming of identity and recognition of community across differences for the accomplishment of shared and progressive ends in the face of an epidemic.

But my point is not that we ever truly "knew" each other, or even ourselves, through the process of video production, nor is it that we desired to. Rather, we projected images of ourselves to the other women in the group who were very different from ourselves ("types" of women with whom we had rarely, if ever, interacted before; we hadn't *needed* to) so as to identify with each other, so as to be able to work together to produce a video which would contribute toward a better picture of the AIDS crisis. This demanded a conscious crafting of the selves we came to the group playing: the Alex-at-WAVE, Sharon-at-WAVE, etc., that I mentioned earlier. In the video we produced for our primary intended audience—urban women of color—we did the same. We tamed our images, prettied them up, and shut parts down (our religion, anger, first language), so that the women we wanted to communicate with would identify enough with us to see and hear our ideas. We misidentified ourselves when we needed to, we misrecognized each other when we had to, and since the project's conclusion, we have come to know each other again, on terms different from those necessary for successful video production.

Because I've returned to New York in the summer of 1993 after two and a half years out of the city, I've had the opportunity to see the women of WAVE again. I've learned a great deal about the misidentifications we made in 1990 to further the cause of communication, community, and video production. I've learned, for instance, that Sharon's "mother-in-law," an HIV-positive, middle-aged woman, who is one of the stars of *We Care,* was, in fact, Sharon's lover. Sharon recently explained to me, over lunch, that she thought that the fundamentalist values of some of the women in the group would have made them reject Sharon's lesbianism. Since Sharon's primary motivation was to produce a useful and powerful videotape about the issues that all care providers share, she misidentified herself as straight (although it's true that she was once married to a man and has two daughters) to allow other prioritized forms of communication and identification to occur successfully. Now that Sharon's lover has died, and the group is considering making another video (dependent upon funding, of course), Sharon wants to express the anger she felt in the denial of her rights to mourn, inherit material goods, and simply take care of her lover because of their socially and legally "illegitimate" relationship. She says she won't buckle down to the pressure of other group member's attitudes this time, because her motivations have changed.

During similar interactions this summer we've also discussed the roles I played to form community with the women in WAVE. Upon viewing a tape I recently produced with my students at Swarthmore, *Safer and Sexier: A College Student's Guide to Safer Sex,* Juanita and Sharon tell me they screamed in amazement, shock, and disbelief. They couldn't believe that goody-goody Alex had made a sexually explicit video, with penises, vaginas, oral and anal sex! All during WAVE I had been so *nice.* What happened? Well, I explained, I was interacting with the group with the pressures of being in charge, yet also wanting to forfeit control. I was the teacher, but I also wanted to let others teach me. I was the white girl, the authority figure— I didn't want to offend. I wanted to please. I wanted to be neutral. I thought that if I had let people know who I *truly* was, everything I believed and valued, we never could have worked as a group. I made an identity that I thought best fit in, that I thought people expected, in order to produce collectively. For example, in my production journal dated April 3 I wrote, "Aida and Carmen identified themselves as Born Again Christians. Their church seems to be the only place in their community where unconditional support is practiced. 'They even accept homosexuality—and their acceptance cures it.' Their ideas about homosexuality worry me a little, but I didn't jump in— I'm not sure if preaching is the right thing now."

These tales of misrecognition and misidentification are important because they point to the contradictions of identity and community politics. Our identities are not stable, but we try to stabilize them in an attempt to interact. We have some control over the performance of our own identities, but we are not in control of how we will be read. Differences of race, class, sexual orientation, neighborhood separate us, even as common ground can be found from which to communicate and produce. In the process of making and viewing AIDS TV we "name" ourselves in a strategic and discursive act that fixes us within a position from which to speak for the duration of a video, this in service of a particular polemic or material goal (PWAs sharing holisitic cures, mothers of PWAs talking about their grief, women with AIDS discussing the effects of their invisibility). Video provides a privileged site, often unavailable in the "real world," where identity can be played with, worked upon, communicated, and interrogated. What does being a PWA mean? What are the shared goals and needs of care givers of PWAs? What are the various ways of being an AIDS activist? Yet, simply because identity is up for debate, discussion, or interpretation never means that it can or wants to be written into stone.

Although I know that my descriptions of identity and community construction through video may come across as hopelessly idealistic, I conclude with a reminder that, in fact, I find this work and its implications to be *realistic* rather than optimistic. I do not believe that the making or watching of AIDS TV turns one into another person, ends the AIDS crisis, or even combats suffering. I have not moved in with the women from WAVE to form a radical video commune, and my friend Jim, as well as Sharon's lover, Marie, and Carmen's husband, Willy, have died. Yet it is also true that all of our lives were profoundly affected by our work on this video project and that our tape fills a small but vitally important gap in available resources about the crisis. Because of our work on the tape, and with each other, our sense of ourselves and our sense of AIDS changed, and the picture of AIDS was altered to include the images that mattered to us. On any particular day, several people who need something from the tape will watch it. On any particular day one of us who made it may watch it to remember, or screen it to share our tape with others. These small gains hold true for each and every tape of the alternative AIDS media. Through video, we make AIDS identities and communities because it is one of the most productive things we know to do.

Identity/Community/Video/1994: The Very Last Conclusion to *AIDS TV*

Wow! I've been mad at Gregg Bordowitz since 1988—six years.

He probably doesn't know it. Why would he? It's not as if we're friends. We hardly know each other. Our words beyond pleasantries have been few. But of course, we know *of* each other. That's New York. The AIDS activist and art scenes. Our intimate community. Close friends of each other's close friends, the Whitney Independent Studio Program, ACT UP, GMHC. He never knew I was angry at him (enough at least to avoid him in social situations for six years), but now I hope that he'll understand how I'm quite suddenly past it.

His video, *Fast Trip, Long Drop* (1994), did it. And time.

In 1988 I was making my third (and last) video for GMHC—a video I hate, rarely mention, never show—*A Test for the Nation: Women, Children, Families, AIDS.* Here's a story that doesn't show up in any of my "revealing" AIDS video writing (understandably: it's about lack of connection, an inability to work together). I showed Gregg a rough cut, and he simply trashed it. Or so my memory of it goes. I can't remember why I was so intimidated—what he said or how he said it—I just remember that I was hurt, and this resulted in making a video that never felt like my own, the end of my involvement with GMHC, and then holding a worthless grudge. For six years. Until tonight, in June 1994, in San Francisco of all places, particularly strange because my grudge against Gregg, my life-that-kind-of-includes-Gregg, feels so New York.

I saw Gregg's new video *Fast Trip,* and it spoke right to me. Past the part of me that has been hurt by the AIDS activist video community, the part that is about small jealousies, petty personal politics, and living in a small community rife with gossip and the potential for funds and fame. Gregg spoke to me with images about death, religion, anger, boredom, confusion, and AIDS. What made me hear him was that many of *his* images were of *my* past.

It started when I saw Jim, out of the corner of my eye, at the ACT UP Kiss-In that I missed because I was in Europe getting away from the AIDS activist and Whitney art scenes that were making me feel crazy and inspired, talented and drab, all at the same time. I saw Jim, and it sparked a moment so fresh that my heart hurt (figure 22). And then I saw face after face that I knew or recognized. And buildings. And books. The signifiers of *Gregg's* "personality" built at the same time, with the same forces pressing in, the same figures being key, as my own. The images and words of his angst, memory, and anger were mine. Ours?

But he has AIDS(!), and I do not(?). He is dying(?), and I am living(!). He has let AIDS and video shape his adult life, and now as he needs to confront the meaning of his own mortality, he finds the same banality that I see. He says that he once believed that collective will, anger, passion could do something. *So did I.* And now it is many years later, and neither of us is twenty-three anymore, although we both were at about the same time, in the same city, with many of the same teachers and friends and influences. And while it is now clear that those videos we made did not save the lives of the faces they so mechanically recorded, and that today, six years and hundreds

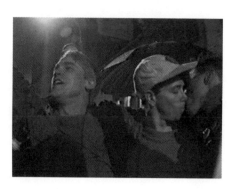

Figure 22   Protesters at
ACT UP Kiss-In, April
1988, Greenwich Village.
Man with hat was mis-
taken for Jim Lamb on
my first viewing, *Fast
Trip, Long Drop* (Gregg
Bordowitz, 1994).

of videos later, another person, Gregg this time, attempts to make sense of
HIV in his body, I am somehow not surprised to see that he remarks upon
his ambivalence about the power of video . . . through video.

Fast Trip, Long Drop marks yet another transformation of this always
adapting movement by being the first meta-AIDS video—mocking, scorning,
questioning the formal codes, media personalities, and angry mottoes that
we produced with so much righteousness such a short time ago. And in
the meantime, Gregg counters this black AIDS video humor with countless
found images of leaps off cliffs, dives off boards, jumps on motorcycles, all
there, I think to represent how quickly he will become nothing more nor less
than history, or at least an image in history.

And I am right there with him: despondent, angry, cynical beyond
belief, scared, sad. Sickened by those early activist video images of dead
people and dead passion that show up in his new work. He uses them in
1994, and I too feel how useless it's been, how naive, how petty. Except . . .

Except that he made this video. And his video speaks to me one
night in San Francisco, of all places, passing over a rickety grudge, making
me think, making me feel, speaking to me like he never would in real life
because we're not really friends, and there, on that screen, even so, he's
speaking things which I find that I need to hear and feel, too, he's recording
and remembering and validating *my* past, and my feelings in 1994. Ah, you
see—community. Identity. AIDS. Video.

He made a video to speak back to AIDS, to speak himself in the face
of AIDS (as AIDS), and he spoke to *me,* affirming my existence, my experience, my reality, even as his images have nothing to do with me (his parents
in Long Island, his HIV-support group), and even though I have changed.
For, in 1994, I'm not the Alex-I-was when many of Gregg's images were shot:
when Jim marched and kissed with a belief in his future. I'm not even the

Alex-from-a-few-pages-back: that straight, white, blah, blah, blah I thought I was at the time. Now, I'm thirty, underemployed, dating a lesbian. (Jim would've been so happy. He always wanted me to be gay like him. And as much as he loved women, he loved lesbians most of all.)

So I find that the power of AIDS video is not that it grants or confirms identity, but precisely that it is more permanent than identity. It holds one vision of reality still and unchanging, even as our sense of ourselves in reality must constantly change. A video document of something that was once real weathers the fickleness of "feelings" and "personality"—holding forever and frozen Jim's kiss and the yellow-blue of New York in summer—to allow us to see and interpret again, with our ever-changing eyes, a past we may have shared. Each time I see Jim's recorded face, I am different; it calls out to different needs, it speaks another version of history to another version of the same woman. A document, in the form of an image from my past, makes my sense of myself and Jim and AIDS newly, because I change even as the image does not.

So maybe I'm only calling up postmodernism's favorite trope: we children of the late century pass off TV and images as if they are memories. But then, I'm not talking about *The Partridge Family* here, but rather about *activist video,* a completely different manner of TV. Alternative AIDS video is made of images of a real place and time where I actually was because I worked hard to be there; I believed in it. These images were taken by someone who sees and saw enough like me to share a political and ideological agenda: to be in a place that matters to me; to videotape it through eyes that see things that I need to know.

I don't confuse video images with reality or memory. I don't confuse the faces locked on videotape with the impermanence of their bodies or identities. I don't mistake the making of allegiances through video with the physical and emotional bonds of friendship. What I do understand, however, is that video images let me remember newly; let Gregg communicate to me complex ideas about the past and the future; remind me that there are others in the world who have been made by AIDS and who struggle to understand this awful fact.

It's the most we can do. It's not enough, this fighting through video. But sometimes (writing tonight, summer of 1994 in San Francisco), it feels like a lot, like it could matter. And then, it does.

NOTES

1 Introduction to *AIDS TV*

1 See Appendix 1, an annotated videography, by Catherine Saalfield.

2 See Jan Zita Grover, "Visible Lesions: Images of People With AIDS," *Afterimage,* Summer 1989, pp. 10–16. Grover provides a timeline of AIDS representation from 1981–88, arguing how gay men, gay media, and gay service organizations were the first to respond to the damning images of AIDS found in the mainstream media, creating, instead, images of AIDS with which gay people could identify "because of shared history and concerns."

3 See, for example, James Meyer, "AIDS and Postmodernism," *Arts Magazine,* April 1992, pp. 60–68; Jeffrey Weeks, "Postmodern AIDS?" in Tessa Boffin and Sunil Gupta, eds., *Ecstatic Anti-Bodies* (London: Rivers Oram Press, 1990), pp. 133–41; Lee Edelman, "The Mirror and the Tank: 'AIDS,' Subjectivity, and the Rhetoric of Activism," in Timothy Murphy and Suzanne Poirier, eds., *Writing AIDS* (New York: Columbia University Press, 1993), pp. 9–38. Murphy writes: "intellectual efforts to theorize the epidemic, its constructions, and its representations, frequently invoke, toward differing ends and with varying degrees of insight and engagement, some notion of the postmodern," pp. 10–11.

4 John Greyson, "Strategic Compromises: AIDS and Alternative Video Practices," in Mark O'Brien and Craig Little, eds., *Reimaging America* (Philadelphia: New Society Publishers, 1990), p. 61.

5 Greyson, pp. 63 and 73.

6 Jean Carlomusto, "Making IT: AIDS Activist Television," *Video Guide,* Nov. 1989, p. 18.

7 Catherine Saalfield, "On the Make," in Martha Gever, John Greyson, and Pratibha Parmar, eds., *Queer Looks: Perspectives on Lesbian and Gay Film and Video* (New York: Routledge, 1993), p. 19.

8 In personal discussions with Ginsburg regarding *AIDS TV.*

9 Timothy Landers, "Bodies and Anti-Bodies: A Crisis in Representation," in Cynthia Schneider and Brian Wallis, eds., *Global Television* (Cambridge, Mass.: MIT Press, 1988), p. 282.

10   Jean Carlomusto in Lorraine Kenny, "Testing the Limits," *Afterimage,* Oct. 1989, p. 7.

11   Todd Gitlin, "Television's Screenings: Hegemony in Transition," in Donald Lazere, ed., *American Media and Mass Culture* (Berkeley: University of California Press, 1987), p. 243.

12   James Kinsella, *Covering the Plague: AIDS and the American Media* (New Brunswick, N.J.: Rutgers University Press, 1989), p. 1.

13   Michael Parenti, *Inventing Reality: The Politics of News Media* (New York: St. Martin's Press, 1993), p. 23.

14   Kinsella, pp. 251, 257.

15   Cook and Colby, "The Mass-Mediated Epidemic: The Politics of AIDS on the Nightly Network News," in Elizabeth Fee and Daniel Fox, eds., *AIDS: The Making of a Chronic Disease* (Berkeley: University of California Press, 1992), p. 86.

16   Randy Shilts, *And the Band Played On* (New York: St. Martin's Press, 1987), p. xxiii.

17   Sandra Elgear and Robyn Hutt, "Some Notes on Collective Production," *Video Guide,* Nov. 1989, p. 20.

18   Gregg Bordowitz, "The AIDS Crisis Is Ridiculous," in Gever et al., eds., *Queer Looks,* p. 212.

19   Jean Carlomusto and Gregg Bordowitz, "Do It!" *Video Guide,* Nov. 1989, p. 22.

20   David Armstrong, *A Trumpet to Arms: Alternative Media in America* (Los Angeles: JP Tarcher, 1981), p. 22.

21   Sean Cubitt, *Timeshift: On Video Culture* (New York: Routledge, 1991), p. 140.

22   See for example, Andrew Arato and Eike Gebhardt, eds., *The Essential Frankfurt School Reader* (New York: Urizen Books, 1978), and Max Horkheimer and Theodor Adorno, *Dialectic of Enlightenment,* trans. John Cumming (New York: Seabury Press, 1972).

23   See, for example, Stuart Hall et al., eds., *Culture, Media, Language* (London: Hutchinson, 1980); James Curran et al. eds., *Mass Communication and Society* (Beverly Hills, Calif.: Sage, 1979), or John Fiske, "British Cultural Studies," in Robert Allen, ed., *Channels of Discourse* (Chapel Hill: University of North Carolina Press, 1987): 254–89.

24   Jacqueline Bobo, "The Color Purple: Black Women as Cultural Readers," in E. Deidre Pribaum, ed., *Female Spectators* (London: Verso, 1988), pp. 90–109.

25   bell hooks, *Yearning: Race, Gender and Cultural Politics* (Boston: South End Press, 1990), p. 6.

26   Jackie Stacey, "Feminine Fascinations," in Christine Gledhill, ed., *Stardom: Industry of Desire* (New York: Routledge, 1991), p. 147.

27   Anne Friedberg, "Identification and the Star," in Christine Gledhill, ed., *Star Signs* (London: BFI, 1982), p. 50.

28   Paula Treichler, "AIDS Narratives on Television," in *Writing AIDS,* pp. 186–87.

29 Faye Ginsburg, "Indigenous Media: Faustian Contract or Global Village?" *Visual Anthropology* 6, no. 1 (1991): 108.
30 E. Ann Kaplan, "Theories of the Feminist Documentary," in Alan Rosenthal, ed., *New Challenges for Documentary* (Berkeley: University of California Press, 1988), p. 80.
31 Manohla Dargis and Amy Taubin, "Double Take," *Village Voice,* Jan. 21, 1992, p. 56.
32 Renee Sabatier, *Blaming Others: Prejudice, Race and Worldwide AIDS* (Philadelphia: New Society Publishers, 1988), p. 123.
33 Jane Delgado, interview, Oct. 1987, in Sabatier, *Blaming Others,* p. 139.
34 José Guiterrez-Gomez and José Vergelin, "Mining the Oro Del Bario," *Video Guide,* Nov. 1989, p. 13.
35 Jan Zita Grover, "Introduction," *AIDS: The Artists' Response,* exhibit at Ohio State University, 1989, p. 3.
36 Ada Gay Griffin, "What's Mine Is Not Mine/What's Mine Is Ours/What's Mine Is Yours/What's Yours Is Yours (Power Sharing and America)," *FELIX,* Spring 1992, p. 15.
37 Barbara Halpern Martineau, "Talking About Our Lives and Experiences: Some Thoughts About Feminism, Documentary and 'Talking Heads,'" in Thomas Waugh, ed., *Show Us Life* (Metuchen, N.J.: Scarecrow Press, 1984), p. 254.
38 Bordowitz, "The AIDS Crisis Is Ridiculous," p. 211.
39 James Miller, introduction, in James Miller, ed., *Fluid Exchanges* (Toronto: University of Toronto Press, 1993).
40 Edelman, p. 27.
41 Jan Zita Grover, "AIDS, Keywords and Cultural Work," in Lawrence Grossberg, Cary Nelson, and Paula Treichler, eds., *Cultural Studies* (New York: Routledge, 1992), p. 239.
42 Hall, "Theoretical Legacies," in Grossberg et al., eds., *Cultural Studies,* p. 285.
43 Timothy Murphy, "Testimony," in *Writing AIDS,* p. 316.

2 A History of the Alternative AIDS Media

1 Lorraine Kenney, "Testing the Limits: An Interview," *Afterimage,* Oct. 1989, p. 7.
2 Robert Stam and Louise Spence, "Colonialism, Racism, and Representation: An Introduction," in Bill Nichols, ed., *Movies and Methods: Volume 2* (Berkeley: University of California Press, 1985), p. 638.
3 David James, *Allegories of Cinema: American Film in the Sixties* (Princeton, N.J.: Princeton University Press, 1989), p. 3.
4 Michael Leigh, "Curiouser and Curiouser," in Scott Murray, ed., *Back and Beyond: Discovering Australian Film and Television* (Sydney: Australian Film Commission, 1988), p. 88.

5   Barbara Halpern Martineau, "Talking About Our Lives and Experiences: Some Thoughts About Feminism, Documentary and 'Talking Heads,'" in Thomas Waugh, ed., *Show Us Life: Toward a History and Aesthetics of the Committed Documentary* (Metuchen, N.J.: Scarecrow Press, 1984), p. 258.

6   Alile Sharon Larkin, "Black Women Film-makers Defining Ourselves: Feminism in Our Own Voice," in E. Deidre Pribaum, ed., *Female Spectators: Looking at Film and Television* (New York: Verso, 1988), p. 158.

7   Ellen Spiro, "Outlaws Through the Lens of Corporate America," *Cinematograph* 4 (1991): 180.

8   James, pp. 6 and 8.

9   Julianne Burton, ed., *Cinema and Social Change in Latin America: Conversations with Filmmakers* (Austin: University of Texas Press, 1986), p. ix.

10 Julianne Burton, "Marginal Cinemas and Mainstream Critical Theory," *Screen,* May-August 1985, p. 66.

11 See "The Resolutions of the Third World Filmmakers Meeting in Algiers, 1973," reprinted in Teshome Gabriel, *Third Cinema in the Third World* (Ann Arbor, Mich.: UMI Research Press, 1982), pp. 105–6, in which it is stated: "The countries enjoying political independence and struggling for varied development are aware of the fact that the struggle against imperialism on the political, economic and social levels is inseparable from its ideological content and that, consequently, action must be taken to seize from imperialism the means to influence ideologically, and forge new methods adapted in content and form to the interests of the struggles of their peoples."

12 Friedrich Engels's terms quoted in Gabriel, p. 9.

13 Fernando Solanas and Octavio Getino, "Toward a Third Cinema," in Coco Fusco, ed., *Reviewing Histories: Selections from New Latin American Cinema* (Buffalo, N.Y.: Hallwalls, 1987), p. 59.

14 James, pp. 95–100.

15 James, pp. 94, 99.

16 James, p. 167.

17 Robert Stam and Ismail Xavier, "Recent Brazilian Cinema: Allegory/Metacinema/ Carnival," *Film Quarterly* 43, no. 3: 17.

18 Emilie de Brigard, "The History of Ethnographic Film," in Paul Hockings, ed., *Principles of Visual Anthropology* (New York: Aldine, 1975), p. 15.

19 Margaret Mead, "Visual Anthropology in a Discipline of Words," in Hockings, ed., *Principles of Visual Anthropology,* p. 8.

20 Faye Ginsburg, "Indigenous Media: Faustian Contract or Global Village," *Visual Anthropology* 6, no. 1 (1991): 97.

21 Claudia Springer, "A Short History of Ethnographic Film," *Independent,* Dec. 1984, p. 14.

22 Jay Ruby, "The Image Mirrored: Reflexivity and the Documentary Film," in Alan

Rosenthal, ed., *New Challenges for Documentary* (Berkeley: University of California Press, 1988), p. 64.

23   David MacDougall, "Beyond Observational Cinema," in Nichols, ed., *Movies and Methods: Volume 2*, p. 282.

24   MacDougall, "Beyond Observational Cinema," in Hockings, ed., *Principles of Visual Anthropology*, p. 122.

25   Eric Barnouw, *Documentary: A History of the Non-Fiction Film* (Oxford: Oxford University Press, 1983), p. 258.

26   Ginsburg, p. 98.

27   Patricia Mellencamp, "Video and the Counterculture," in Cynthia Schneider and Brian Wallis, eds., *Global Television* (New York: Wedge Press, 1988), p. 200.

28   Hans Magnus Enzenberger, "Constituents of a Theory of Media," in Michael Roloff, ed., *The Consciousness Industry: On Literature, Politics and the Media* (New York: Seabury Press, 1974), p. 97.

29   Paul Ryan, "Guerrilla Strategy and Cybernetic Theory," *Radical Software* (Spring 1971), quoted in Stuart Marshall, "Video—From Art to Independence," *Screen* 26, no. 2 (1985): 67.

30   Mellencamp, pp. 199–200.

31   John Downing, *Radical Media: The Political Experience of Alternative Communication* (Boston: South End Press, 1984), pp. 128–29.

32   Larkin, p. 157.

33   Roger House, "Bedford-Stuyvesant: Voices from the Neighborhood," *Afterimage*, Summer 1991, p. 3.

34   Julia Lesage, "Political Aesthetics of Feminist Documentary Films," *Quarterly Review of Film Studies*, Fall 1978, p. 511.

35   Mary Ann Doane, Patricia Mellencamp, and Linda Williams, "Feminist Film Criticism: An Introduction," in Doane, Mellencamp, and Williams, eds., *Re-Vision* (Los Angeles: AFI, 1984), p. 4.

36   B. Ruby Rich, "In the Name of Feminist Film Criticism," in Nichols, ed., *Movies and Methods: Volume 2*, p. 342.

37   See Sean Cubitt, *Timeshift: On Video Culture* (New York: Routledge, 1991), chap. 1, "The Discontinuity Announcer," pp. 1–20; Todd Gitlin, *Inside Prime Time* (New York: Pantheon, 1985), p. 84; Larry Kirkman, "Videos: Democratic Media," *Foundation News*, May-June, 1993, pp. 43–45.

38   Ellen Spiro, "What to Wear on Your Video Activist Outing (Because the Whole World Is Watching): A Camcordist's Manifesto," *Independent*, May 1991, p. 22.

39   Karen Hirsch, "Do Environmental Films Help the Environment? Here are Some That Are," *Independent*, Jan.-Feb. 1993, p. 36.

40   See Janet Sorensen, "News With A View," *Afterimage*, May 1991, p. 3, and Richard Thompson, "Dismything Objectivity," *Independent*, June 1990, pp. 12–15.

41   A good deal of the specific information for this timeline comes from five sources

about AIDS representation in the mainstream media: Jan Zita Grover's "Visible Lesions: Images of People With AIDS," *Afterimage,* Summer 1989, pp. 10–16; James Kinsella's *Covering the Plague* (New Brunswick, N.J.: Rutgers University Press, 1989); Randy Shilts's *And the Band Played On* (New York: St. Martin's Press, 1987); Timothy Cook and David Colby's "The Mass-Mediated Epidemic: The Politics of AIDS on the Nightly Network News," in Elizabeth Fee and Daniel Fox, eds., *AIDS: The Making of a Chronic Disease* (Berkeley: University of California Press, 1992), pp. 84–124; and Paula Treichler's "AIDS, Gender and Biomedical Discourse," in Douglas Crimp, ed., *AIDS: Cultural Analysis/Cultural Activism* (Cambridge, Mass.: MIT Press, 1988), pp. 31–70.

42   Kinsella, p. 52.
43   Kinsella, p. 61.
44   Kinsella, pp. 127–28.
45   Cook and Colby, pp. 93–95.
46   Grover, p. 12.
47   Kinsella, pp. 73, 33.
48   Kinsella, p. 127.
49   Kinsella, quoting a Midwestern newspaper editor, p. 74.
50   Cook and Colby, pp. 99–102.
51   Grover, p. 12.
52   Grover, p. 12.
53   Grover, p. 12.
54   Treichler, p. 243.
55   Shilts, p. 513.
56   Grover, p. 13.
57   Crimp discusses Helms's amendment in depth in "How to Have Promiscuity in an Epidemic," in Crimp, ed., *AIDS: Cultural Analysis/Cultural Activism,* pp. 259–65. He includes a good portion of the senator's remarks, including this opening of the amendment: "Purpose: To prohibit the use of any funds provided under this Act to the Centers for Disease Control from being used to provide AIDS education information, or prevention materials and activities that promote, encourage, or condone homosexual activities or the intravenous use of illegal drugs."
58   Jean Carlomusto, "Focusing on Women: Video as Activism," in the ACT UP/NY Women and AIDS Book Group, eds., *Women, AIDS and Activism* (Boston: South End Press, 1990), pp. 215–18, and Kenney, "Testing the Limits: An Interview."
59   Kinsella, p. 156.
60   See Media Network's *Seeing Through AIDS* (New York: Media Guide, 1989).
61   Rich, p. 357.
62   Catherine Saalfield, "On the Make: Activist Video Collectives," in Martha Gever, John Greyson, and Pratibha Parmar, eds., *Queer Looks: Perspectives on Lesbian and Gay Film and Video* (New York: Routledge, 1993), p. 27.
63   Saalfield, p. 26.

64   Saalfield, p. 31.
65   Saalfield, pp. 31, 27.
66   Renee Tajima and Ernesto de la Vega, *Retooling for Diversity* (New York: Ford Foundation, 1993), p. 4.
67   Tajima and de la Vega, p. 1.
68   Tajima and de la Vega, p. 23.
69   Tajima and de la Vega, p. 26.

3   The Politics of Mimesis

1   John Greyson, "Parma Violets for Wayland Flowers," in James Miller, ed., *Fluid Exchanges* (Toronto: University of Toronto Press, 1992), p. 135.
2   Trinh T. Minh-ha, "The Totalizing Quest of Meaning," in Michael Renov, ed., *Theorizing Documentary* (New York: Routledge, 1993), p. 98.
3   Bill Nichols, *Representing Reality* (Bloomington: Indiana University Press, 1991), p. 17.
4   Claire Johnston, "Women's Cinema as Counter Cinema," in Claire Johnston, ed., *Notes on Women's Cinema* (London: Society for Education in Film and Television, 1973), p. 28.
5   E. Ann Kaplan, "Theories and Strategies of the Feminist Documentary," in Alan Rosenthal, ed., *New Challenges for Documentary* (Berkeley: University of California Press, 1988), p. 80.
6   Kobena Mercer, "Recoding Narratives of Race and Nation," *Independent,* Jan.-Feb. 1989, p. 23.
7   Barbara Halpern Martineau, "Talking About Our Lives and Experiences," in Thomas Waugh, ed., *"Show Us Life"* (Metuchen, N.J.: Scarecrow Press, 1984), p. 26.
8   Fernando Birri, "Cinema and Underdevelopment," in Michael Chanan, ed., *Twenty-five Years of New Latin American Cinema* (London: BFI, 1983), p. 12.
9   Fee and Fox, Introduction, in Fee and Fox, eds., *AIDS: The Making of a Chronic Disease*, p. 5.
10   Margaret Morse, "The Television News Personality and Credibility: Reflections on the News in Transition," in Tania Modleski, ed., *Studies in Entertainment: Critical Approaches to Mass Culture* (Bloomington: Indiana University Press, 1986), p. 55.
11   Richard Collins, "Seeing Is Believing: The Ideology of Naturalism," in John Corner, ed., *Documentary and the Mass Media* (London: Arnold, 1986), p. 130.
12   Stuart Hall, "Culture, the Media and the 'Ideological Effect,'" in James Curran et al. eds., *Mass Communication and Society* (London: Arnold, 1977), p. 345.
13   Paul Willemen, "On Realism in Cinema," in John Ellis, ed., *Screen Reader 1* (London: Society for Education in Film and Television, 1977), p. 57.
14   Cindy Patton, *Sex and Germs: The Politics of AIDS* (Boston: South End Press,

1985), p. 11, writes extensively about how the modern concept of "germs" has been used to discriminate against people on the basis of race, class, gender, and other markers of difference: "dirt and germs serve an important symbolic role in the social organization of difference." Feminist scholars writing about AIDS, like Paula Treichler, "AIDS, Gender and Biomedical Discourse," p. 193, also discuss the ways that AIDS feeds already operating understandings of illness: "the real and imagined links between women's bodies and disease—especially infections and sexually transmitted diseases—are many and complex, and have a history reaching back many centuries." Much recent scholarship in gay studies has made similar claims for the gay body. See Jeffrey Weeks, *Sexuality and Its Discontents: Meanings, Myths and Modern Sexualities* (London: Routledge, 1985), and Michel Foucault, *The History of Sexuality* (New York: Vintage Books, 1980).

15 Robert Stam, "Television News and Its Spectator," in E. Ann Kaplan, ed., *Regarding Television* (Los Angeles: AFI, 1983), p. 39.

16 Dziga Vertov, "Kino-Eye to Radio Eye," in Annette Michelson, ed., *Kino-Eye: The Writings of Dziga Vertov* (Berkeley: University of California Press, 1984), p. 87.

17 Catherine Saalfield and Ray Navarro, "Not Just Black and White: AIDS Media and People of Color," *Independent,* July 1989, p. 18.

18 Dai Vaughn, "Television Documentary Usage," in Rosenthal, ed., *New Challenges for Documentary,* p. 37.

19 Catherine Belsey, *Critical Practices* (New York: Metheun, 1980), p. 51.

20 Iris Davis, M.D. relays an anecdote in "No Names and No Pictures," in *Women, AIDS and Activism,* p. 97, in which her naive suggestion to a female AIDS patient to try and give a newspaper interview was met with an emphatic, "No."

21 Gregg Bordowitz and Jean Carlomusto, "Do It!" *Video Guide* 10, nos. 3, 4 (1989): 22.

22 Cindy Patton, "Safe Sex and the Pornographic Vernacular," in Bad Object-Choices, eds., *How Do I Look? Queer Film and Video* (Seattle: Bay Press, 1991), pp. 44–45.

23 Bordowitz and Carlomusto, p. 22.

4 The Pleasure and Power of Seeing Science

1 Michel Foucault, *The History of Sexuality: Volume I* (New York: Vintage Books, 1980), p. 48.

2 Brian Winston, "The Documentary Film as Scientific Inscription," in Michael Renov. ed., *Theorizing Documentary* (New York: Routledge, 1993), pp. 37–57. Direct quotation is from an earlier draft, presented at the University of Ohio Film Conference, p. 4.

3 See Trinh T. Minh-ha, "Documentary Is/Not a Name," *October* 52 (Spring 1990): 76–97, and Stuart Hall, "Media Power: The Double Bind," in Alan Rosenthal, ed., *New Challenges for Documentary* (Berkeley: University of California Press, 1988), pp. 357–64.

4 See Stanley Aronowitz, *Science as Power: Discourse and Ideology in Modern Society* (Minneapolis: University of Minnesota Press, 1988).

5 Dorothy Nelkin, *Selling Science* (New York: W. H. Freeman, 1987), p. 34.

6 Foucault, p. 44.

7 Emily Martin, "Science and Women's Bodies: Forms of Anthropological Knowledge," in Mary Jacobus, E. F. Keller, and Sally Shuttleworth, eds., *Body/Politics: Women and the Discourses of Science* (New York: Routledge, 1990), p. 69.

8 Evelyn Fox Keller, *Reflections on Gender and Society* (New Haven, Conn.: Yale University Press, 1985), p. 18.

9 Susanna Hornig, "Television's *NOVA* and the Constitution of Scientific Truth," *Critical Studies in Mass Communications,* March 1990, p. 12.

10 Christian Metz, "Story/Discourse," in Bill Nichols, ed., *Movies and Methods: Volume 2* (Berkeley: University of California Press, 1985), p. 548.

11 Stuart Hall, "Culture, the Media, and 'the Ideological Effect,'" in James Curran et al., eds., *Mass Communication and Society* (London: Arnold, 1977), p. 342.

12 Judith Williamson, "Every Virus Tells a Story: The Meaning of HIV and AIDS," in Erica Carter and Simon Watney, eds., *Taking Liberties: AIDS and Cultural Politics* (London: Serpent's Tail, 1989), p. 69.

13 Jean Baudrillard, "The Precession of Simulacra," in Brian Wallis, ed., *Art After Modernism: Rethinking Representation* (New York: New Museum of Contemporary Art, 1984), p. 254.

14 Baudrillard, p. 253.

15 Nelkin, p. 71.

16 Williamson, p. 77.

17 Williamson, p. 78.

18 Treichler, "AIDS, Gender, and Biomedical Discourse," in Elizabeth Fee and Daniel Fox, eds., *AIDS: The Burden of History* (Berkeley: University of California Press, 1988), p. 200.

19 Simon Watney, *Policing Desire* (Minneapolis: University of Minnesota Press, 1987), p. 28.

20 Anne Karpf, *Doctoring the Media* (London: Routledge, 1988), p. 51.

21 Hall, "Media Power," pp. 359–60.

22 Metz, p. 547.

23 Ludmilla Jordanova, *Sexual Visions: Images of Gender in Science and Medicine Between the Eighteenth and Twentieth Centuries* (Madison: University of Wisconsin Press, 1988), p. 87.

24 Donna Haraway, *Primate Visions* (New York: Routledge, 1989), p. 179.

25 Gregory Ulmer, *Teletheory: Grammatology in the Age of Video* (New York: Routledge, 1989), p. 7.

26 Williamson, p. 77.

27 Judith Newton, "Feminism and Anxiety in *Alien*," in Annette Kuhn, ed., *Alien Zone* (London: Verso, 1990), p. 85.

28 Barbara Creed, "Gynesis, Postmodernism, and the Science Fiction Horror Film," in Kuhn, ed., *Alien Zone*, p. 214.

29 Patton, *Inventing AIDS* (New York: Routledge, 1990), p. 55.

30 Jordanova, p. 150.

31 See Renee Sabatier, *Blaming Others* (Philadelphia: New Society Publishers, 1988) and the ACT UP/NY Women and AIDS Book Group, *Women, AIDS and Activism* (Boston: South End Press, 1990).

32 See the AIDS Discrimination Unit of the New York City Commission on Human Rights, *AIDS and People of Color: The Discriminatory Impact* (New York: Commission on Human Rights, 1987).

33 Elizabeth Fee, "Critiques of Modern Science: The Relationship to Feminism and Other Radical Epistemologies," in Ruth Bleir, ed., *Feminist Approaches to Science* (New York: Pergamon Press, 1986), p. 47.

5   Containing and Unleashing the Threat

1 Simon Watney, *Policing Desire* (Minneapolis: University of Minnesota Press, 1987), p. 33.

2 See the excellent discussion of safer sex and cleaning works in Cynthia Chris, "Transmission Issues for Women," in the ACT UP/NY Women and AIDS Book Group, eds., *Women, AIDS and Activism* (Boston: South End Press, 1990), pp. 17–26, or in Cindy Patton and Janis Kelly, *Making It: A Woman's Guide to Sex in the Age of AIDS* (Ithaca, N.Y.: Firebrand Books, 1988).

3 See Gena Corea, *The Invisible Epidemic: The Story of Women and AIDS* (New York: Harper Collins, 1992).

4 Paula Treichler, "AIDS, Gender, and Biomedical Discourse," in Elizabeth Fee and Daniel Fox, eds., *AIDS: The Burdens of History* (Berkeley: University of California Press, 1988), p. 232.

5 Sunny Rumsey, "Communities Under Siege," in Ines Rieder and Patricia Ruppelt, eds., *AIDS: The Women* (San Francisco: Cleis Press, 1988), p. 188.

6 See Corea, esp. pp. 8–18, for a careful discussion of sexism within the medical establishment and the painstaking work by women to get women's relationship to the disease taken seriously.

7 Mary Guinan and Ann Hardy, "Epidemiology of AIDS in Women in the United States," *JAMA* 257, no. 15: 2039–42.

8 See Treichler's "AIDS: Gender, and Biomedical Discourse," for detailed descriptions of this new onslaught of reportage.

9 "AIDS: Changing the Rules" was produced by an independent production company, AIDSFilms, and aired on PBS, Sept. 30, 1987. "AIDS Hits Home: A CBS News Special" was produced by CBS News and aired, Oct. 22, 1986. "Donahue: AIDS Ward," was produced by NBC and aired in Nov. 1986. "Life, Death and AIDS: An NBC News Special" was produced by NBC News and aired, Jan. 21, 1986.

10   In "How Do Women Live?" in *Women, AIDS and Activism*, pp. 6–9, Chris writes
      about the many controls of women's sexuality that are enacted currently in our
      culture. She explains that the U.S. Supreme Court's 1989 *Webster* decision is
      only the most blatant form of these social controls which also include lack of
      100 percent safe birth control, lack of family planning education, discrimination
      against lesbian mothering, education of poor women and teenagers, and pervasive
      patriarchal thinking on women's sexuality.

11   Raymond Williams, *Television: Technology and Cultural Form* (New York:
      Schocken Books, 1975), p. 40.

12   Watney, p. 42.

13   Sander Gilman, "AIDS and Syphilis: The Iconography of Disease," in Douglas
      Crimp, ed., *AIDS: Cultural Analysis/Cultural Activism* (Cambridge, Mass.: MIT
      Press, 1988), p. 107.

14   In discussions with John Hoffman from AIDSFilms about my criticisms of this
      film, he explained that Beverly Johnson *was* uncomfortable with this material
      and that she was difficult to direct. This problem was intensified by a very tight
      shooting schedule, which meant that they did not have the luxury to retake her
      performance to smooth out all the ripples I later analyzed as *intended*. Neverthe-
      less, I believe that our somewhat conflicting stories about the meanings of these
      pauses are in the end not that distinct. Whatever the producers' intentions (or
      Johnson's), what has been caught through the camera and allowed to air on PBS
      is an image of a woman in conflict about how to perform a liberated and safe
      sexuality.

15   Robin Gorna, "Delightful Visions: From Anti-Porn to Eroticizing Safer Sex," in
      Lynne Segal and Mary McIntosh, eds., *Sex Exposed: Sexuality and the Pornogra-
      phy Debate* (New Brunswick, N.J.: Rutgers University Press, 1993), p. 175.

16   In *Inventing AIDS* (New York: Routledge, Chapman and Hall, 1990), p. 47, Cindy
      Patton writes how the "Heterosexual AIDS Panic" was based upon very pro-
      scriptive ideas about straight people's sexuality: "penile-vaginal intercourse is
      the hegemonic and identity-creating act, the meaning of safe sex shifted toward
      abstinence, monogamy, or the use of condoms."

17   Treichler, "AIDS, Homophobia and Biomedical Discourse: An Epidemic of Signi-
      fication," in Crimp, ed., *AIDS: Cultural Activism/Cultural Analysis,* p. 67.

18   Chris, "Transmission Issues for Women," pp. 19–23.

19   Watney writes about the way that "morality" has been used as both justification
      to punish the "unacceptable" people who are infected with HIV (through legisla-
      tion and regulation about sexuality, education, and drug use) (esp. pp. 3, 43, 127)
      and to explain why certain "immoral" people are ill (p. 148).

20   Cindy Patton discusses how the rhetoric of the New Right has been fueled by
      AIDS in *Sex and Germs* (Boston: South End Press, 1985), p. 98. And Lynne Segal
      writes in "Lessons from the Front," in Erica Carter and Simon Watney, eds.,
      Taking Liberties (London: Serpent's Tail, 1989), pp. 133, 135: "AIDS has fueled the

already growing New Right backlash against gay liberation and sexual permissiveness, against women's equality and abortion rights, and against the feminist
rejection of all forms of male domination. . . . The onset of AIDS gave this pro-
family, anti-sexual permissiveness rhetoric an apparent legitimacy, not simply in
the name of conservative morality but also in the name of medical wisdom."

21 Gorna, p. 183.

22 Patton writes in *Sex and Germs*, p. 12, how only white men are "believed to be
in control of their sexuality."

23 Elizabeth Fee, "Sin Versus Science: Venereal Disease in Twentieth-Century Baltimore," in Fee and Fox, eds., *AIDS: The Burdens of History*, p. 127.

24 The discussion of women, race, and AIDS always focuses upon the need for
culturally specific educational materials. Renee Sabatier, in *Prejudice, Race and
Worldwide AIDS* (Philadelphia: New Society Publishers, 1988), devotes a chapter
to this issue. Several of the articles in *Women, AIDS and Activism* are also dedicated to this important principle, including an entire section, "Race, Women and
AIDS," documenting the needs of women from specific communities of color.

25 Dooley Worth, "Minority Women and AIDS: Culture, Race and Gender," in
Douglas Feldman, ed., *Culture and AIDS: The Global Pandemic* (New York:
Praeger, 1990), pp. 111–36. See also "Race, Women and AIDS," in *Women, AIDS
and Activism*, pp. 81–112.

26 Lurie writes in her article "Teenagers," pp. 136–37, that the Board of Regents of
New York State, for example, has a policy which states that it "views the use
of condoms as extremely high-risk behavior. The view that condoms should or
can be used as a way to reduce the risk of transmission of AIDS should not
be supported." In a review of eighteen curricula nationwide, Lurie reports that
one-fourth of them "did not address abstinence or condom use."

27 Crimp, "How to Have Promiscuity in an Epidemic," in Crimp, ed., *AIDS: Cultural
Analysis/Cultural Activism*, p. 268.

28 Brian Goldfarb, "Video Activism and Critical Pedagogy: Sexuality at the End of
the Rainbow," *Afterimage*, May 1993, p. 6.

29 Goldfarb, p. 4.

30 Anthony Pinching and Donald Jeffries, "AIDS and HTLV-III/LAV Infection: Consequences for Obstetrics and Perinatal Medicine," *British Journal of Obstetrics
and Gynecology* 92:1211–17.

31 See Risa Denenberg, "Pregnant Women and HIV," in *Women, AIDS and Activism*, pp. 159–64, Angela Davis, "Racism, Birth Control, and Reproductive Rights,"
and Marlene Gerber Fried, "Abortion and Sterilization in the Third World," in
Marlene Fried, ed., *From Abortion to Reproductive Freedom* (Boston: South End
Press, 1990), pp. 15–26 and pp. 63–64.

32 AIDS Discrimination Unit, *AIDS and People of Color: The Discriminatory Impact*
(New York: Commission on Human Rights, 1987).

33 Patton, *Inventing AIDS*, p. 108.

34 Priscilla Alexander, "Prostitutes Are Being Scapegoated for Heterosexual AIDS," in Frederique Delacost and Priscilla Alexander, eds., *Sex Work* (San Francisco: Cleis Press, 1987), pp. 248–65.

35 Patton writes about Americans' inability to see African AIDS as akin to our own in her chapter "Inventing 'African AIDS,' " in *Inventing AIDS*. Other useful discussions of this phenomenon can be found in Paula Treichler, "AIDS and HIV Infection in the Third World: A First World Chronicle," in Barbara Kruger and Phil Mariani, eds., *Remaking History* (Seattle: Bay Press, 1989), pp. 31–86, or in Simon Watney, "Missionary Positions: AIDS, Africa and Race," in Russell Ferguson et al., eds., *Out There* (New York: New Museum of Contemporary Art, 1990), pp. 89–106.

36 Zoe Leonard, "Lesbians in the AIDS Crisis," in *Women, AIDS and Activism*, pp. 113–18.

37 Lee Chiaramonte, "Lesbian Safety and AIDS: The Very Last Fairy Tale," *Visibilities*, Jan.-Feb. 1988, p. 5.

38 Leonard, "Lesbians in the AIDS Crisis," pp. 115–16.

39 Chiaramonte, pp. 5–6.

40 Gorna, p. 174.

41 See Margaret Morse, "Sports on Television," in E. Ann Kaplan, ed., *Regarding Television* (Los Angeles: AFI, 1983), pp. 44–66. In a complex argument Morse attempts to use the psychoanalytic framework of feminist discussions of images of women to think about the potential psychic pleasures evoked when television spectators regard men's bodies.

42 Bill Nichols, *Representing Reality* (Bloomington: Indiana University Press, 1991), p. 178.

43 Mary Ann Doane, *The Desire to Desire: The Woman's Film of the 1940s* (Bloomington: Indiana University Press, 1987), p. 40.

44 Nichols, *Representing Reality*, p. 31.

6 WAVE: A Case Study

1 Terry Eagleton, *Marxism and Literary Criticism* (Berkeley: University of California Press, 1976), p. 60.

2 Janet Wolff, *The Social Production of Art* (New York: St. Martin's Press, 1981), p. 30.

3 Wolff, p. 40.

4 For writing that explains the Birmingham School's development of their position regarding ethnographic research, see Dorothy Hobson et al., eds., *Culture, Media, Language* (London: Hutchinson, 1980); Tony Bennett et al., eds., *Popular Television and Film: A Reader* (London: BFI, 1981), and John Fiske, "British Cultural Studies and Television," in Robert Allen, ed., *Channels of Discourse* (Chapel Hill: University of North Carolina Press, 1987), pp. 254–90. For examples of this

theory put into action, see esp. Angela McRobbie and Mica Nava, eds., *Gender and Generation* (London: Macmillan, 1984).

5   Douglas Crimp, "Introduction: Cultural Analysis/Cultural Activism," in Crimp, ed., *AIDS Cultural Analysis/Cultural Activism* (Cambridge, Mass.: MIT Press, 1988), pp. 4–6.

6   Douglas Crimp, *AIDS Demo/Graphics* (Seattle: Bay Press, 1990), p. 19.

7   WAVE received preproduction and production grants from the New York Council for the Humanities totaling $19,500; grants for $500 from the Astraea Fund for Women; $1,500 from ArtMatters; a postproduction, in-kind editing grant from Women Make Movies; a $5,000 distribution grant from the New York State Council on the Arts; and a $1,000 contribution from a private funder.

8   Frances Negrón-Muntaner, "The Ethics of Community Media: A Filmmaker Confronts the Contradictions of Producing Media about and for a Community Where She Is Both an Insider and Outsider," *Independent*, May 1992, p. 20.

9   Annie Goldson, "Color-Develop Normal or Multicultural Politics Dissected," *FELIX*, Spring 1992, pp. 120–21.

10   Michelle Valladares, "Guarding Our Own Best Interests or Parallel Lines/ Connecting Tongues," *FELIX*, Spring 1992, p. 44.

11   Negrón-Muntaner, p. 20.

12   Dooley Worth, "Minority Women and AIDS: Culture, Race and Gender," in Douglas Feldman, ed., *Culture and AIDS: The Global Pandemic* (New York: Praeger, 1990), p. 126.

13   Renee Sabatier, *Blaming Others: Prejudice, Race and Worldwide AIDS* (Philadelphia: New Society Publishers, 1988), p. 7.

14   Catherine Saalfield and Ray Navarro, "Not Just Black and White: AIDS Media and People of Color," *Independent*, July 1989, p. 18.

15   Sabatier, p. 5.

16   The original "Weekly Schedule":

Week 1: *Introductions.* Introduce ourselves to each other. Introduction to the camera. How it works; its parts. Watch *Mildred Pearson*, BATF's community-produced video, and AIDSFilms' *Vida, Seriously Fresh*, and *Are You with Me?*

Week 2: *Videotape "Hellos"; Women and AIDS in the Media.* Each group member will briefly introduce herself and will have the opportunity to tape someone else's introduction. Watch *Women and AIDS* and *Life, Death and AIDS*, narrated by Tom Brokaw.

Week 3: *Plan videotape introducing the group's meeting space; Representation of AIDS in minority communities.* Discuss various methods useful to describe a place on tape. Watch *AIDS in the Barrio* and *DiAna's Hair Ego.*

Week 4: *Shoot "Meeting Space"*

Week 5: *Plan tape about neighborhood in Brooklyn; Representation of AIDS in Minority Communities.* How can we best show life in a neighborhood in Brooklyn? Watch *AIDS Is About Secrets.*

Week 6: *Representation of AIDS in Minority Communities.* Watch *Se Met Ko.*

Week 7: *Shoot "Brooklyn Neighborhood"*

Week 8: *Plan Role Plays: The Soap Opera Format.* What are difficult situations that can occur between people confronting AIDS? Watch *Ojos Que No Ven.*

Week 9: *Shoot "Role Plays"*

Week 10: *Guest Speaker: Representation of Women and Disease*

Week 11: *Plan Self-Portraits.* How would you like to see yourself represented on video? Watch *Her Giveaway* and *Safe Sex Slut.*

Week 12: *Guest Speakers.* Amber Hollibaugh and Alisa Lebow screen *Women and Children Last.*

Week 13: *Shoot "Self-Portraits"*

Week 14: *Edit "Self-Portraits"*

Week 15: *Plan Final Project; Community Produced AIDS Media.* What do we want to say? What do people need to know? Guest speakers from Testing the Limits screen tape.

Week 16: *Plan Final Project; AIDS Activist Video.* Speaker from DIVA TV.

Week 17: *Plan Final Project; AIDS Art Video.* View video by Tom Kalin.

Weeks 18–19: *Shoot Final Project.*

Weeks 20–21: *Edit Final Project.*

Week 22: *Screen Final Video/Party*

17 Sabatier, p. 7.

18 Trinh T. Minh-ha, "Outside In Inside Out," in Jim Pine and Paul Willemen, eds., *Questions of Third Cinema* (London: BFI, 1989), p. 145.

19 Cindy Patton, *Inventing AIDS* (New York: Routledge, Chapman and Hall, 1990), pp. 1–25.

20 Crimp, "Introduction: Cultural Analysis/Cultural Activism," p. 12.

21 Thomas Waugh, "Introduction," in Waugh, ed., *"Show Us Life"* (Metuchen, N.J.: Scarecrow Press, 1984), p. xiii.

22 Dziga Vertov, "Kino-Eye to Radio-Eye," in Annette Michelson, ed., *Kino-Eye: The Writings of Dziga Vertov* (Berkeley: University of California Press, 1984), p. 29.

23 Octavio Getino and Fernando Solanas, "Towards a Third Cinema," in Coco Fusco, ed., *Reviewing Histories* (Buffalo, N.Y.: Hallwalls, 1987), p. 76.

24 John Downing, *Radical Media* (Boston: South End Press, 1984), p. 138.

25 Bernice Johnson Reagon and Mark O'Brien, "Introduction: Personal Impulses, Social Intentions," in Reagon and O'Brien, eds., *Reimaging America: The Arts of Social Change* (Philadelphia: New Society Publishers, 1990), p. 14.

26 Lucy Lippard, "Hanging Onto Baby, Heating Up the Bathwater," in Reagon and O'Brien, eds., *Reimaging America,* p. 230.

27 Teshome Gabriel, "Third Cinema as Guardian of Popular Memory: Towards a Third Aesthetics," in Pines and Willemen, eds., *Questions of Third Cinema,* p. 60.

28 For example, *We Care* has been screened at the Department of Housing Preservation and Development Health Fair, NYU's Department of Cinema Studies, the

Brooklyn AIDS Task Force, the Broadway Women's Shelter, Empire State College, the Departments of Health in Manhattan and Queens, St. Mary's Medical Center, the Monica House Women's Shelter, Visiting Nurses, Rockaway Home Attendants, the East New York Avenue Community Center, the Hacer Hispanic Women's Center, the Ridgewood Bushwick Senior Citizen Attends, the National Congress of Neighborhood Women, Gay Men's Health Crisis, etc. It has been screened at the Whitney Museum, the Brooklyn Museum, the Museo del Barrio, the Women in the Director's Chair Festival, and Donnell Library's Meet the Maker Program. More than 700 copies of the tape have been distributed to AIDS service organizations, colleges, and individuals.

29   Burton, "Marginal Cinemas and Mainstream Critical Theory," *Screen* 2, nos. 3–4 (1985): 12.

30   Getino and Solanas, p. 79.

31   Barbara Halpern-Martineau, "Talking About Our Lives and Experiences," in Waugh, ed., "*Show Us Life,*" p. 254.

7   Identity, Community, and Alternative AIDS Video

1   Douglas Crimp, "AIDS Demo/Graphics," in Allan Klusacek and Ken Morrison, eds., *A Leap in the Dark: AIDS, Art and Contemporary Cultures* (Montreal: Vehicule Press, 1992), p. 53.

2   bell hooks, *Yearning: Race, Gender, and Cultural Politics* (Boston: South End Press, 1990), p. 22.

3   For example, here are just a few of the many titles which identify the tape's intended audience: *Doctors, Liars and Women, We Are Not Republicans, Facing Our Fears: Mental Health Professionals Speak Out, AIDS in the Black Community, AIDS in the Barrio, Black People Get AIDS Too, Drugs and AIDS: An Appeal to Users, Women and AIDS, PWA Power,* and *Talking with Teens.* See Videography for further information.

4   Dennis Altman, "AIDS and the Reconceptualization of Homosexuality," in Klusacek and Morrison, eds., *A Leap in the Dark,* p. 36.

5   In a conversation with Saalfield about *AIDS TV.*

BIBLIOGRAPHY

ACT UP/NY Women and AIDS Book Group. *Women, AIDS and Activism*. Boston: South End Press, 1990.

Adler, Peter, and Patricia Adler, eds. *Journal of Contemporary Ethnography: Special Issue on Ethnography and AIDS*. London: Sage Publications, 1990.

AIDS Discrimination Unit of the New York City Commission on Human Rights. *AIDS and People of Color: The Discriminatory Impact*. New York: Commission on Human Rights, 1987.

Alexander, Priscilla. "Prostitutes Are Being Scapegoated for Heterosexual AIDS." *Sex Work: Writings by Women in the Sex Industry*. Ed. Frederique Delacost and Priscilla Alexander. San Francisco: Cleis Press, 1987: 248–65.

Altman, Dennis. "AIDS and the Reconceptualization of Homosexuality." *A Leap in the Dark*. Ed. Allan Klusacek and Ken Morrison. Montreal: Vehicule Press, 1992: 32–46.

Amaro, Hortensia. "Women's Reproductive Rights in the Age of AIDS." *From Abortion Rights to Reproductive Freedom*. Ed. Marlene Gerber Fried. Boston: South End Press, 1990: 245–54.

Andrade-Watkins, Claire, and Mbye Cham, eds. *Blackframes: Critical Perspectives on Black Independent Cinema*. Cambridge, Mass.: MIT Press, 1988.

Armes, Roy. *On Video*. London: Routledge, 1988.

Armstrong, David. *A Trumpet to Arms: Alternative Media in America*. Los Angeles: JP Tarcher, 1981.

Aronowitz, Stanley. *Science as Power: Discourse and Ideology in Modern Society*. Minneapolis: University of Minnesota Press, 1988.

Bad Object Choices, ed. *How Do I Look? Queer Film and Video*. Seattle: Bay Press, 1991.

Barnouw, Erik. *Documentary: A History of the Non-Fiction Film*. New York: Oxford University Press, 1983.

Baudrillard, Jean. "The Precession of the Simulacra." *Art After Modernism: Rethinking Representation*. Ed. Brian Wallis. New York: New Museum of Contemporary Art, 1984.

Belsey, Catherine. *Critical Practices*. New York: Metheun, 1980.

Birri, Fernando. "Cinema and Underdevelopment." *Twenty-five Years of New Latin American Cinema*. Ed. Michael Chanan. London: British Film Institute, 1983: 9–12.

Bleir, Ruth, ed. *Feminist Approaches to Science*. New York: Pergamon Press, 1986.

Bobo, Jacqueline. *"The Color Purple:* Black Women as Cultural Readers." *Female Spectators*. Ed. E. Deidre Pribaum. London: Verso, 1988: 90–109.

Bordowitz, Gregg. "Picture a Coalition." *AIDS: Cultural Analysis/Cultural Activism*. Ed. Douglas Crimp. Cambridge, Mass.: MIT Press, 1988: 183–96.

———. "The AIDS Crisis Is Ridiculous." *Queer Looks*. Ed. Martha Gever, John Greyson, and Pratibha Parmar. New York: Routledge, 1993: 209–24.

Bordowitz, Gregg, and Jean Carlomusto. "Do It." *Video Guide* 10, no. 3–4 (1989): 22.

Bourne, St. Clair. "Bright Moments: The Black Journal Series." *Independent,* May 1988: 10–13.

Brandt, Alan. "AIDS: From Social History to Social Policy." *AIDS: The Burdens of History*. Ed. Elizabeth Fee and Daniel Fox. Berkeley: University of California Press, 1988: 147–71.

Brigard, Emilie de. "The History of Ethnographic Film." *Principles of Visual Anthropology*. Ed. Paul Hockings. New York: Aldine, 1975: 13–43.

Burton, Julianne. "Marginal Cinemas and Mainstream Critical Theory." *Screen* 2, no. 3–4 (1985): 2–21.

———, ed. *Cinema and Social Change in Latin America: Conversations with Filmmakers*. Austin: University of Texas Press, 1986.

Carlomusto, Jean. "Making It: AIDS Activist Television." *Video Guide* 10, no. 3–4 (1989): 18.

———. "Focusing on Women: Video as Activism." *Women, AIDS and Activism*. Ed. ACT UP/NY Women and AIDS Book Group. Boston: South End Press, 1990: 215–18.

Carroll, Noel. *The Philosophy of Horror*. New York: Routledge, 1990.

Chanan, Michael, ed. *Twenty-five Years of New Latin American Cinema*. London: British Film Institute, 1983.

Chiaramonte, Lee. "Lesbian Safety and AIDS: The Very Last Fairy Tale." *Visibilities*, Jan.–Feb. 1988, pp. 4–7.

Chris, Cynthia. "Against the Law: Sex Workers Speak." *Afterimage*, Summer 1991: 8.

———. "Documents and Counter-Documents: AIDS Activist Video at the Crossroads." *Afterimage*, Nov. 1994: 6–8.

———. "Transmission Issues for Women." *Women, AIDS and Activism*. Ed. ACT UP/NY Women and AIDS Book Group. Boston: South End Press, 1991: 17–26.

Collins, Richard. "Seeing Is Believing: The Ideology of Naturalism." *Documentary and the Mass Media*. Ed. John Corner. London: Arnold, 1986: 125–40.

Cook, Timothy, and David Colby. "The Mass-Mediated Epidemic: The Politics of AIDS on the Nightly Network News." *AIDS: The Making of a Chronic Disease.* Ed. Elizabeth Fox and Daniel Fee. Berkeley: University of California Press, 1992: 84–124.

Corea, Gena. *The Invisible Epidemic: The Story of Women and AIDS.* New York: Harper Collins, 1992.

Creed, Barbara. "Gynesis, Postmodernism and the Science Fiction Horror Film." *Alien Zone.* Ed. Annette Kuhn. London: Verso, 1990: 214–18.

Crimp, Douglas. "Introduction." *AIDS: Cultural Analysis/Cultural Activism.* Ed. Douglas Crimp. Cambridge, Mass.: MIT Press, 1988: 3–16.

———. "How to Have Promiscuity in an Epidemic." *AIDS: Cultural Analysis/Cultural Activism.* Ed. Douglas Crimp. Cambridge, Mass.: MIT Press, 1988: 237–71.

———. "AIDS Demo/Graphics." *A Leap in the Dark: AIDS, Art and Contemporary Cultures.* Ed. Allan Klusacek and Ken Morrison. Montreal: Vehicule Press, 1992: 47–57.

Crimp, Douglas, with Adam Rolston. *AIDS: Demo/Graphics.* Seattle: Bay Press, 1990.

Cubitt, Sean. *Timeshift: On Video Culture.* New York: Routledge, 1991.

Cvetovich, Ann. "Video, AIDS, and Activism." *Afterimage,* Sept. 1991: 8–11.

Dargis, Manohla, and Amy Taubin. "Double Take." *Village Voice,* Jan. 21, 1992: 56.

Davis, Angela. "Racism, Birth Control, and Reproductive Rights." *From Abortion to Reproductive Freedom.* Ed. Marlene Gerber Fried. Boston: South End Press, 1990: 15–26.

Denenberg, Risa. "Pregnant Women and HIV." *Women, AIDS and Activism.* Ed. ACT UP/NY Women and AIDS Book Group. Boston: South End Press, 1991: 159–64.

Doane, Mary Ann. *The Desire to Desire: The Woman's Film of the 1940s.* Bloomington: Indiana University Press, 1987.

Downing, John. *Radical Media: The Political Experience of Alternative Communication.* Boston: South End Press, 1984.

Eagleton, Terry. *Marxism and Literary Criticism.* Berkeley: University of California Press, 1976.

Edelman, Lee. "The Mirror and the Tank: 'AIDS,' Subjectivity, and the Rhetoric of Activism." *Writing AIDS.* Ed. Timothy Murphy and Suzanne Poirier. New York: Columbia University Press, 1993: 9–38.

Elgear, Sandra, and Robyn Hutt. "Some Notes on Collective Production." *Video Guide* 10, no. 3–4: 20–21.

Ellis, John, ed. *Cinema/Ideology/Politics.* London: Society for Education in Film and Television, 1977.

Enzenberger, Hans Magnus. "Constituents of a Theory of the Media." *The Consciousness Industry: On Literature, Politics and the Media.* Ed. Michael Roloff. New York: Seabury Press, 1974: 95–128.

Fee, Elizabeth. "Sin Versus Science: Venereal Disease in Twentieth-Century Baltimore." *AIDS: The Burdens of History.* Ed. Elizabeth Fee and Daniel Fox. Berkeley: University of California Press, 1988: 121–46.

———. "Critiques of Modern Science: The Relationship of Feminism to Other Radical Epistemologies." *Feminist Approaches to Science.* Ed. Ruth Bleir. London: Macmillan, 1986.

Fee, Elizabeth, and Daniel Fox. *AIDS: The Making of a Chronic Disease.* Berkeley: University of California Press, 1992.

Ferguson, Russell, Martha Gever, Trinh T. Minh-ha, and Cornel West, eds. *Out There: Marginality and Contemporary Culture.* New York: New Museum of Contemporary Art, 1990.

Fiske, John. "British Cultural Studies and Television." *Channels of Discourse: Television and Contemporary Criticism.* Ed. Robert Allen. Chapel Hill: University of North Carolina Press, 1987: 254–90.

Foucault, Michel. *The History of Sexuality: Volume I.* New York: Vintage Books, 1980.

Fox, Daniel, and Elizabeth Fee, eds. *AIDS: The Burden of History.* Berkeley: University of California Press, 1988.

Friedberg, Ann. "Identification and the Star." *Star Signs.* Ed. Christine Gledhill. London: British Film Institute, 1982.

Friedman, Sharon, Sharon Dunwoody, and Carol Rogers, eds. *Scientists and Journalists.* New York: Free Press, 1986.

Fusco, Coco, ed. *Reviewing Histories: Selections from New Latin American Cinema.* Buffalo, N.Y.: Hallwalls, 1987.

Gabriel, Teshome. *Third Cinema in the Third World: The Aesthetics of Liberation.* Ann Arbor, Mich.: UMI Research Press, 1982.

———. "Third Cinema as Guardian of Popular Memory: Towards a Third Aesthetics." In *Questions of Third Cinema.* Ed. Jim Pines and Paul Willemen. London: British Film Institute, 1989: 53–64.

Getino, Octavio, and Fernando Solanas. "Towards a Third Cinema." *Reviewing Histories.* Ed. Coco Fusco. Buffalo, N.Y.: Hallwalls, 1987: 56–81.

Gever, Martha. "Pictures of Sickness: Stuart Marshall's *Bright Eyes.*" *AIDS: Cultural Activism/Cultural Analysis.* Ed. Douglas Crimp. Cambridge, Mass.: MIT Press, 1988: 109–26.

———. "The Names We Give Ourselves." *Out There.* Ed. Russell Ferguson et al. New York: New Museum of Contemporary Art, 1990: 191–202.

Gilman, Sander. "AIDS and Syphilis: The Iconography of Disease." *AIDS: Cultural Analysis/Cultural Activism.* Ed. Douglas Crimp. Cambridge, Mass.: MIT Press, 1988: 87–108.

Ginsburg, Faye. "Indigenous Media: Faustian Contract or Global Village?" *Visual Anthropology* 6, no. 1 (1991): 94–113.

Gitlin, Todd. *Inside Prime Time.* New York: Pantheon, 1985.

———. "Television's Screenings: Hegemony in Transition." *American Media and Mass Culture: Left Perspectives.* Ed. Donald Lazere. Berkeley: University of California Press, 1987: 240–65.

Gledhill, Christine. "Recent Developments in Feminist Film Criticism." *Quarterly Review of Film Studies* 3, no. 4 (1978): 458–93.

Goldfarb, Brian. "Video Activism and Critical Pedagogy: Sexuality at the End of the Rainbow." *Afterimage,* May 1993: 4–8.

Goldson, Annie. "Color-Develop Normal or Multicultural Politics Dissected." *FELIX* 1, no. 2 (Spring 1992): 10–13.

Gorna, Robin. "Delightful Visions: From Anti-Porn to Eroticizing Safer Sex." *Sex Exposed: Sexuality and the Pornography Debate.* Ed. Lynne Segal and Mary McIntosh. New Brunswick, N.J.: Rutgers University Press, 1993: 169–83.

Greyson, John. "Strategic Compromises: AIDS and Alternative Video Practices." *Reimaging America: The Arts of Social Change.* Ed. Mark O'Brien and Craig Little. Philadelphia: New Society Publishers, 1990: 60–74.

———. "Parma Violets for Wayland Flowers." *Fluid Exchanges.* Ed. James Miller. Toronto: University of Toronto Press, 1992: 135–45.

Griffin, Ada Gay. "What's Mine Is Not Mine/What's Mine Is Ours/What's Mine Is Yours/What's Yours Is Yours (Power Sharing and America)." *FELIX* 1, no. 2 (Spring 1992): 14–17.

Grimshaw, Roger, Dorothy Hobson, and Paul Willis. "Introduction to Ethnographic Studies at the Centre." In *Culture, Media, Language.* Ed. Hobson et al. London: Hutchinson, 1980: 73–77.

Gross, Larry. "The Ethics of (Mis)Representation." *Image Ethics: The Moral Rights of Subjects in Photographs, Film and Television.* Ed. John Stuart Katz, Larry Gross, and Jay Ruby. New York: Oxford University Press, 1988: 188–202.

Grover, Jan Zita. "AIDS: Keywords." *AIDS: Cultural Analysis/Cultural Activism.* Ed. Douglas Crimp. Cambridge, Mass.: MIT Press, 1988: 17–30.

———. "Introduction to AIDS: The Artists' Response." *Exhibit Guide: AIDS: The Artists' Response.* Ed. Jan Zita Grover. Columbus: Ohio State University, 1989: 2–7.

———. "Visible Lesions: Images of the PWA." *Afterimage* 17, no. 1 (1989): 10–16.

———. "AIDS, Keywords and Cultural Work." *Cultural Studies.* Ed. Grossberg et al. New York: Routledge, 1992: 227–33.

Hall, Stuart. "Culture, Media and the 'Ideological Effect.'" *Mass Communication and Society.* Ed. James Curran et al. London: Arnold, 1977: 315–48.

———. "Introduction to Media Studies at the Centre." *Culture, Media, Language.* Ed. Dorothy Hobson, Stuart Hall, Andrew Lowe, and Paul Willis. London: Hutchinson, 1980: 117–21.

———. "The Rediscovery of 'Ideology': Return of the Repressed in Media Studies." *Culture, Society and the Media.* Ed. Michael Gurevitch et al. London: Metheun, 1982: 56–90.

———. "Media Power: The Double Bind." *New Challenges for Documentary.* Ed. Alan Rosenthal. Berkeley: University of California Press, 1988: 357–64.

———. "The Whites of Their Eyes: Racist Ideologies and the Media." *The Media*

Reader. Ed. Manuel Alvarado and John Thompson. London: British Film Institute, 1990: 7–23.

———. "Theoretical Legacies." *Cultural Studies.* Ed. Grossberg et al. New York: Routledge, 1992: 277–85.

Halleck, DeeDee. "Watch Out Dick Tracy! Popular Video in the Wake of the *Exxon Valdez.*" *Technoculture.* Ed. Constance Penley and Andrew Ross. Minneapolis: University of Minnesota Press, 1991: 211–30.

Hanson, Jarice. *Understanding Video: Applications, Impact, and Theory.* London: Sage Publications, 1987.

Harding, Sandra. *The Science Question in Feminism.* Ithaca, N.Y.: Cornell University Press, 1986.

Hardy, Ann, and Mary Guinan. "Epidemiology of AIDS in Women in the United States." *JAMA* 257, no. 15 (1987): 2039–42.

Harraway, Donna. *Primate Visions: Gender, Race and Nature in the World of Modern Science.* New York: Routledge, 1989.

Hirsch, Karen. "Do Environmental Films Help the Environment? Here Are Some That Are." *Independent,* Jan.–Feb. 1993: 36–40.

hooks, bell. *Yearning: Race, Gender, and Cultural Politics.* Boston: South End Press, 1990.

———. *Black Looks.* Boston: South End Press, 1991.

Hornig, Susanna. "Television's *NOVA* and the Construction of Scientific Truth." *Critical Studies in Mass Communication* 7 (March 1990): 11–23.

Horrigan, Bill. "Notes on AIDS and Its Combattants: An Appreciation." *Theorizing Documentary.* Ed. Michael Renov. New York: Routledge, 1993: 164–73.

House, Roger. "Bedford-Stuyvesant: Voices from the Neighborhood." *Afterimage,* Summer 1991: 3.

Institute, Panos. *AIDS and the Third World.* Philadelphia: New Society Publishers, 1989.

James, David. *Allegories of Cinema: American Film in the Sixties.* Princeton, N.J.: Princeton University Press, 1989.

Jeffries, Donald, and Anthony Pinching. "AIDS and HTLV-II/LAV Infection: Consequences for Obstetrics and Perinatal Medicine." *British Journal of Obstetrics and Gynecology* 92 (1985): 1211–17.

Johnston, Claire, ed. *Notes on Women's Cinema.* London: Society for Education in Film and Television, 1973.

Jordanova, Ludmilla. *Sexual Visions: Images of Gender in Science and Medicine Between the Eighteenth and Twentieth Centuries.* Madison: University of Wisconsin Press, 1988.

Kalin, Tom. "Flesh Histories." *VIEWS: The Journal of Photography in New England* 11, no. 3 (1990): 3–7.

Kaplan, E. Ann. "Theories and Strategies of the Feminist Documentary." *New Chal-*

lenges for Documentary. Ed. Alan Rosenthal. Berkeley: University of California Press, 1988: 78–102.

Karpf, Anne. *Doctoring the Media: The Reporting of Health and Medicine.* London: Routledge, 1988.

Keller, Evelyn Fox. *Reflections on Gender and Society.* New Haven, Conn.: Yale University Press, 1985.

Kellner, Douglas. "Public Access Television: Alternative Views." *Making Waves: The Politics of Communications.* Ed. Radical Science Collective. London: Free Association Books, 1985: 79–92.

Kelly, Janis, and Cindy Patton. *Making It: A Woman's Guide to Sex in the Age of AIDS.* Ithaca, N.Y.: Firebrand Books, 1987.

Kenny, Lorraine. "Testing the Limits: An Interview." *Afterimage* 17, no. 3 (1989): 4–7.

————. "Traveling Theory: The Cultural Politics of Race and Representation/An Interview with Kobena Mercer." *Afterimage* 18, no. 2 (1990): 7–9.

Kinsella, James. *Covering the Plague: AIDS and the American Media.* New Brunswick, N.J.: Rutgers University Press, 1989.

Kirkman, Larry. "Videos: Democratic Media." *Foundation News* 34, no. 3 (May–June, 1993): 43–45.

Klusacek, Allan, and Ken Morrison, eds. *A Leap in the Dark: AIDS, Art and Contemporary Cultures.* Montreal: Vehicule Press, 1992.

Landers, Timothy. "Bodies and Anti-Bodies: A Crisis in Representation." *Global Television.* Ed. Cynthia Schneider and Brian Wallis. Cambridge, Mass.: MIT Press, 1988: 281–300.

Larkin, Alile Sharon. "Black Women Film-makers Defining Ourselves: Feminism in Our Own Voice." *Female Spectators: Looking at Film and Television.* Ed. E. Deirdre Pribaum. London: Verso, 1988: 157–73.

Leigh, Michael. "Curiouser and Curiouser." *Back and Beyond: Discovering Australian Film and Television.* Ed. Scott Murray. Sydney: Australian Film Council, 1988: 79–88.

Leonard, Zoe. "Lesbians in the AIDS Crisis." *Women, AIDS and Activism.* Eds. ACT UP/NY Women and AIDS Book Group. Boston: South End Press, 1990: 113–18.

Leonard, Zoe, and Polly Thistlethwaite. "Prostitution and HIV Infection." *Women, AIDS and Activism.* Ed. ACT UP/NY Women and AIDS Book Group. Boston: South End Press, 1990: 177–86.

Lesage, Julia. "The Political Aesthetics of the Feminist Documentary Film." *Quarterly Review of Film Studies,* Fall 1978: 507–23.

Lippard, Lucy. "Hanging Onto Baby, Heating Up the Bathwater." *Reimaging America.* Ed. Mark O'Brien and Craig Little. Philadelphia: New Society Publishers, 1990: 227–33.

Loewinger, Larry. "Hi-8: High Powered, Low Priced." *Independent,* May 1991: 25–27.

Lurie, Rachel. "Teenagers." *Women, AIDS and Activism.* Ed. ACT UP/NY Women and AIDS Book Group. Boston: South End Press, 1990: 135–38.

MacDougall, David. "Beyond Observational Cinema." *Movies and Methods: Volume 2.* Ed. Bill Nichols. Berkeley: University of California Press, 1985: 274–86.

———. "Media Friend or Media Foe?" *Visual Anthropology* 1, no. 1 (1989): 54–58.

McGarry, Eileen. "Documentary, Realism, and Women's Cinema." *Women and Film* 2, no. 7 (1975): 50–57.

Mariani, Phil, and Barbara Kruger, eds. *Remaking History.* Seattle: Bay Press, 1989.

Marshall, Stuart. "Video—From Art to Independence." *Screen* 26, no. 2 (1985): 66–72.

Martin, Emily. "Science and Women's Bodies: Forms of Anthropological Knowledge." *Body/Politics: Women and the Discourses of Science.* Ed. Evelyn Fox Keller, Sally Shuttleworth, and Mary Jacobus. New York: Routledge, 1990: 69–82.

Martineau, Barbara Halpern. "Talking About Our Lives and Experiences: Some Thoughts About Feminism, Documentary, and 'Talking Heads.'" *"Show Us Life."* Ed. Thomas Waugh. Metuchen, N.J.: Scarecrow Press, 1984: 252–73.

Mead, Margaret. "Visual Anthropology in a Discipline of Words." *Principles of Visual Anthropology.* Ed. Paul Hockings. New York: Aldine, 1975: 3–14.

Media Network. *Seeing Through AIDS.* New York: Media Guide, 1989.

Mellencamp, Patricia. "Video and the Counterculture." *Global Television.* Ed. Cynthia Schneider and Brian Wallis. Cambridge, Mass.: MIT Press, 1988: 199–224.

Mellencamp, Patricia, Linda Williams, and Mary Ann Doane, eds. *Re-Vision: Essays in Feminist Film Criticism.* Los Angeles: American Film Institute, 1984.

Mercer, Kobena. "Recoding Narratives of Race and Gender." *Independent,* Jan.–Feb. 1989: 19–26.

Metz, Christian. "Story/Discourse." In *Movies and Methods: Volume 2.* Ed. Bill Nichols. Berkeley: University of California Press, 1985: 543–48.

Meyer, James. "AIDS and Postmodernism." *Arts Magazine* 66, no. 8 (April 1992): 60–68.

Michaels, Eric. "How To Look at Us Looking at the Yanomami Looking at Us." *The Mirror Cracked.* Ed. Jay Ruby. Philadelphia: University of Pennsylvania Press, 1982: 133–46.

Miller, James, ed. *Fluid Exchanges: Artists and Critics in the AIDS Crisis.* Toronto: University of Toronto Press, 1993.

Morse, Margaret. "Sports on Television." *Regarding Television.* Ed. E. Ann Kaplan. Los Angeles: American Film Institute, 1983: 44–66.

———. "The Television News Personality and Credibility: Reflections on the News in Transition." *Studies in Entertainment: Critical Approaches to Mass Culture.* Ed. Tania Modleski. Bloomington: Indiana University Press, 1986: 55–79.

Murphy, Timothy. "Testimony." *Writing AIDS.* Ed. Timothy Murphy and Suzanne Poirier. New York: Columbia University Press, 1993: 306–20.

Murphy, Timothy, and Suzanne Poirier, eds. *Writing AIDS: Gay Literature, Language and Analysis.* New York: Columbia University Press, 1993.

Narboni, Jean, and Jean-Louis Comolli. "Cinema/Ideology/Criticism." *Screen Reader*

1: *Cinema/Ideology/Politics*. Ed. John Ellis. London: Society for Education in Film and Television, 1977: 2–11.

Navarro, Ray, and Catherine Saalfield. "Not Just Black and White: AIDS Media and People of Color." *Independent,* July 1989: 18–23.

Negrón-Muntaner, Frances. "The Ethics of Community Media: A Filmmaker Confronts the Contradictions of Producing Media About and for a Community Where She Is Both an Insider and Outsider." *Independent,* May 1991: 20–24.

Nelkin, Dorothy. *Selling Science: How the Press Covers Science and Technology.* New York: W. H. Freeman, 1987.

Newton, Judith. "Feminism and Anxiety in *Alien*." *Alien Zone.* Ed. Annette Kuhn. London: Verso, 1990: 82–90.

Nichols, Bill. *Ideology and the Image.* Berkeley: University of California Press, 1981.

———. *Representing Reality.* Bloomington: Indiana University Press, 1991.

Parenti, Michael. *Inventing Reality: The Politics of News Media.* New York: St. Martin's Press, 1993.

Patton, Cindy. *Sex and Germs: The Politics of AIDS.* Boston: South End Press, 1985.

———. *Inventing AIDS.* New York: Routledge, Chapman and Hall, 1990.

———. "Safe Sex and the Pornographic Vernacular." *How Do I Look? Queer Film and Video.* Ed. Bad Object Choices. Seattle: Bay Press, 1991: 31–64.

———. "Women at Risk From/In Discourse." *Women and AIDS: Psychological Perspectives.* Ed. Corinne Squire. London: Sage Publications, 1993: 165–87.

Ports, Suki. "Needed (For Women and Children)." *AIDS: Cultural Analysis/Cultural Activism.* Ed. Douglas Crimp. Cambridge, Mass.: MIT Press, 1988: 169–76.

Pryluck, Calvin. "Ultimately We Are All Outsiders: The Ethics of Documentary Filmmaking." *New Challenges for Documentary.* Ed. Alan Rosenthal. Berkeley: University of California Press, 1988: 255–68.

Reagon, Berenice Johnson, and Mark O'Brien. "Introduction: Personal Impulses, Social Intentions." In *Reimaging America: The Arts of Social Change.* Ed. Berenice Johnson Reagon and Mark O'Brien. Philadelphia: New Society Publishers, 1990: 1–13.

Rich, B. Ruby. "In the Name of Feminist Film Criticism." *Movies and Methods: Volume 2.* Ed. Bill Nichols. Berkeley: University of California Press, 1985: 340–58.

Rosenberg, Jan. *Women's Reflections: The Feminist Film Movement.* Ann Arbor, Mich.: UMI Research Press, 1983.

Rosenthal, Alan, ed. *New Challenges for Documentary.* Berkeley: University of California Press, 1988.

Rubenstein, Anna. "Seeing Through AIDS: Media Activists Join Forces with NYC Department of Health." *Independent,* Jan.–Feb. 1993: 13–15.

Ruby, Jay. "The Image Mirrored: Reflexivity and the Documentary Film." *New Challenges for Documentary.* Ed. Alan Rosenthal. Berkeley: University of California Press, 1988: 64–77.

————, ed. *A Crack in the Mirror: Reflexive Perspectives in Anthropology.* Philadelphia: University of Pennsylvania Press, 1982.

Rumsey, Sunny. "Communities Under Seige." *AIDS: The Women.* Ed. Ines Rieder and Patricia Ruppelt. San Francisco: Cleis Press, 1988: 187–90.

Ruppelt, Patricia, and Ines Rieder, eds. *AIDS: The Women.* San Francisco: Cleis Press, 1988.

Saalfield, Catherine. "On the Make: Activist Video Collectives." *Queer Looks: Perspectives on Lesbian and Gay Film and Video.* Ed. Martha Gever, John Greyson, and Pratibha Parmar. New York: Routledge, 1993: 21–37.

Sabatier, Renee. *Blaming Others: Prejudice, Race and Worldwide AIDS.* Philadelphia: New Society Publishers, 1988.

Segal, Lynne. "Lessons from the Past: Feminism, Sexual Politics and the Challenge of AIDS." *Taking Liberties.* Ed. Erica Carter and Simon Watney. London: Serpent's Tail, 1989: 133–46.

Shilts, Randy. *And the Band Played On: Politics, People and the AIDS Epidemic.* New York: St. Martin's Press, 1987.

Sorensen, Janet. "News With a View." *Afterimage,* May 1991: 3.

Spence, Louise, and Robert Stam. "Colonialism, Racism and Representation: An Introduction." *Movies and Methods: Volume 2.* Ed. Bill Nichols. Berkeley: University of California Press, 1985: 632–49.

Spiro, Ellen. "Outlaws Through the Lens of Corporate America." *Cinematograph* 4 (1991): 180–83.

————. "What to Wear on Your Video Activist Outing (Because the Whole World Is Watching): A Camcorderist's Manifesto." *Independent,* May 1991: 22–24.

Springer, Claudia. "A Short History of Ethnographic Film." *Independent,* Dec. 1984: 13–18.

Squire, Corrine, ed. *Women and AIDS: Psychological Perspectives.* London: Sage Publications, 1993.

Stacey, Jackie. "Feminine Fascinations: Forms of Identification in Star-Audience Relations." *Stardom: Industry of Desire.* Ed. Christine Gledhill. New York: Routledge, 1991: 141–66.

Stam, Robert. "Television News and Its Spectator." *Regarding Television: Critical Approaches—An Anthology.* Ed. E. Ann Kaplan. Los Angeles: American Film Institute, 1983: 23–43.

Tajima, Renee, and Ernesto de la Vega. *Retooling for Diversity.* New York: Ford Foundation, 1993.

Thompson, Richard. "Dismything Objectivity." *Independent,* June 1990: 12–15.

Treichler, Paula. "AIDS, Gender, and Biomedical Discourse." *AIDS: The Burdens of History.* Ed. Elizabeth Fee and Daniel Fox. Berkeley: University of California Press, 1988: 190–266.

————. "AIDS, Homophobia, and Biomedical Discourse: An Epidemic of Signification." *AIDS: Cultural Analysis/Cultural Activism.* Ed. Douglas Crimp. Cambridge, Mass.: MIT Press, 1988: 31–70.

———. "AIDS and HIV Infection in the Third World: A First World Chronicle." *Remaking History.* Ed. Barbara Kruger and Phil Mariani. Seattle: Bay Press, 1989: 31–86.

———. "How to Have Theory in an Epidemic: The Evolution of AIDS Treatment and Activism." *Technoculture.* Ed. Constance Penley and Andrew Ross. Minneapolis: University of Minnesota Press, 1991: 57–106.

———. "AIDS Narratives on Television: Whose Story?" *Writing AIDS.* Ed. Timothy Murphy and Suzanne Poirier. New York: Columbia University Press, 1993: 161–99.

Trinh, Minh-ha T. "Outside In Inside Out." *Questions of Third Cinema.* Ed. Jim Pines and Paul Willemen. London: British Film Institute, 1989: 133–49.

———. "Documentary Is Not a Name." *October* 52 (Spring 1990): 76–97.

———. "The Totalizing Quest of Meaning." *Theorizing Documentary.* Ed. Michael Renov. New York: Routledge, 1993: 90–107.

Tytell, John. "The Broken Curcuit." *William S. Burroughs at the Front: Critical Reception, 1959-1989.* Ed. Jennie Skerl and Robin Lyndenberg. Carbondale: Southern Illinois University Press, 1991: 149–58.

Ulmer, Gregory. *Teletheory: Grammatology in the Age of Video.* New York: Routledge, 1989.

Valladares, Michelle. "Guarding Our Own Best Interests or Parallel Lines/Connecting Tongues." *FELIX* 1, no. 2 (Spring 1992): 42–44.

Vaughn, Dai. "Television Documentary Usage." In *New Challenges for Documentary.* Ed. Alan Rosenthal. Berkeley: University of California Press, 1988: 34–47.

Vergelin, Jose, and Jose Gutierrez-Gomez "Mining the Oro Del Bario." *Video Guide* 10, no. 3–4 (1989): 13.

Vertov, Dziga. "Kino-eye to Radio-Eye." *Kino-Eye: The Writings of Dziga Vertov.* Ed. Annette Michelson. Berkeley: University of California Press, 1984: 85–91.

Wallis, Brian, and Cynthia Schneider, eds. *Global Television.* Cambridge, Mass.: MIT Press, 1988.

Watney, Simon. *Policing Desire.* Minneapolis: University of Minnesota Press, 1987.

———. "Missionary Positions: AIDS, Africa and Race." *Out There.* Ed. Russell Ferguson et al. New York: New Museum of Contemporary Art, 1990: 89–106.

Watney, Simon, and Erica Carter. eds. *Taking Liberties: AIDS and Cultural Politics.* London: Serpent's Tail, 1989.

Waugh, Thomas. "Introduction: Why Documentary Filmmakers Keep Trying to Change the World, or Why People Changing the World Keep Making Documentaries." *"Show Us Life": Toward a History and Aesthetics of the Committed Documentary.* Ed. Thomas Waugh. Metuchen, N.J.: Scarecrow Press, 1984: xi–xxvii.

Weed, Elizabeth, and Naomi Schor, eds. *differences: Special Issue on Life and Death in Sexuality: Reproductive Technologies and AIDS.* Bloomington: Indiana University Press, 1989.

Weeks, Jeffrey. "Postmodern AIDS?" *Ecstatic Anti-Bodies.* Ed. Tessa Boffin and Sunil Gupta. London: Rivers Oram Press, 1990: 133–41.

West, Cornel. "Black Culture and Postmodernism." *Remaking History*. Ed. Barbara Kruger and Phil Mariani. Seattle: Bay Press, 1989: 87–96.

Willemen, Paul. "On Realism in the Cinema." *Screen Reader 1: Cinema/Ideology/Politics*. Ed. John Ellis. London: Society for Education in Film and Television, 1977: 47–54.

Willemen, Paul, and Jim Pines, eds. *Questions of Third Cinema*. London: British Film Institute, 1989.

Williams, Raymond. *Television: Technology and Cultural Form*. New York: Schocken Books, 1975.

Williamson, Judith. "Every Virus Tells a Story: The Meaning of HIV and AIDS." *Taking Liberties*. Ed. Erica Carter and Simon Watney. London: Serpent's Tail, 1989: 69–80.

Winston, Brian. "The Documentary Film as Scientific Inscription." *Theorizing Documentary*. Ed. Michael Renov. New York: Routledge, 1993: 37–57.

Wolff, Janet. *The Social Production of Art*. New York: St. Martin's Press, 1981.

Worth, Dooley. "Minority Women and AIDS: Culture, Race and Gender." *Culture and AIDS: The Global Pandemic*. Ed. Douglas Feldman. New York: Praeger, 1990: 111–36.

Xavier, Ismael, and Robert Stam. "Allegory/Metacinema/Carnival." *Film Quarterly* 43, no. 3 (1988): 15–30.

Young, Colin. "Observational Cinema." *Principles of Visual Anthropology*. Ed. Paul Hockings. New York: Aldine. 1975: 65–80.

VIDEOGRAPHY

by Catherine Saalfield

Introduction

Gently they go, the beautiful, the tender, the kind. Quietly they go, the intelligent, the witty, the brave. I know. But I do not approve. And I am not resigned. —Edna St. Vincent Millay

Collaboratively and collectively, I have been producing AIDS videos for seven years. My closest work partner died four years ago, and many other comrades have "crossed over" since then. Still more of my brilliant, inspirational friends are HIV-positive. So, all of my AIDS work—my life at this point in time—is dedicated to those I know and love who are living with HIV in their blood and those who have already been stolen from this precious earthly existence. We have been robbed. HIV is the quintessential virus. It attacks the body's very defense against viruses. Against this intimate landscape, I persevere. I proceed with great faith, relentless frustration, and the trenchant challenge of an ever-growing sense of desperation. We must insist on struggle. This war has already claimed far too many.

Seeing Through AIDS

Because making apologies that nobody gives a shit about, and because failing to sing my song, finally, finally, got on my absolute last nerve, I pick up my sword, I lift up my shield, and I stay ready for war, because now I live ready for a whole lot more than that. —June Jordan

The following videography complements this book's overall effort to develop a vocabulary for media literacy in the age of AIDS. Most communities are saturated with only the rampant misrepresentations and outright lies about HIV spewed by commercially driven network television. However, activists and artists who make AIDS tapes are resisting and refuting these dangerous constructs; we are just picking up our swords and lifting up our shields. The dispossessed are building a multimedia arsenal which transcends individual creative experiences. These weapons must be disseminated if they are to function, since a comprehensive approach to video production, distribution, facilitation, criticism, and counterproduction can unleash the power of independent media. The consequent use of tapes is fundamentally the ends and the means of making them.

What do different people get out of seeing these pieces? How can viewers absorb life-changing information in an empowering way which allows them to actually integrate the information into their daily routines? What is missing from the available material? How does a tape effectively present characters with which viewers can identify? How can producers and facilitators use disagreement with both narrative and documentary representations to the viewer's advantage? Why is media such a profound and powerful resource in HIV-prevention efforts? How has the quality of life for some HIV-positive people been improved or enhanced by independently produced media? These are a few open questions for producers, curators, facilitators, media users, and media viewers alike.

Many of these questions have been answered in the selective context of film and video festivals—primarily those featuring avant-garde or lesbian and gay work—which have been inundated by AIDS media for almost ten years. However, until recently, quality media had not been reaching the hardest-hit communities with the same vigor or intensity. Now, through the efforts of countless producers, community-based organizers, and media consultants, culturally specific media about HIV is being seen and used regularly by health-care workers and people with HIV in their own immediate and familiar settings. For example, in 1989 the Chicano gay activist video-maker Ray Navarro teamed up with New York's Media Network. Together, they addressed the abundance of work and the dearth of community-based screenings by initiating media workshops at the Brooklyn AIDS Task Force and The Hub in the South Bronx. Unanimous enthusiasm confirmed the demand for AIDS media in embattled communities. The two workshops attracted 123 participants. Ninety percent were people of color; 85 percent had seen two or fewer of the tapes screened; nearly 80 percent said they would incorporate AIDS media into their educational and counseling efforts.

After Ray's death in 1990, I joined Media Network in the launching of a second round, fine-tuning and expanding the model. Currently in its fourth year, the interactive "Seeing Through AIDS" Media Workshops for care providers and community workers now take place primarily in hospitals and community centers, about three times a month, all over the HIV epicenter that is New York City. We took the name of the workshop from the 1989 Media Network directory of film and video on AIDS, *Seeing Through AIDS*, because it explicitly communicates the goal of our project, which is to imagine beyond the crisis without ignoring the multifaceted obstacles along the way. The workshops are resourceful and optimistic. We use audiovisual material to move the dialogue forward.

In the workshops we have developed a complement to the generally academic notion of "media literacy" education by advocating and teaching "media use." Participants see clips of Hollywood films and analyze how these movies construct their viewers. They talk about how the characters on the screen dictate the viewer's place in the world. They reject stereotypes and delve beneath clichés. When viewers are critical of mainstream representations, they become more demanding of culturally appropriate and accurate representations of themselves and others. They demand a known world, expressions of lived experience. If they do not find it, they want to explain how and where it went wrong. And then they want to create their own. In a vehemently racist and homophobic society, mediamaking, media literacy, and media use are often conditions for survival.

In the "Seeing Through AIDS" workshops, each facilitator brings her own style to the process, but what remains consistent throughout is our commitment to addressing the attendant issues of AIDS. We are not scientists or medical professionals. We focus on poverty, power issues in relationships, racism, homophobia, culturally specific modes of communication in families, the negotiation of safer sex in potentially dangerous situations, drug use and addiction of all kinds, death and dying, grief, the stigma associated with drug use and that of being lesbian or gay, the value and simultaneous devaluation of motherhood, and so forth.

AIDS is clearly not a simulated space, an external plane of being, a TV show. But AIDS media can have a relationship to the processes of prevention education, behavior modification, and identity formation. HIV has compounded a multitude of social, political, emotional, sexual, mental, financial, and physical issues, on both individual and global levels. For these reasons, media can help us untangle and prioritize these challenges and feelings. HIV education that ignores these realities is useless. Without acknowledgment of these factors, an AIDS video will make no sense at all. In any case, without acknowledging these realities, the AIDS crisis will not end.

To get to the heart of such demands, "Seeing Through AIDS" facilitators apply the Pablo Friere model of interactive teaching. We encourage participants to examine their own lives. They testify to the personal and professional impact HIV has had on them. The most effective education comes from identifying with and exploring the individual experiences of participants, facilitators, and the people who appear in the videos. Health-care providers come with an enormous amount of experience and their own survival skills. This premise dictates the passion of video producers and media literacy educators nationwide. As well, this understanding is the foundation from which people with HIV/AIDS and their care providers can most profoundly affect the course of the epidemic.

Using This Videography

Independent media, or "alternative media," is no more perfect than its mainstream counterpart. To get the most out of any media experience, viewers must talk back, agree and disagree, analyze, and appreciate. When we practice critical viewing, we arm ourselves to expect better for ourselves, to expect more from omnipotent and powerful institutions. We are barraged by media messages which can sap us of needed energy. Yet delving into the power of media and making it our own also can rejuvenate a passion for genuine interaction and social justice. Contrasting independent media with network television and Hollywood movies invariably fosters empowerment. Remarkably, the overwhelming majority of work included in the videography is produced by and for the same people. This is self-representation at its best since material emerging from the communities for which it is intended results in more accurate and effective imagery. Various national and state institutions also provide valuable materials which were either commissioned to appropriate independent makers or supervised by members of the target audience. For example, some of the tapes listed below were produced by the United Nations, the Centers for Disease Control, several Africa-U.S. partnerships, and the National Film Board of Canada.

There are numerous strategies for using culturally sensitive media in education, counseling, and outreach. During a group support meeting or in a classroom, most tapes are too long to be shown in their entirety and still allow time for discussion. In that case, a presenter/facilitator can excerpt from two to fifteen minutes of a selected piece and fill up the hour by asking viewers to provide endings to narratives, to take on characters and role-play negotiations, or simply to talk about the issues the tape raises and how the viewers have responded in similar situations. Tapes can be used in classrooms, waiting rooms, support groups, prisons, community centers, mobile vans, drug treatment centers, homes, testing sites, clinics, and hospitals. One of the most effective uses of HIV material is in one-on-one counseling. A videotape can trigger personal reflection on taboo subjects like sexuality, death and dying, or any sort of drug use.

"Seeing Through AIDS" has been successful in part because the New York City Department of Health maintains an AIDS resources lending library with more than 350 tapes on HIV/AIDS available for free loan. In the workshops, facilitators always refer to various titles which are immediately accessible to the participants and can be borrowed for two weeks at a time. If you are located in New York, call the Lending Library at (212) 693-1065 and make an appointment to visit, or pick up one of their comprehensive guides (DOH HIV Support Services, 225 Broadway, 23rd Floor, New York, NY 10007). The library also offers a variety of print resources on all the most up-to-date protocols, community-based programs, courses of treatment, and so forth. Of course, not every city has such an effective service. The New York City DOH Support Services library can provide referrals for resources in other cities, such as the AIDS Library of Philadelphia. Also, Media Network maintains the *Seeing Through AIDS* video guide (Media Network, 39 West 14th St., Suite 403, New York, NY 10011. Phone (212) 929-2663. Fax (212) 929-2732).

Since the field of AIDS media is growing alongside the pandemic, it is impossible to be completely updated on the most recent developments. Each year since the virus took hold, every aspect of the disease has changed considerably, from demographics to safer-sex practices, science to statistics, treatments to the very language we use to understand and explain the horror of this crisis. Although many tapes are capable of enduring for many years despite these changes, some become obsolete very quickly. This videography primarily includes material produced between 1988 and 1993. (Videos are generally produced in much less time than it takes to publish a book!) So even if only one or two pieces are referred to in the following list, be sure to ask distributors about other new titles they carry and other new work they may be aware of.

Because of the severity of the crisis, some producers and production companies have focused solely or primarily on HIV/AIDS in their work, pumping out up-to-date material according to standardized production schedules. These include the thirteen-part Toronto *Living With AIDS* show, AIDSFilms, ACT UP/NY's weekly public access program *AIDS Community TV,* and the Gay Men's Health Crisis weekly *Living With AIDS* cable show which includes regular caring segments and timely medical news. Another place to check listings is at film and video festivals, especially those concentrating on community-based and gay and lesbian media. These festivals often program the short, innovative, personal, and occasionally less accessible media that is being created by independent producers and collectives around the globe.

The videography includes many genres: educational, documentary, drama, animation, experimental, public service announcement (PSA), and explicit safer sex. The videos cover a multitude of subjects, including activism, coping, counseling, criminal justice system/inmates, family communication, health-care providers, hemophilia, heterosexuals, homelessness, immigration, international, media and representation, men who have sex with men, pediatrics, people with HIV/AIDS, prevention/harm reduction, safer sex, stigma/discrimination, substance use, women, women who have sex with women, and youth. The target audiences run the gamut from community-based health workers to PWA/HIVs, and include young people, women, substance users, volunteers/caregivers, parents, health-care providers, inmates, activists, immigrants, and people of all sexual preferences. Some pieces are shot on film and some on video, but all are available on VHS for rental or sale.

The works listed below were chosen for a variety of reasons. First of all, most pieces referred to in this book are included in the listing. The additional titles also represent tools proven effective in HIV/AIDS education, counseling, and outreach. Keep in mind that material which does not fully resonate with some viewers can still be useful for tapping into the highly emotional, often taboo, and usually important individual or community issues of their own. Ask "How is this different from your experience? What is your experience?" And you can always choose a different tape. With its diverse selection, this videography should provide the reader a feel for the breadth and depth of the field of AIDS media production in the United States and abroad.

The entries are organized according to the following form: title, director(s); producer(s); production company, date. Length. Language. Description. (Distributor.) All tapes are in English unless otherwise noted. Address, phone, and fax for each distributor follow at the end of the entire listing. Rates for rental and sale of various formats are not included. Contact distributors for this information. The sale price for most half-hour tapes on VHS format ranges from $20 to $100. Keep in mind that many distributors maintain a sliding-scale fee for underfunded community-based organizations, religious institutions, grassroots groups, and other types of AIDS projects. You can, and should, request a free preview copy of a tape before you rent or buy it.

AIDS media should never be an end in itself. The material must be previewed, evaluated, selected, and facilitated. In short, it must be mediated again to be most useful. Production of AIDS media is at a crossroads right now. In some ways, now more than ever, the challenge is to get anyone to listen. As life with HIV gets more embedded in the grain of our global experience, mediamakers and media users will continue to fight to make sense and make change.

New York City, Summer 1994

Absolutely Positive, Peter Adair; Janet Cole; Adair Films, 1991. 90 mins. Here the filmmaker, a white gay man, weaves a riveting tapestry of thirteen diverse personal testimonies by HIV-positive people, including himself. The powerful portraits include an African American single mother reflecting on stigma and fear expressed by the congregation at her neighborhood church, a young, HIV-negative Puerto Rican mother demonstrating love and support for her husband who has the virus, and the award-winning black gay videomaker Marlon Riggs. (Frameline.)

ACT TV—Public Access Series, James Wentzy; DIVA TV, 1992–94. 30 minutes per show. ACT TV continues the grassroots, activist documentation and counter-surveillance work of ACT UP/NY's video collective, DIVA TV (Damned Interfering Video Activist Television). Produced out of ACT UP/NY's offices, this series updates New York City's activist community on monthly actions, medical research and development, and strategy meetings. (ACT UP/NY.)

Acting Up for Prisoners, Eric Slade, Mic Sweeney; 1992. 26 mins. ACT UP/San Francisco activists, including previously incarcerated women, HIV-positive women, and others, successfully forced authorities to take action in the Frontera Women's Prison. Consisting primarily of talking heads, this tape covers many issues, including the activist pressure on the system which effectively made a difference in prison attitudes and prisoner rights, the ways in which women with HIV are treated inside, and how they feel about support from the outside. (Mic Sweeney (415) 552–2751; Eric Slade (415) 665–3661.)

AIDS in the Barrio: Eso No Me Pasa a Mi, Frances Negron, Peter Biella; Alba Martinez and Frances Negron; David Haas, executive producer, 1989. 30 mins. Spanish/English. An excellent, enduring film documenting how AIDS has impacted one Puerto Rican community in Philadelphia. Focuses on drug use, homophobia, and sexism as three issues exacerbated by, and exacerbating, the AIDS crisis. Although it lacks a gay character, the film is especially strong on gender-role stereotyping, mythologies, and assumptions. (Cinema Guild.)

AIDS Is About Secrets, Sandra Elkin; HIV Center for Clinical and Behavioral Studies, 1989. 37 mins. This soap opera-style video is targeted at heterosexual African American women who are sex partners of IV drug users (IVDUs). Represents the life situations of four women and dramatizes the behaviors which place sex partners of IVDUs at risk. Powerfully demonstrates obstacles to staying clean and issues of self-esteem, support, trust, and monogamy—both within marriage and with boyfriends. Very effective for excerpting. (HIV Center for Clinical and Behavioral Studies.)

AIDS—Life at Stake, Heather E. Edmondson; Arnold C. Mayer, Jr.; Kenya Red Cross, 1992. 37 mins. This drama tells the story of Onesimus Safari, who leaves his small village promising to find a job and build a beautiful home for his new wife, Hannah. Once in Nairobi, Safari struggles to earn a living and spends nights out with different women, returning to his wife in the village on the weekends. He falls sick shortly after Hannah gives birth to their first child. The story is left open-ended after a doctor explains that Safari contracted HIV from unprotected sex. If Safari has infected Hannah, then the baby may also be infected, since HIV can be passed from mother to child. (DSR.)

AIDS: Me and My Baby, Sandra Elkin; HIV Center for Clinical and Behavioral Studies, 1988. 23 mins. Employs the accessible soap opera format to convey dense information. Targets black and Latino communities, with an emphasis placed upon heterosexual sex. Good information on testing, transmission, and safer sex for hetero-sexuals. Unfortunately, homosexuality is represented inaccurately; the only men who have sex with men are in prison. Needs to be accompanied by a speaker who can provide additional information. Study guide available. (HIV Center for Clinical and Behavioral Studies.)

AIDS: Not Us, Harry Howard; The Media Group, Inc.; HIV Center for Clinical and Behavioral Studies, 1989. 36 mins. Engaging and entertaining, this tape is geared toward black and Latino urban youth. Focuses on five young men living in New York City's housing projects who depict individuals as members of a group struggling with drugs, AIDS, venereal disease, machismo, prostitution, sexual activity, and con-dom use (includes a demonstration). Interactions reveal peer pressure experienced by young men to be sexually active and to gain esteem by dealing drugs. Through rap, humor, and creative self-expression, provides models for communication about the difficult issues related to HIV/AIDS. One guy humorously coaches his younger sister on condom negotiation with her new older boyfriend. The gay character, presented in a relationship, realistically confronts his friend's homophobia. (Film Library.)

(An) Other Love Story: Women and AIDS, Gabrielle Micallef, Debbie Douglas, 1990. 30 mins. Taking place in a multiracial and multicultural lesbian community in Toronto, this fictional narrative revolves around the issues that arise for two lovers when one of them is advised by her doctor to test for HIV. An HIV-positive friend tells her own compelling story of fear, disclosure, and isolation, imploring people to take

the risks seriously. Although at times the acting is not so great, the tape is invaluable since very little AIDS media exists for and about lesbians. A didactic thread is provided throughout by a man asking women passersby what they think about HIV and its impact on their own lives. (V Tape.)

Are You With Me? M. Neema Barnette; AIDSFilms, 1989. 17 mins. Well-made, dramatic narrative. When a young woman in an African American urban community dies of AIDS, a divorced mother encourages her teenage daughter to take precautions. The teenager confronts her boyfriend in a useful modeling of behavior. Meanwhile, in her own relationship with a man, the mother finds it hard to practice what she preaches. Study guide available. (Select Media.)

Belinda, Anne Lewis Johnson; Appalshop, 1992. 29 mins. Portrait of Belinda Mason, a native of eastern Kentucky, and, in her words, "a small-town journalist, a young mother, a reliable Tupperware party guest," until she became infected with HIV in 1987. She decided to go public with her status and spent the rest of her life as a powerful advocate for AIDS prevention, education, treatment, and human rights. Her activism took her to Washington, D.C., where she was chosen to serve on President Bush's National Commission on AIDS. In a presentation to members of the Southern Baptist convention, she says, "People ask me if I think AIDS is a punishment from God. I can't pretend to fathom what God is thinking, but maybe we should look at AIDS as a test, not for the people who are infected, but for the rest of us." Study guide available. (Appalshop.)

Between Friends, Severo Perez; Buffy Bunting, 1990. 25 mins. Spanish/English. Dramatizes the story of a few typical days in the lives of several young Chicanos in San Francisco. Brings home consequences of teens' choices about sex and drugs when a young girl finds out her mother has AIDS. The girl, who is sexually active and uses drugs, fears that she, too, may be infected with the virus. Provides information on HIV transmission and prevention and stresses the importance of safer sex or abstinence. Study guide available. (San Francisco Study Center.)

Bleach, Teach and Outreach, Ray Navarro, Catherine Saalfield; GMHC, 1988. 28 mins. Upbeat and accessible, this video examines the volatile political debate surrounding the implementation of a needle exchange and education program in New York City. Yolanda Serrano from the Association for Drug Abuse Prevention and Treatment (ADAPT) describes the pilot needle-exchange program as "really encompassing everything from getting people into detox, drug free treatment, counseling for HIV antibody testing, distribution of condoms, education, and counseling on safer-sex practices." The tape argues that the exchange program is the initial link to get intravenous drug users in touch with a network of services which can lead to treatment. (GMHC.)

BOLO! BOLO! Gita Saxena, Ian Rashid; Toronto's *Living With AIDS* Show, 1991. 30 mins. Including an interview with British photographer Sunil Gupta, this tape examines AIDS and the South Asian community. Employs visually engaging imagery, music, and art (both ancient and contemporary). Because of exceptionally mild depictions of gay men caressing, this tape led to Toronto's thirteen-part *Living With AIDS* show being discontinued from cablecast. (V Tape.)

Caring for Infants and Toddlers with HIV Infection; Children's Welfare League of America, 1990. 21 mins. Three families share their stories about living with HIV-positive children. This video teaches guardians—natural parents, foster care parents, grandparents, and others—about ways to tend to the special needs of infected children. Addresses custody issues, death and dying, HIV-negative siblings, letting go, medical issues, and loving. The issue of pediatric AIDS is presented from the many perspectives of the care-giving team, including siblings, parents, guardians, doctors, and social workers. (Children's Welfare League of America.)

Caring Segments, Juanita Mohammed; GMHC, 1993. This series, produced for the GMHC *Living with AIDS* show, comprises short portraits of care givers, those who do everything from cleaning to shopping to talking and holding to "just being there." Parents and other relatives, lovers, friends, social workers, and other care providers relay their stories of obstacles, love, and pain. Integrating activist footage and still photographs, these shorts present powerful and important images of the HIV community. One wonderful segment called "Two Men and a Baby" shows a gay man and his lover bringing up his HIV-positive niece after his sister has died of AIDS. (GMHC.)

Clips, Debbie Sundhal; Nan Kinney; Fatale Video, 1989. 30 mins. Safer-sex porn for lesbians, in three ten-minute vignettes: one artsy anal masturbation fantasy; one couple having fun with dental dams, scarves, and blindfolds; and the celebrated female ejaculation short, starring Fanny Fatale and her glassine dildo. (Blush Entertainment.)

Condomnation, Anne Chamberlain; 1992. 8 mins. An artsy montage, this tape debunks some myths about AIDS and addresses lesbian invisibility in the crisis. An HIV-positive lesbian who got infected by unprotected sex with a woman who has already died provides voice-over narration. Images of latex, dental dams, plastic wrap, condoms, hands, and fists abound. (Anne Chamberlain.)

Current Flow, Jean Carlomusto; GMHC, 1989. 4 mins. This sexually explicit short is designed to educate lesbians on safer-sex practices, including the use of dental dams, vibrators, and mutual masturbation with sex toys. Safer-sex toys are laid out on the coffee table next to the couch where two women have sex, providing many examples of what is safe and possible for women who have sex with other women. (GMHC.)

DHPG Mon Amour, Carl Michael George; 1989. 12 mins. A powerful documentary portrait of a day in the life of Joe Walsh and his lover, David Conover, a PWA who takes the drug DHPG (gansiclovir) to combat cytomegalovirus. The camera follows Joe leaving work, shopping for groceries, and cooking dinner. Meanwhile, David goes through the elaborate ritual of injecting DHPG, which he did once a day until he lost his sight. After blindness set in, Joe had to infuse David three times daily until David's death on September 1, 1989. The film's narration—David describing the edited footage to Joe—combines personal remembrances with commentary on the importance of PWAs taking control of their lives and their medical treatment. (Drift Distribution.)

DiAna's Hair Ego: AIDS Info Up Front, Ellen Spiro; Ego Video, 1989. 30 mins. Responding to the lack of AIDS education provided by local and state health agencies, cosmetologist DiAna DiAna and Dr. Bambi Sumpter took on the task of educating their community in Columbia, South Carolina. This provocative, humorous, and empowering tape documents the ensuing growth of the South Carolina AIDS Education Network. Operating out of DiAna's beauty salon, SCAEN is an inspiring model of grassroots community organizing. DiAna's salon offers free condoms and sex-positive AIDS information. Accessible and entertaining, this tape could be used to stimulate discussion in any college, community center, or hair salon. (Video Data Bank [and] Women Make Movies.)

Doctors, Liars and Women, Jean Carlomusto, Maria Maggenti; GMHC, 1988. 22 mins. In January 1988 the Women's Committee of ACT UP/NY organized a protest against *Cosmopolitan* magazine for publishing an article which offered dangerously misleading information on the risks of unprotected heterosexual sex. Documents the Women's Committee's planning before the action, their meeting with the article's author, Dr. Robert Gould, the subsequent demonstration outside the magazine's offices, and the mainstream media coverage of the debate. Serves as a "how to" guide for direct action and embodies the role of video in activist efforts. (GMHC.)

El Abrazo (The Embrace), Diana Coryat; Pregones Touring Puerto Rican Theater Collection, 1990. 30 mins. Spanish/English. Documents a theatrical performance about a family confronting AIDS; punctuated with question and answer sessions and interviews with audience participants. Meant to be turned off at several points to encourage viewers to assume the roles of the screen characters and solve dilemmas. Bilingual study guide available. (Pregones.)

The Faces of AIDS, Frances Reid; Family Health International AIDSTECH/ AIDSCAP, 1993. 20 mins. Documents the courageous personal and emotional experiences of women and men with HIV/AIDS in Cameroon and Zimbabwe. Speakers address issues of shame, stigma, rejection, fear, pain, and abandonment in order to combat denial and despair, challenge stereotypes, and encourage support for HIV-positive people. Also presents strong testimonies from professional care providers and family members. Ultimately focuses on the children of Zimbabwe and Cameroon, many of whom are orphans because of the ravages of AIDS. This moving and intimate piece makes a powerful case for prevention education and hope. Study guide available. (Media for Development International.)

Fast Trip, Long Drop, Gregg Bordowitz; 1994. 54 minutes. The extraordinary diary of Alter Allesman (Yiddish for Everyman), this fictitious tape embodies the many guises of the activist, artist, and educator who directed it. Allesman is a character who insists on the nihilistic, utopian, and darkly comic responses available to everyone living with AIDS. The result is a triumphant declaration of freedom from any definition of living with AIDS. A stunning narrative of one man's revelations drawn from sex, parents, history, daily routines, drug treatment, and learning how to drive in New York City. Archival footage of car crashes, disasters, and daredevil stunts appear throughout, provoking a meditation on the notion of risk. Bordowitz mines his own Jewish cultural history in search of ethical criteria to face the loss and despair caused by the AIDS pandemic. (Drift Distribution.)

Fear of Disclosure, Phil Zwickler, David Wojnarowicz; Fear of Disclosure Project, 1990. 5 mins. Targeted at gay men, this tape challenges the "sexual apartheid" of the HIV-positive and the HIV-status-unknown (or negative). Voice-over narration syncs up with men dancing together in gold lamé skivvies, as the film provocatively explores the emotionally charged act of revealing one's positive status to a potential lover. An evocative narration contrasts fear of rejection with fear of "contamination." Works well to trigger group discussion or as one component of a safer-sex video series. (Fear of Disclosure [and] Testing the Limits.)

Fighting Chance, Richard Fung; Toronto's *Living With AIDS* Show, 1990. 30 mins. This upbeat documentary features interviews with four HIV-positive gay Asian men from San Francisco, Boston, and Vancouver, as well as interviews with people from the Gay Asian AIDS project. Deals with social, political, and cultural responses to issues such as transmission, death and dying, Asian stereotypes, relationships, family and friends, the impact of immigration policy, traditional Chinese medicine, disclosure, and more. (V Tape.)

Fighting for Our Lives, Center for Women's Policy Studies, 1990. 29 mins. Women constitute the fastest-growing group of people with AIDS in the United States, and women of color make up at least three-quarters of those infected. Profiled here are women living with HIV as well as service providers, care givers, and advocates. Rather than detailing the facts of HIV transmission or giving extensive statistics on women and AIDS, this remarkable program focuses on how women are taking action in their own communities to reduce the epidemic in women. (Women Make Movies.)

Fighting in Southwest Louisiana, Peter Friedman; 1991. 28 mins. An engaging, moving portrait of an HIV-positive gay mailman in southwest Louisiana. The viewer accompanies him on his daily routine, delivering mail and chatting with his neighbors. He tells of coming out as a teenager, relates his successful but painful struggle to get his job back after being fired illegally, and discusses his community's response to his lover's death and his own fight against AIDS. (Filmmakers Library.)

The Forgotten People: Latinas with AIDS, Hector Galan; KCET and Centers for Disease Control National AIDS Information Clearinghouse, 1990. 29 mins. Spanish/English. A personal look at four HIV-positive Latina women who were infected through IV drug use and another woman who was infected by unprotected sex with her drug-using husband. Three sisters, all HIV-positive, are shown with their mother and teenage sons. Useful for discussions about family communication, death, and grief. The goal of the video is to prevent the spread of AIDS in the Latino community, specifically targeting drug users and their families. (CDC National AIDS Information Clearinghouse.)

Grid-Lock: Women and the Politics of AIDS, Beth Wichterich; 1993. 27 mins. Documents the chronology of activism which led the Centers for Disease Control (CDC) to change their internationally recognized AIDS definition to include some medical manifestations of HIV illness in women. Although consisting primarily of talking heads, this tape integrates images from a mountaintop memorial gathering for the director's gay male friend who died of AIDS-related complications. (Beth Wichterich.)

Hard to Get, Alisa Lebow; New York City Commission on Human Rights, 1991. 30 mins. Narrated by actress Ruby Dee, this tape is good for use in the workplace. Entertainingly debunks myths about HIV transmission, casual contact, and other workplace worries. Intercut with great old black-and-white film clips. (New York City Commission on Human Rights.)

He Left Me His Strength, Sherry Busbee, Merle Jawitz; Busbee, Jawitz, Sheila Ward, John Bassinger; Downtown Community TV, 1989. 13 mins. Profiles an inspirational mother who turned her own personal loss into a bold AIDS educational campaign. When Mildred Pearson's son died, she resolved to educate her community about AIDS by telling her story in churches, hospitals, and other community-based settings. She also formed a support group, Mother's Love, for mothers of adult children who are HIV-positive. (April Productions.)

Heart of the Matter, Gini Retticker, Amber Hollibaugh; 1993. 56 mins. A truly powerful and empowering documentary about AIDS from women's perspectives. Explores the traps women face as they confront sexual double standards, racial myths and racism, and the prevalent desire to please others. Janice Jirau, who died of AIDS-related complications in October 1993, provides the core of wisdom and passion that permeates this invaluable film. Without any support from her husband's family, she loved and cared for him until he died. However, her sons, sisters, and mother rally around her with love and food. They sustain her through her illness. Includes footage of Janice's many compelling public appearances, her personal and spiritual development, her relationship with the black church, her support groups, her determination, and her contagious appetite for life. (Also available: the thirteen-minute trailer, *Women and Children Last,* in which Janice shares insights on women's socialization, solidarity, and strength.) (First Run Features.)

Her Giveaway, Mona Smith; 1988. 20 mins. Explores Carol Lafavor's personal journey with AIDS and the impact of AIDS on Native American communities.

With rare and intimate insights, Carol discusses how she was exposed to HIV, her experiences of living as a lesbian with AIDS, and how her illness has changed her relationships with her daughter, her extended family, her community, and her friends. The tape addresses mythologies about Native Americans with respect to sexuality, IV drug use, and AIDS. Traditional images and music augment the educational narrative and underscore the spiritual and holistic perspective with which Carol approaches her positive status. Excellent for anyone interested in self-empowerment and healing strategies. (Minnesota Indian Affairs Council [and] Women Make Movies.)

I'm You, You're Me: Women Surviving Prison, Living with AIDS, Debra Levine, Catherine Saalfield; 1992. 28 mins. Documents HIV-positive women making the transition from prison to independent living by intimately following developments in a weekly support group on the outside. ACE—the inmate AIDS peer Counseling and Education organization—was founded in 1989 at the Bedford Hills Maximum Security Correctional Facility for women in New York State. In 1992, previously incarcerated women began ACE OUT, which consists of a hotline, educational workshops and presentations, support groups, a buddy system, and medical and legal intervention for women being released. In this tape the women of ACE OUT tackle numerous complicated issues head-on, sharing survival skills and hope. (Women Make Movies [and] Women's Prison Association.)

Identities, Nino Rodriguez; 1991. 7 mins. A man with AIDS says a lot in this short tape, although he rarely speaks. Examining moments between speech, this tape pictures thought, preparation, exhaling, tears, visual pleas, and confident communications. (Nino Rodriguez.)

(In)Visible Women, Marina Alvarez, Ellen Spiro; Fear of Disclosure Project, 1991. 30 mins. Spanish/English. Through community education, art, and activism, three HIV-positive Latinas challenge notions of female invisibility and political complacency in the face of the epidemic. Engaging and moving, this documentary focuses on Marina Alvarez, the dynamic AIDS educator and mother from the South Bronx; Jeannie Pedjko, the passionate Chicago-based ACT UP activist; and Irma McLaren, the beautiful dancer and AIDS educator. The women stress self-reliance, family support, and women's solidarity, and they urge women with AIDS to speak out. (Fear of Disclosure [and] Women Make Movies.)

It is what it is . . . Gregg Bordowitz; GMHC, 1993. 60 mins. A multiracial group of teenagers presents both the myths (while dressed in fake noses and mustaches) and truths (while dressed as themselves) about identity, homophobia, and HIV/AIDS. This tape can be divided into three twenty-minute segments for easy classroom use. High-energy and right on, the breadth of issues addressed is impressive and the repetition useful. Also includes three short dramatic segments: a young gay man coming out to his sister, two lesbians getting harassed on a beach, and a straight couple negotiating safer sex. Study guide available. (GMHC.)

It's Not Easy, Faustin J. Misanvu; John Riber, 1991. 48 mins. Career and family are going well for Suna, a young African business executive. At the beginning of this engaging drama, he is given an important promotion at his manufacturing company, and his wife, Serra, is pregnant with their first child. But everything changes when his newborn son is found to be infected with HIV. Employers, coworkers, and neighbors learn to become allies instead of enemies in the battle for life. (DSR.)

Karate Kids, Derek Lamb; Lamb, Michael Scott, Peter Dalgish, Christopher Lowry; National Film Board of Canada and Street Kids International, 1990. 20 mins. Aimed at the 100 million homeless children of the world, this animation is set in a colorful marketplace where homeless children of different ages, sexes, and races earn their living by shining shoes, washing car windows, juggling, or stealing, while being preyed upon by wealthy, seedy male adults who lure them into heterosexual or homosexual sex in cars or alleys in exchange for money or goods. The film centers on the story of Pedro, a tiny juggler, Mario, a pickpocket, and Karate and Rosa, a young couple who live in an abandoned house and take care of the kids. Karate warns against HIV transmission through unprotected sex and teaches the kids about condom use. Deals frankly with anti-gay bias and care for people with AIDS. Addresses some of society's taboos such as anal sex and sex-for-survival. (National Film Board of Canada.)

Kecia, Peter Von Puttkamer; Gryphon Productions, Ltd., 1992. 30 mins. An articulate and dynamic Native American teenage woman, Kecia Larkin, discusses her experience on the streets and how her HIV-positive status has changed her life. The tape shows her relationships with her mother, brother, and community. Now an AIDS educator, working primarily on reservations, Kecia compellingly imparts invaluable information, analysis, and hope to viewers. (Gryphon Productions.)

Keep Your Laws Off My Body, Catherine Saalfield, Zoe Leonard; 1990. 13 mins. Black-and-white images of a lesbian couple at home juxtaposed with police in riot gear in the streets during an ACT UP demonstration. The image is overlaid periodically with summarized legislation which seeks to limit our bodily freedoms, including abortion and reproductive rights laws, the Helms amendments, sodomy cases, obscenity, pornography, and prostitution laws. (Women Make Movies.)

Kissing Doesn't Kill; Gran Fury Collective, 1990. Four 30-second spots. Protesting homophobia and governmental neglect in the AIDS crisis, same-sex couples make out in a take-off on the multiracial Benetton clothing ads. These slick, thirty-second, public service announcements are edited to different styles of music, but they all have the same message: "Kissing Doesn't Kill, Corporate Greed and Government Indifference Make AIDS a Political Crisis." These PSAs work well as one component in a comprehensive HIV/AIDS video series. (Drift Distribution.)

Latex and Lace, Laird Sutton, Janet Taylor, Dolores Bishop; Exodus Trust, 1988. 22 mins. This explicit safer-sex tape for women begins with lesbian, straight, and bisexual women talking about AIDS, and then a number of them take part in a women-only "safer-sex party" (i.e., sex and latex). (Multi-Focus, Inc.)

Le Ravissement, Charline Boudreau; 1992. 4 mins. Like an old black-and-white Hollywood flick, the gates open on a high-style affair, and the man in the tux, cruising the stunning blond, is, of course, a butch dyke who seduces and plays . . . safe. Cigars and latex abound. (Charline Boudreau.)

Like a Prayer, DIVA TV, 1991. 29 mins. Produced by the activist video collective of ACT UP/NY called DIVA TV (Damned Interfering Activist Television), this tape analyzes the collaborative demonstration "Stop the Church" by WHAM! (Women's Health Action and Mobilization) and ACT UP/NY on December 10, 1990, against Cardinal John O'Connor and the Roman Catholic Church's murderous stand on abortion rights, safer sex, and homosexuality. (ACT UP/NY [and] Printed Matter.)

Mi Hermano, Edgar Michael Bravo; American Red Cross, 1990. 30 mins. Spanish/English. This story of a working-class Mexican-American family, shocked to silence by the sudden AIDS-related death of the eldest son, is presented through the eyes of the youngest son, who desperately tries to learn just what killed his brother. The father refuses to talk about AIDS and blames the surviving (and pregnant) young wife for having infected his son. She, in turn, struggles with the news that she is infected and possibly will give birth to a sick baby. Excellent in its cultural specificity, visual quality, and a very careful and nuanced presentation of the possible hidden bisexual behavior of the son who has died. The film ends in a moment of nonverbal communication when the new baby boy tests negative. The grandfather welcomes the young mother into the family and finally begins to learn about AIDS. (American Red Cross.)

Mildred Pearson: When You Love a Person, Yannick Durand; Brooklyn AIDS Task Force, 1988. 9 mins. Mildred Pearson is an African American woman who, after her son died of AIDS, dedicated herself to raising consciousness about HIV infection and PWAs within her community. She demonstrated constant and unconditional support for her son. Emotionally engaging, the tape shows how grief turned into action, discussion, and empowerment. Especially useful in small workshops and training sessions for people doing grassroots education, counseling, and outreach. It is also useful in any series that deals with volunteerism. Should be supplemented with current information about transmission and resources for PWAs. (Brooklyn AIDS Task Force.)

My Body's My Business, Vivian Kleinman; 1992. 18 mins. Shot mostly on the streets, this powerful tape speaks from prostitutes to prostitutes. Combines interviews as well as documentation of safer-sex training on the job and some visual collages. Great safer-sex techniques are demonstrated, and then women discuss the pros and cons of trying them with or without the consent of the johns. How much money would you accept to have sex without a condom? (Fear of Disclosure.)

Native Americans, Two Spirits and HIV; American Indian Community House, Wee Wah and Bar Che Ampe, and DIVA TV, 1991. 12 mins. By foregrounding lesbians, gays, and people with AIDS, this talking-heads tape (shot mostly at a conference) affirms that lesbians and gays have always been a recognized and vital component of Native American culture. Addresses spirituality, violence against women, intravenous drug use, and HIV/AIDS education in the community. (American Indian Community House.)

No Rewind: Teenagers Speak Out on HIV/AIDS Awareness, Paula Mozen; No Excuses Productions, 1992. 23 mins. This fast-paced video educating teenagers about HIV gives young people the opportunity to speak for themselves in interviews and peer-group discussions. Promotes safer sex and abstinence. Frank and intimate, HIV-positive youth show that it is worth it to take care of yourself now because "in life there is no rewind." Study guide available. (No Excuses Productions.)

Non, Je Ne Regrette Rien (No Regret), Marlon Riggs; Fear of Disclosure Project, 1992. 30 mins. An artist/activist exploration of HIV, identity, and mortality among videomaker Riggs and his peers and colleagues, this tape focuses on stigma and the process of disclosure in the African American community. Five inspiring HIV-positive black gay men discuss their families, personal survival skills, and fears in this sensitive documentary, constructed with song, poetry, and the participants' personal photographs. The tape is dedicated to Donald Woods, who courageously reflects on his own experiences and also appears periodically reciting some of his powerful poems. The video's director, one of the leading innovators in gay and lesbian media production, directly addresses some of his own concerns about living with AIDS in this articulate and riveting video. (Fear of Disclosure.)

Ojos Que No Ven/Eyes That Fail to See, Jose Gutierrez-Gomez, Jose Vergelin; Adinfinitum Films, 1987. 51 mins. Spanish/English. This early film uses the popular and compelling narrative format of the *telenovela* to illuminate the effects of AIDS on a cross-section of the Latino community in Northern California. Different families and individual characters address complex issues such as sexual practice, sexual identity, and drug use in the family. Touches upon safer sex, male homosexuality and bisexuality, and does well representing several Spanish-language idioms. Allows for the development of an elaborate story encouraging honesty and cultural survival as well as self-criticism within the Latino community. An excellent example of the ways in which community media can serve as a relevant and significant means for conveying crucial information. Study guide available. (Latino AIDS Project.)

One Foot on a Banana Peel, the Other Foot in the Grave (Secrets from the Dolly Madison Room), Juan Botas, Lucas Platt, Joanne Howard, Jonathan Demme, Ed Saxon; 1993. 80 mins. Shot over many months as if the camera were just another member of the group, this tape takes place entirely within a doctor's office where a number of HIV-positive men (including Botas) come for their regular treatments. Incredibly personal and intimate, this documentary allows for all the joking, sadness, fears, and hopes of the patients as they take their injections, conduct spontaneous treatment teach-ins, and reflect directly to the camera on their life experiences. (Clínica Estético.)

Part of Me, Juanita Mohammed, Alisa Lebow; GMHC, 1993. 12 mins. A short documentary portrait of Alida "Lilly" Gonzalez, a charismatic Latina lesbian mother in recovery from drug use. Fixing up her new apartment with her children and friends, Lilly talks intimately about accepting her sexual identity and her HIV status with positive energy and confidence. Part of the GMHC series of Caring Segments. (GMHC.)

Party! Charles Sessoms; Laverne Berry; AIDSFilms, 1993. 25 mins. Targets self-identified black gay men and addresses particular barriers they face in reducing their risk for HIV by practicing safer sex. The main storyline revolves around the party's host, Paul. During the course of the party Paul must decide how to respond to his boyfriend Brian's pressure to have sex without using a condom. Meanwhile, Paul's guests discuss a number of scenarios related to practicing safer sex, including negotiating condom use, relapse, eroticizing safer sex, frottage, self-esteem, empowerment, and peer support. Study guide available. (Gay Men of African Descent—GMAD.)

Party Safe! with Bambi and DiAna, Ellen Spiro; 1992. 25 mins. In this sequel to *DiAna's Hair Ego,* DiAna and her partner, Bambi Sumpter, travel from South Carolina to New York, Chicago, Los Angeles, and Toronto, where they hold safer-sex informational parties (often in people's homes), complete with ingenious games guaranteed to make the participants more comfortable in imagining, talking about, and carrying through with their decisions about sex. Includes explicit and frank discussions about human relationships. Clearly articulated and important perspective on AIDS. (Video Data Bank [and] Women Make Movies.)

Pediatric AIDS: A Time of Crisis, Pierce Atkins; Association for the Care of Children's Health, 1989. 23 mins. Focuses on the experiences of participants in a support group for parents of children with HIV at Albert Einstein College of Medicine in New York City. A moving account of how the disease affects entire families, this documentary stresses the importance of support, health services, and planning for child placement. Presents some members outside the hospital setting in more intimate and comfortable environments. Haydee and Pedro, an articulate, emotional, and compelling couple, express their fears, guilt, grief, and struggle around impossible dreams, social stigmatization, the positive status of their baby girl, and their love for one another. Can be used as a client education piece in a variety of settings, not only to teach about pediatric HIV disease. (Association for the Care of Children's Health.)

Pitimi San Gado (Millet Without a Guardian); Haitian Teens Confront AIDS, 1992. 29 mins. Introduced by a young narrator in a production studio, this dramatic narrative was researched, written, directed, acted, and edited by Haitian teenagers in New York City. Members of one family are challenged by the eldest son's positive status, which has been the source of gossip around the neighborhood before the family even found out. In an ultimately supportive, strong, and hopeful context, this tape covers issues like racism, immigration, assimilation, the stigma of HIV, and quality of life. (Partners in Health.)

Positively Women, Nalini Singh; 1993. 30 mins. Shot in Bombay, Madras, Calcutta, and Delhi, this documentary employs compelling and intimate talking-head interviews (with many faces obscured because of stigma), voice-over presentation of invaluable information (with simultaneous English translations), and creatively photographed street scenes. One million people in India are estimated to be HIV-positive, according to a U.N. study. Because of strict marital and gender-based social codes, many women feel incapable of insisting on condom use or sexual dialogue with their husbands. The women ask rhetorically, "Who exercises control over physical relations?" They relate stories of beatings for refusing to have sex, men drinking too much, and difficult interpersonal communications. However, since 1992, courageous women have been holding support groups in the Rajastan, learning how to talk with their husbands about sex, monogamy, condoms, and rape. (United Nations Development Programme.)

Prostitutes, Risk and AIDS, Alexandra Juhasz, Jean Carlomusto; GMHC, 1988. 28 mins. Examines the scapegoating of prostitutes for HIV/AIDS and other sexually transmitted diseases (STDs) in the heterosexual community. Also analyzes the media image distortion of who is really at risk for HIV infection. (GMHC.)

Prowling by Night, Gwendolyn; National Film Board of Canada, 1991. 10 mins. Produced for the Canadian series, Five Feminist Minutes, this animation demonstrates the difficulty of engaging in safer-sex education on the streets. Working girls (past and present) speak about the problems with police and other obstacles to doing their jobs right. Meanwhile, outreach workers talk to sex workers about police harassment. (National Film Board of Canada.)

PWA Power, Gregg Bordowitz, Jean Carlomusto; GMHC, 1988. 28 mins. Aimed at individuals recently diagnosed with AIDS. Inspiring and powerful portraits contextualize the birth of the People with AIDS self-empowerment movement and provide useful information about how to deal with day-to-day emotional issues, discrimination, and quality-of-life issues. (GMHC.)

Reframing AIDS, Pratibha Parmar; 1987. 30 mins. Produced by a South Asian lesbian living in England, this video analyzes AIDS in relation to race, gender, social standing, and sexual orientation by interviewing different people about their opinions and feelings. Portrays a wide range of people—Asian, black, white, gay, straight, and lesbian. Political and social aspects of the AIDS crisis are stressed over scientific and medical information. Useful to compare and contrast with mainstream media approaches to HIV. (Video Data Bank.)

Reunion, Jamal Joseph; Laverne Berry; AIDSFilms, 1993. 30 mins. Focuses on the impact of HIV on the lives of three African American brothers who come together during a family reunion at their mother's home. This slick and well-written drama examines how each of the brothers responds to safer sex and the AIDS epidemic and how their responses affect their relationships with their partners, their families, and one another. Excellent scene with women encouraging each other to stick to their decisions about using condoms. Also includes three useful scenes of negotiation: one where an HIV-positive man talks with his wife in bed; one in which the woman suggests not using a condom and the man insists; one in which the couple fights about using protection. (Select Media.)

Safe Is Desire, Debi Sundhal; Nan Kinney; Fatale Productions, 1993. 45 mins. In this dramatic pornography, Allie and Dione are in love, but safer-sex issues threaten their new relationship. They visit a San Francisco sex club where they see lesbian sex, 1990s' style, in a lust-filled orgy scene, a delightfully playful demonstration by the Safe Sex Sluts, and other downright kinky—as well as safe—kinds of lesbian sex. Well-shot, scripted, and performed, this tape challenges negative attitudes and ignorance about safer sex for lesbians (Blush Entertainment.)

Safe Love, Lori Ayers, Eric N. Duran, Ellen V. Shapiro; Fusion Artists, Inc., 1993. 27 mins. The nitty-gritty about safer sex in the age of AIDS. Primary focus is on the experiences of HIV-positive women (including one co-director) and what they have learned that enables them to have satisfying sexual lives. Random on-the-street interviews with younger and older women reveal current attitudes, misconceptions, and fears regarding safer sex. Interviews with health-care professionals and footage of women participating in safer-sex seminars complete the emotional and educational perspective. How have women's dating habits changed? What do they consider safe? Do they follow their own rules? What do they tell their children? And more. (Fusion Artists.)

Safe Sex Slut, Carol Leigh; 1987. 2½ mins. This tape, made at a cable-access TV center in Arizona, is a quasi-music video featuring Carol Leigh (aka Scarlot Harlot). Ms. Leigh, a self-avowed prostitutes' rights advocate and AIDS activist, sings about having great safer sex. Funny, rambunctious, and full of quirky video tricks, the tape portrays sex in a positive, lusty, and safe way. There are very few tapes made by women for women and about women that deal with safer sex and sexual empowerment which are also funny and friendly. This tape is a rare find. (Video Data Bank.)

Safer and Sexier: A College Student's Guide to Safer Sex; the Lay-Techs Entertainment Group, 1993. 18 mins. Collectively produced by college students and their professor. Funny, up-front, and entertaining, this tape speaks from young people to young people in their own language, using dramatic and realistic scenes. Condoms, latex, and model behavior abound. (Alexandra Juhasz.)

Safer Sex Shorts (various directors); Gregg Bordowitz and Jean Carlomusto; GMHC, 1989–90. 4 mins each. Six tapes—"Current Flow," "Car Service," "Midnight Snack," "Something Fierce," "Gotstobeadrag," and "Steam Clean"—make up *Safer Sex Shorts.* These sexually explicit dramatic videos illustrate and eroticize safer-sex activities. They can play an effective role in safer-sex workshops for gays and lesbians. (GMHC.)

SaferSister, Maria Perez, Wellington Love; 1992. 30 seconds each. Spanish/English. These four thirty-second public service announcements (two in English, the same two in Spanish) draw attention to the fact that lesbians and women who have sex with other women are always depicted as not having sex, not having much sex, or not having to have safer sex. These PSA's include sexy shots of body parts, latex, and the words "safe sex." They get the juices flowing when used in a longer program of AIDS videos. (Wellington Love.)

Se Met Ko, Patricia Benoit; Haitian Women's Program, American Friends Service Committee, 1989. 28 mins. Creole/English. A very accessible tape designed for the Haitian community as an introduction to AIDS issues. Using the *telenovela* format and likable characters, this tape provides insights into how AIDS information is communicated among family members and within a community. Although this tape is accurate and believable regarding safer sex, condoms, and casual contact, it does not deal with the social and cultural stigmas placed on IV drug users and gay men. (American Friends Service Committee.)

The Second Epidemic, Amber Hollibaugh; New York City Commission on Human Rights, 1989. 27 mins. This documentary positions itself squarely within the lives of those most affected by the AIDS crisis—the HIV-infected, their friends, lovers, family members, and care providers. Portrays the power and resistance of people with AIDS, as well as the experiences of those who have been discriminated against because they were perceived to have the illness. Brings its viewers to a clearer understanding of the crisis by identifying and analyzing AIDS discrimination. Provides good examples of compassionate, nondiscriminatory responses to AIDS in various communities. (New York City Commission on Human Rights.)

Seize Control of the FDA, Gregg Bordowitz, Jean Carlomusto; GMHC, 1988. 28 mins. Documents AIDS activists in the October 1988 seizure of the Food and Drug Administration building in Rockville, Maryland. Arms the viewer with necessary information to counter and analyze mainstream broadcast media. As an example of how to engage in direct action, this tape is valuable for people outside the immediate circle of street activists. Since the information provided is often dense, this tape should be supplemented by a speaker or written materials. (GMHC.)

Seriously Fresh, Reggie Life; AIDSFilms, 1989. 28 mins. A drama about four guys in an all-black basketball-playing posse who find out that their neighborhood hero, Kenny, has AIDS. This discovery throws them into a morning-long, intense conversation at the basketball court, filled with individual flashbacks which show how each is dealing with issues such as drug use, condom negotiation with sexual partners, and casual sex with other men. The award-winning film's gem is when Jazzy Jay, the group's rapper, role-plays with himself in the bathroom mirror while his little brother listens and looks on through a door crack. Jazzy tries different ways to convince his girlfriend that they should "put a cap on Jimmy" when they are making love. Also, one of the heterosexually identified young men tells his positive friend that he sometimes has sex with other men. Study guide available. (Select Media.)

Silverlake Life: The View from Here, Peter Friedman; Tom Joslin, Jane Weiner, Doug Block; Silverlake Productions, 1993. 77 mins. When Mark Massi and his lover, Tom Joslin, discovered they both were infected with HIV, Tom decided to document the progress of the disease on videotape. Personal and at times confrontational, this devastatingly real chronicle encourages a more immediate understanding of AIDS in viewers by detailing the agony of living with this disease. The vivid portrait intercuts interviews with family members and footage from an earlier film about what it feels like to be gay. The mundaneness of everyday life is reframed in the face of imminent death, where separation from society only magnifies the pain. Neither voyeuristic nor cathartic, the film offers a profound opportunity to witness life with AIDS and the horror of death. (Zeitgeist Films.)

Simple Courage: An Historical Portrait for the Age of AIDS, Stephanie Castillo; Hawai'i Public Television, 1992. 60 mins. Presents a valuable historical precedent to the handling of the AIDS epidemic in the United States. With complex yet accessible storytelling, this film examines the political, social, cultural, and religious forces that brought about the lifetime banishment of some 8,000 people with leprosy, mostly native Hawaiians. Central to this tragic tale is the hope and dignity brought to the sufferers by Belgian missionary priest Father Damien de Veuster, whose tireless efforts during the later nineteenth century made sure that these forsaken people were not forgotten. Moving and powerful, the account is told through writings and testimonies of those who were banished as well as historians, and the letters of Father Damien. Especially useful connections to AIDS in regard to patient care, isolation, social stigma, and the consequent shame of those infected. (Filmmakers Library.)

Snow Job: The Media Hysteria of AIDS, Barbara Hammer; 1986. 8 mins. The mainstream media's reaction to the crisis is revealed through this collage of AIDS representations from the popular press. Here, distortion and misinformation amount to a "snow job" promoting homophobia, discrimination, and repression of lesbian and gay people. Employs a formal device of repeated and computer-generated snow patterns and formations. One of the few experimental tapes made by a woman about AIDS, this works well in a series of alternative media representations. (Video Data Bank [and] Barbara Hammer.)

So Sad, So Sorry, So What, Jane Gilloolly; 1990. 27 mins. Filmed during three months in 1988, this is a moving portrait of Joanne, a 28-year-old white woman, recovering drug user, single mother, and person with HIV. Fragments of song and conversation—tape-recorded during her prerelease from prison—weave Joanne's life story from her troubled childhood home and the beginning of her experiments with drugs at age eight, to her rebellious and painful youth, adult drug addiction, prostitution, and incarceration. Soft black-and-white photographs of Joanne, her two-year-old son, her family home, and the correctional institution slowly appear and fade into shadow. (Fanlight Productions.)

Steam Clean, Richard Fung; GMHC, 1990. 2 mins. Numerous Asian language translations. This sexy invitation into a busy gay bathhouse recuperates that space as erotic and legitimate and affirms the East Asian man as a desiring subject. Part of the GMHC series of Safer Sex Shorts. (GMHC.)

Stop the Church, Robert Hillferty; 1990, 28 mins. Documents the planning and execution of WHAM! and ACT UP's controversial "Stop the Church" demonstration at St. Patrick's Cathedral in December 1989. Provides an inside look at the organization of the demonstration, including debates within the group about whether or not church services should be disrupted. The tape was supposed to air nationally on PBS's *P.O.V.* series but was censored in the wake of the controversy about Marlon Riggs's *Tongues Untied.* (Frameline.)

Target City Hall, DIVA TV, 1989. 28 mins. The first tape produced by those Damned Interfering Video Activists (DIVA TV) exhibits a wide range of styles and statements on ACT UP's massive demonstration at New York's City Hall on March 28, 1989, to protest state-level governmental negligence in the AIDS crisis. Begins with a poignant music video of new activists being trained in civil disobedience. Segues into an intimate portrait of one large affinity group called CHER, in which passionate first-timers glowingly support each other in a committed battle against the system. The final section, called "L.A.P.I.T." (Lesbian Activists Producing Innovative Television), emphasizes the role of ACT UP's women and deconstructs the media hype stemming from the illegal strip searches they endured in jail. (ACT UP/NY [and] Printed Matter Bookstore.)

A Test for the Nation: Women, Children, Families, AIDS, Alexandra Juhasz; GMHC, 1988. 25 mins. This well-edited video includes pro-and-con interviews with doctors and HIV-positive women about AIDS and abortion rights. Points out, among other things, the coercion of HIV-positive women into having abortions, despite the fact that only 20–30 percent of babies born to HIV-positive women develop their own antibodies and ultimately test positive for the virus. Provocatively presents HIV-positive women, their families, and care providers confronting this challenge and the risk. (GMHC.)

Testing the Limits: NYC, Testing the Limits Collective, 1987. 28 mins. An important historical document, this collectively produced tape emerged from inside the birth of AIDS activism in NYC. Reflects the impact of AIDS on many aspects of daily life—jobs, housing, health care, family, nutrition. Challenged with increasing social problems, communities undertook innovative and far-reaching solutions, including everything from direct action and civil disobedience to community-based drug trials. With its broad scope—covering demonstrations, speak-outs, and street actions from March until October 1987—the tape catalogs the inadequate responses of federal, state, and city governments, as well as the strong responses by people infected and affected, desperate and outraged. (Testing the Limits.)

Thinking About Death, Gregg Bordowitz; GMHC, 1991. 26 mins. Presenting many perspectives on death and dying, this tape includes diverse people and diverse views. HIV-positive and HIV-negative, younger and older people, doctors and pastors, provide a useful introduction to conversations about this difficult—if not taboo—subject. The strongest moment is when an African American pastor tells about how she helped an isolated and angry hospitalized woman "make her transition peacefully." Speakers address issues such as family relationships, spirituality, health-care proxies, funerals and cremation, letting people go, letting oneself go, etc. (GMHC.)

This Is a Dental Dam, Suzanne Wright; DIVA TV, 1989. 1 min. In this cute commercial, the hands of two women at a dinner table demonstrate how to cut a condom into a latex barrier for women having oral sex with other women. This psa is included in the hour-long, live cablecast, "We Interrupt This Program," the Kitchen's contribution to "A Day Without Art." (The Kitchen.)

This Is Not an AIDS Advertisement, Isaac Julien; 1987. 10 mins. A slick, technologically playful music video that functions as a sort of commercial for gay male sexual desire and romance. Shot on film in Venice and London, with scenes of men kissing, playing, holding flowers, and flirting, the film focuses on a black-and-white couple. The music has a funk beat and explicit lyrics about sexuality and sexual desire. The conclusive refrain suggests "Feel no guilt in your desire." Created as a challenge to the "hegemony of the dominant media advertisements in Britain," subversive power lies in a shrewd appropriation and use of well-known advertising motifs and techniques—water, extreme close-ups, rapid editing—toward very different ends than usual. (Frameline.)

Too Close for Comfort, Peg Campbell; Gay Hawley, Wild Ginger Productions and National Film Board of Canada, 1990. 27 mins. While David is working at the local video store, he overhears his friend Nick being fired because he is HIV-positive. Word spreads quickly in the small town. David and his friends are challenged by their fear of AIDS, homophobia, and prejudice. Engaging, well-produced, and well-written, this drama deals frankly and thoroughly with discrimination against gay men and lesbians. Should be supplemented with basic information about HIV transmission, prevention, and support strategies. Study guide available. (ETR Associates.)

Untitled, John Sanborn, Mary Perillo; Alive from Off Center, 1989. 10 mins. Against a fluid and compelling backdrop of black-and-white photographs, dancer Bill T. Jones performs an extraordinary tribute to his lover, Arnie Zane, who died of AIDS-related complications in 1988. The spoken and written word provide a simply profound and sincere texture. (The Kitchen.)

Vida, Lourdes Portillo; AIDSFilms, 1989. 18 mins. Spanish/English. This excellent narrative film presents Elsie, a young Latina single mother struggling with her fear of AIDS. Two experiences coincide in Elsie's life which help drive home the importance of protection. She finds out that her neighbor is HIV-positive, and her savvy best friend implores her to bring up condom use with her new boyfriend. Elsie is caught between a traditionally passive woman's role and her need to stand up for herself against any sort of abuse, whether from men or from her own domineering mother. This *telenovela* successfully models both HIV prevention and self-empowerment. Employing an entirely bilingual cast, the producers created two separate films, one in Spanish and one in English. Comes with a bilingual discussion guide. (Select Media.)

Viva Eu! Tania Cypriano; 1989. 18 mins. Portuguese/English. An extraordinary portrait of the exuberant Brazilian artist Wilton Braga, one of the first people in Brazil to be diagnosed with HIV. His birthday party, full of other unique and inspiring artists, provides the stage for Braga's carefree dancing. He proudly displays his embattled but thriving body, speckled with hundreds of purple Kaposi Sarcoma lesions. Combining direct interviews, cinema verité, and fantasy enactments, this wonderfully eclectic and intimate montage celebrates Braga's life and work. (Tania Cypriano.)

Voices from the Front, Testing the Limits Collective, 1992. 60 mins. An award-winning broadcast documentary that maps out issues relevant to an activist movement which has expanded in size and scope as the epidemic has grown. Now, HIV disproportionately affects people of color, gay men, women, intravenous drug users, sex workers, and undocumented immigrants. A comprehensive sequel to *Testing the Limits: NYC,* this tape frames AIDS within the context of preexisting social problems—from discrimination and prejudice-related violence to people's lack of access to housing, health care, child care, and drug treatment. Examines pharmaceutical industry profiteering and documents medical personnel shortages, drug trials, and the denial of health care to millions of U.S. residents. Makes the case for a national health-care system and offers an impressive record of AIDS activism in the United States. (Frameline.)

Voices of Positive Women, Darien Taylor, Michael Balser; 1992. 27 mins. Testifying to the impact of AIDS on women, this tape unravels many of the more prevalent stereotypes. Diverse women speak candidly and articulately about their responses to diagnosis and the ways their lives have changed. (V Tape.)

   A WAVE Taster, Women's AIDS Video Enterprise, 1990. 33 mins. This collectively produced tape documents the group's previous six-month process of making the tape *We Care.* Group dialogue and individual commentary re-create the history of how seven women came together as strangers. They became a family which refused to disassemble upon completion of their initial task. Perhaps the most remarkable trait of this piece is how accurately the group's life process and testimony is mirrored in the making of its first tape. Effectively models a community uniting to create both AIDS education materials and internal support systems. (Brooklyn AIDS Task Force.)

   We Care: A Video for Care Providers of People Affected by AIDS, Women's AIDS Video Enterprise, 1990. 33 mins. Targeted at low-income women of color, this tape was collectively produced by WAVE, an unusual "video support group" sponsored by the Brooklyn AIDS Task Force (see above). For six months, seven women met to talk and learn about AIDS and video. The result is a rich grassroots effort which documents many challenges that AIDS presents to care-givers and which rebukes many common myths about HIV/AIDS. One HIV-positive member provides an intimate tour of her home while she speaks of daily life with the virus, demonstrating how things have changed for her and her family. Also includes interviews with a doctor, a volunteer, and several educators. The women not only speak about men's resistance to condom use and the need to face death realistically, but also offer resources and referrals. (Brooklyn AIDS Task Force.)

   With Loving Arms, Children's Welfare League of America, 1989. 18 mins. Spanish/French/English. Profiles five HIV-positive children and their natural and foster families. Carefully designed to assist in the recruitment of foster parents for HIV-infected children, this tape honestly illustrates the serious challenges for loving parents, grandparents, and other guardians. Ada Setal, the grandmother and guardian of four young children, speaks through her tears about the pain of letting go. The baby Angela has died. As Angela's siblings search through a photo album for her image, Ada asks, "Where is Angela?" Their tiny voices answer, "In the heart." This tape brings to light the issues of pediatric AIDS in a positive and moving way and can be used in a wide range of educational programs dealing with pediatrics, family communication, coping strategies, or death and dying. (Children's Welfare League of America.)

   Women and AIDS, Alexandra Juhasz, Jean Carlomusto; GMHC, 1988. 28 mins. Women have been dying of AIDS since at least 1981. This was effectively denied by the press, media, and government until 1986, when shocking increases in the numbers made it more difficult to continue to perpetuate depictions of AIDS as a deserved plague attacking gay men, Haitians, and IV drug users. This tape challenges the continuing media misrepresentations of the dangers of AIDS to white middle-class women. It also points out that women of color have been largely overlooked by the mainstream media in its reporting on AIDS, even though women of color are the fastest-growing group of HIV-infected people. Focuses on the concerns of poor people of color and IV drug users through interviews with HIV-infected women, women active in AIDS care, and women on the streets. Includes safer-sex and clean works demonstrations. (GMHC.)

Women and AIDS: A Survival Kit; California AIDS Clearinghouse, 1988. 22 mins. Provides a well-balanced overview of HIV disease, focusing on the particular cultural and social factors that affect women. Features vignettes illustrating approaches to effective communication concerning safer sex and condom use. Includes a demonstration of how to clean IV drug needles with bleach. Two women with AIDS talk candidly about transmission issues and their personal experiences with the virus. (California AIDS Clearinghouse.)

Women and Children Last. See *Heart of the Matter.*

Women, Children and AIDS, Jane Wagner; San Francisco AIDS Foundation, 1987. 30 mins. Documents the goals and findings of California-based research projects about women, children, and AIDS. Includes a short presentation by former U.S. Surgeon General C. Everett Koop. Addresses antibody testing, donor insemination, drug use, psychosocial issues, and health-care needs. Deals with transmission by means of unprotected heterosexual sex, a mother to her fetus, sharing unclean needles, and blood transfusions, but does not provide information about risks or prevention for women who have sex with women. Should be complemented with a speaker or written material. (San Francisco AIDS Foundation.)

Work Your Body: Options for People Who Are HIV-Positive, Gregg Bordowitz, Jean Carlomusto; GMHC, 1988. 28 mins. Health-care providers and HIV-positive men present a strong case for getting the HIV antibody test and discuss how the results can affect people's daily lives. Provides upbeat, empowering examples of how to take care of yourself after diagnosis. Factual and personal information is provided in a friendly, conversational manner that makes the material accessible to almost any audience. Denise Ribble, a community health nurse, discusses nutrition and quality-of-life issues for people who are positive. John Robles, a former IV drug user, elaborates on his HIV status in a manner which is both down-to-earth and philosophical. Michael Callen, a PWA, talks about how to assess treatment options and what exactly HIV sero-positivity means. (GMHC.)

Zero Patience, John Greyson; Anna Stratton, Louise Garfield, Zero Patience Productions, 1993. 100 minutes. This timely and eccentric musical feature serves up water ballet, dancing jungle animals, and singing bottoms to explore the politics of AIDS scapegoating. Sir Richard Francis Burton, the 170-year-old Victorian sexologist and explorer, is producing a sensationalistic museum display about Patient Zero, the French-Canadian flight attendant accused of bringing AIDS to North America. There is only one hitch: the ghost of Patient Zero is back in town, and he is determined to stop the display and prove his innocence. Antagonistic and yet attracted to one another, Patient Zero and Burton encounter other AIDS pariahs—the ACT UP media committee, a chain-smoking Green Monkey, and the tiara-wearing Miss HIV. Together, they sing, swim, and sashay their way through the mass media's hysterical headlines, fighting back and refusing the blame. (Cineplex Odeon.)

Distributors

ACT UP/NY, 135 W. 29th St. (10th floor), New York, NY 10001. 212-564-2437.

American Friends Service Committee, Information Services, 15 Rutherford Pl., New York, NY 10003. 212-598-0972.

American Indian Community House, 404 Lafayette St., New York, NY 10013. 212-598-0100.

American Red Cross, Bookstore Department of Greater New York, 150 Amsterdam Ave., New York, NY 10023. 212-875-2196.

Appalshop, 306 Madison St., Whitesburg, KY 41858. 606-633-0108, 800-1545-7467.

April Productions, 236 East 5th St., #4D, New York, NY 10003. 212-473-3143.

Association for the Care of Children's Health, 7910 Woodmont Ave., Suite 300, Bethesda, MD 20814. 301-654-6549.

Blush Entertainment, 526 Castro St., San Francisco, CA 94109. 415-861-4723, 800-845-4617.

Boudreau, Charline, 935 Marie-Anne East, Montreal, Quebec H2J 2B2, Canada. 514-598-7653.

Brooklyn AIDS Task Force, Attn.: Yannick Durand, 465 Dean St., Brooklyn, NY 11217. 718-783-0883.

California AIDS Clearinghouse, P.O. Box 1830, Santa Cruz, CA 95061. 800-258-9090.

CDC National AIDS Information Clearinghouse, P.O. Box 6003, Rockville, MD 20849-6003. 800-458-5231.

Chamberlain, Anne, 618-457-8061.

Children's Welfare League of America, Publications Dept., 440 First St. NW, Suite 310, Washington, DC 20001. 202-638-2952.

Cinema Guild, 1697 Broadway, Suite 803, New York, NY 10019. 212-246-5522. (fax 212-246-5525.)

Cineplex Odeon, 1303 Young St., Toronto, Ontario M4T 2Y9, Canada. 416-323-6600.

Clínica Estético, 127 West 24th St., 7th floor, New York, NY 10011. 212-807-6800.

Cypriano, Tania, 212-691-5303.

Drift Distribution, 611 Broadway, #742, New York, NY 10012. 212-254-4118. (fax 212-254-3154.)

DSR, Inc., 9111 Guilford Rd., #100, Columbia, MD 21046. 301-490-3500. (fax 301-490-4146.)

ETR Associates, P.O. Box 1830, Santa Cruz, CA 95061-1830. 800-321-4407.

Fanlight Productions, 47 Halifax St., Boston, MA 02130. 800-937-4113.

Fear of Disclosure Project, Jonathan Lee. 212-292-2690.

Film Library, Clare Walsh Associates, 22 Florida Ave., Staten Island, NY 10305. 718-720-4488.

Filmmakers Library, 124 East 40th St., Suite 901, New York, NY 11016. 212-808-4980. (fax 212-808-4983.)

First Run Features, 153 Waverly Pl., New York, NY 10014. 212-243-0600. (fax 212-989-7649.)

Frameline, P.O. Box 14792, San Francisco, CA 94114. 415-861-5245.

Fusion Artists, Inc., 222 East 5th St., New York, NY 10003. 212-475-6228.

Gay Men of African Descent—GMAD, 666 Broadway, Suite 520, New York, NY 10012. 212-420-0773. (fax 212-982-3321.)

Gay Men's Health Crisis (GMHC), 129 West 20th St., New York, NY 10011. 212-337-3558.

Gryphon Productions, P.O. Box 53505, 984 West Broadway, Vancouver, British Columbia V5Z 4M6, Canada. 604-983-0079.

Hammer, Barbara, 5700 Florence Terr., Oakland, CA 94661. 415-654-3006.

HIV Center for Clinical and Behavioral Studies, 722 West 168th St., New York, NY 10032. 212-960-2432.

Juhasz, Alexandra, Film/Video Department, Pitzer College, 1050 Mills Ave., Claremont, CA 91711. 909-621-8555

The Kitchen, 512 West 19th St., New York, NY 10011. 212-255-5793. (fax 212-645-4258.)

Latino AIDS Project, 2401 24th St., San Francisco, CA 94110. 415-647-5450.

Love, Wellington, P.O. Box 382, Prince St. Station, New York, NY 10012.

Media for Development International, P.O. Box 281, Columbia, MD 21045. (fax 410-730-8322.)

Minnesota Indian Affairs Council, AIDS Taskforce, 127 University, St. Paul, MN 55155. 612-296-3611.

National Film Board of Canada, 22 D Hollywood Ave., Ho-ho-kus, NJ 07423. 800-542-2164.

New York City Commission on Human Rights, 40 Rector St., New York, NY 10006. 212-306-7450.

No Excuses Productions, 3703 Rhoda Ave., Oakland, CA 94602. 510-530-3247.

Partners in Health, 875 Main St., Fifth Floor, Cambridge, MA 02139. 617-661-4564.

Pregones, 295 St. Ann's Ave., Bronx, NY 10454. 718-585-1202.

Printed Matter Bookstore, 77 Wooster St., New York, NY 10012. 212-925-0325. (fax 212-925-0464.)

Rodriguez, Nino, 1147 North Clark St., West Hollywood, CA 90069. 310-657-1725.

San Francisco AIDS Foundation, 333 Valencia St., P.O. Box 6182, San Francisco, CA 94101. 415-861-3397.

San Francisco Study Center, 1095 Market St., #602, San Francisco, CA 94103. 415-626-1650.

Select Media, 477 Broome St., #42, New York, NY 10013. 212-431-8923.

Testing the Limits, 39 West 14th St., Suite 402, New York, NY 10010. 212-229-2863.

United Nations Development Programme, PDR Productions, Inc., 219 East 44th St., New York, NY 10017. 212-986-2020.

V Tape, 401 Richmond St. West, Suite 452, Toronto, Ontario M5V 3A8, Canada. 416-351-1317. (fax: 416-351-1509.)

183 Bathurst, Main Floor, Toronto, Ontario M5T 2RF, Canada. 514-499-9840.

Video Data Bank, School of the Art Institute, 280 South Columbus, Chicago, IL 60603. 312-443-3793.

Wichterich, Beth, 1902B Robbins Pl., Austin, TX 78705.

Women Make Movies, 462 Broadway, Suite 501, New York, NY 10013. 212-925-0606.

Women's Prison Association, 110 Second Ave., New York, NY 10003. 212-674-1163. (fax 212-677-1981.)

Zeitgeist Films, 247 Center St., New York, NY 10013. 212-274-1989. (fax: 212-274-1644.)

INDEX

Alexandra Juhasz is Assistant Professor of Film/Video
at Pitzer College.
Catherine Saalfield is an independent video producer
and activist. She writes on media, AIDS, and lesbian
and gay issues for various publications.

Library of Congress Cataloging-in-Publication Data
Juhasz, Alexandra.
AIDS TV : identity, community, and alternative video /
Alexandra Juhasz, with a videography by Catherine
Saalfield.
Includes bibliographical references and index.
ISBN 0-8223-1683-8 (cloth : alk. paper). — ISBN
0-8223-1695-1 (paperback : alk. paper)
    1. AIDS (Disease) in mass media.   I. Saalfield,
Catherine.   II. Title.
P96.A39J84   1995
362.1'969792—dc20   95-20385 CIP